INTRAVENOUS ANESTHESIA
and ANALGESIA

INTRAVENOUS ANESTHESIA and ANALGESIA

Guenter Corssen, M.D.

Professor Emeritus of Anesthesiology
The University of Alabama
School of Medicine
Birmingham, Alabama
President, Central Arizona Anesthesiology, Ltd.
Scottsdale, Arizona

J.G. Reves, M.D.

Professor of Anesthesiology
Director, Division of Cardio-Thoracic Anesthesia
Duke University
School of Medicine
Durham, North Carolina

Theodore H. Stanley, M.D.

Professor of Anesthesiology
The University of Utah
School of Medicine
Salt Lake City, Utah

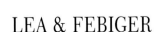 *Philadelphia*

1988

Lea & Febiger
600 Washington Square
Philadelphia, PA   19106-4198
U.S.A.
(215) 922-1330

Library of Congress Cataloging-in-Publication Data

Corssen, Guenter.

  Intravenous anesthesia and analgesia.
  Includes index.
  1. Intravenous anesthesia. 2. Analgesia.
3. Anesthetics. I. Reves, J.G. II. Stanley,
Theodore H. (Theodore Henry), 1940-   . III. Title.
[DNLM: 1. Analgesia–methods. 2. Anesthesia, Intravenous
–methods.   WO 285 C826i]
RD85.I6C67   1987   617'.962   86-21123
ISBN 0-8121-1074-9

PRINTED IN THE UNITED STATES OF AMERICA

Print number: 5   4   3   2   1

IN MEMORY OF THE FATHER OF INTRAVENOUS ANESTHESIA,
JOHN S. LUNDY, M.D., MENTOR, TEACHER AND FRIEND.
HIS GUIDANCE AND CONTINUING INSPIRATION
WERE INVALUABLE TO US.

FOREWORD

It is just over 30 years since I published the monograph "Thiopentone and other Thiobarbiturates." This work reflected anesthetic practice on both sides of the Atlantic in the mid-1950s and reviewed the pharmacology of the available intravenous anesthetic drugs. As its name implied, it concentrated entirely on thiobarbiturates—simply because no other drugs were in clinical use at that time. It did make a brief mention of methohexital, but this drug had not at that stage come into clinical practice. In 1956 there was no mention of the benzodiazepines or the phenothiazines and only very brief mention of the opioids. Reference was made to the 1947 paper by Neff and his co-workers on the nitrous oxide-oxygen and curare combination and to the British equivalent paper by Mushin and his colleagues from Cardiff in 1949, which described the use of parenteral meperidine during anesthesia. These two papers undoubtedly heralded the beginning of the widespread use of analgesics, and particularly of opioids, in anesthesia. Neither of the groups of authors could possibly have foreseen their importance in modern intravenous anesthesia as is set out so clearly in this textbook. Even a decade ago it would have come as a surprise for one to find that the second chapter in the book was dealing not with the barbiturates, but with the narcotics, and that their chemistry and clinical use should take precedence to those of the barbiturates. This is the current state of play.

As stated early in this book, "Many intravenous anesthetic agents have collapsed. Few have been resuscitated." This statement certainly applies to the thiobarbiturates (Ch. 6), of which only two have survived, but it also applies to such compounds as propanidid, Althesin, and hydroxydione. The future of intravenous anesthesia is based on a balanced technique, whether one calls this dissociative anesthesia (Ch. 7) or neurolept (Ch. 8), with perhaps an increasing role by the benzodiazepines (Ch. 9). These, and the "defunct" drugs referred to previously, are fully discussed in this textbook, which even includes a chapter on intravenous alcohol. All these give readers a sound foundation for further advances in this field, such as total intravenous anesthesia.

John W. Dundee, M.D., Ph.D.
Professor of Anaesthetics
The Queen's University of Belfast
Northern Ireland

PREFACE

This book is a summary of current knowledge in the field of intravenous anesthesia and analgesia, and provides the practicing anesthesiologist, nurse anesthetist, general practitioner, and dentist with detailed information regarding the use of intravenous agents and the techniques employed in inducing and maintaining anesthesia and analgesia during surgery. The monograph also addresses young physicians and medical students who have had some exposure to the specialty of anesthesiology and would like to learn more about the parenteral use of hypnotics, tranquilizers, anesthetics, and analgesics to provide sedation, painlessness, and sleep.

The various steps in the evolution of intravenous anesthesia and analgesia to its present status are presented in a special section, with additional historic events, specific for each drug, reflected in the major chapters. Particular emphasis is placed on pharmacokinetics and drug metabolism, which only recently have been recognized as playing an important role in regard to the clinical pharmacologic spectrum of intravenously administered drugs; the benzodiazepines especially are now available in increasing numbers for use in preanesthetic medications and for induction of anesthesia.

We intended to present a comprehensive view of the principles and practices of intravenous anesthesia, and placed special weight and importance on the continuing widespread use of ultra-short acting barbiturates and non-barbiturate compounds; we paid particular attention to those drugs with sedative and analgesic properties that not only induce sleep but also maintain an appropriate anesthetic state, either as the sole agent or by supplementation with general anesthetics.

Much discussion concerns the relatively new concept of "dissociative" anesthesia and its implementation as an unusually safe approach to the anesthetic management of certain patient groups. Pediatric and geriatric patients as well as individuals in shock or shocklike states benefit by its use in that total CNS depression is avoided and vital body functions are minimally affected. Neuroleptanesthesia and neuroleptanalgesia are also thoroughly examined as to their value and suitability for pain control during major, prolonged, and traumatic surgical procedures. The question as to the preference of employing the fixed mixture of the neuroleptic, droperidol, and the narcotic, fentanyl, to establish the neuroleptanalgesic and anesthetic state versus separate administration of these drugs, as is the custom in European countries, is critically examined.

While attempting to determine the boundaries and limitations of intravenous anesthesia and being fully aware that the "ideal" intravenous anesthetic has still not been found, we decided to expand the scope of the book by adding recent research findings and clinical information with the intravenous use of high doses of fentanyl and its congeners, sufentanil and alfentanil, to produce "complete" anesthesia. Because of the success of this method of providing satisfactory pain control to cardiovascular surgical patients with markedly reduced reserves and to other surgical candidates without significant cardiovascular impairment, we believe the up-to-date appraisal of the method with regard to safe dose ranges, safeguards, possible hazards, and complications may be welcomed by the reader.

We hope that this book fulfills its purpose in contributing to the progress of the specialty of anesthesiology by serving as a useful guide to all contemporary practitioners in this field who are interested in the proper use of barbiturates and non-barbiturates, and of dissociative, neuroleptanalgesic, and narcotic drugs, to achieve optimal conditions for the surgical intervention and well-being of patients under our care.

Scottsdale, Arizona   Guenter Corssen
Durham, North Carolina   J.G. Reves
Salt Lake City, Utah   Theodore H. Stanley

ACKNOWLEDGMENTS

We wish to express our sincere appreciation to Lester C. Mark, M.D., Professor Emeritus of Anesthesiology, College of Physicians & Surgeons of Columbia University, for expert contributions and help in the preparation of this monograph. We also are indebted to Laraine Visser, Institute of Anesthesiology, Erasmus University Rotterdam, The Netherlands, for valuable editorial work. Special mention should be given to our secretaries, Kathy Elgar (Phoenix), Laraine Goss (Durham), and Candace Newby (Salt Lake City), without whose technical skill it would have been impossible to complete this work. Particular thanks are expressed to our wives, Anne Corssen, Virginia Reves, and Mary Ann Stanley, who indirectly helped to bring our efforts in writing this book to a conclusion by willingly sacrificing many weeks and months of family life while continuously lending support and inspiration. Finally, we would like to acknowledge with gratitude the cooperative and enthusiastic spirit with which the publisher, Lea & Febiger, proceeded in producing the book.

CONTENTS

Chapter 1

PAST, PRESENT, AND FUTURE OF INTRAVENOUS ANESTHESIA

Many notable past achievements have led to the current practice of anesthesia. The history of intravenous anesthetics has been marked by false starts, as ideas and drugs have been developed and discarded over the past 325 years. As with all medical advances, each new step was taken because prior advances had been made. For example, without the understanding that William Harvey gave Christopher Wren regarding blood and its circulation, the idea of intravenous administration of drugs could not have been conceived in 1657.[1] Ideas are worthless without the development of appropriate equipment (currently termed technologic advancement); for the practice of intravenous drug administration to prosper, the quill and bladder of Wren's day had to be replaced in the early 1850s by the hypodermic hollow needle and glass syringe. These devices were developed by Francis Rynd, Alexander Wood, and Charles Pravaz.[2–4] Thus, the history of intravenous anesthesia is one of ideas, drugs, technology, and, crucially, the innovative investigator, who combined these elements with his own curiosity and courage to try something new. Regrettably, any review of the development of the use of intravenous anesthesia omits most of the biochemists who have devoted years of their lives in chemistry laboratories to the development of compounds that clinicians administer. Similarly, many engineers devised the tools that facilitate the administration of intravenous drugs; for example, the Teflon-coated catheters or computer-driven infusion pumps. Also, there must be clinicians and other persons whose endeavors have inadvertently been omitted. This chapter is therefore incomplete, and those individuals whose major, essential contributions to our present practice of anesthesia go unrecognized deserve our apologies.

The reader is referred to two excellent treatises that catalogue the progress of intravenous anesthesia. The first reference is the scholarly book by Charles R. Adams of the Mayo Clinic, friend and colleague of John Lundy. Printed in 1944, this work contains a detailed review of the history and science of intravenous anesthesia; Adams details those developments of the early 1900s when so much was learned.[5] Adams died, at age 49 years, soon after the publication of his valuable work. A second, more current book (1974), co-authored by John W. Dundee and Gordon M. Wyant, stands as a superb complement to that of Adams.[6] Dundee and Wyant compiled the history of, and more importantly added their own vast clinical experience to, the evaluation of many new intravenous drugs. Their text is an important contribution to our understanding of old and new

1

compounds. There are other historic sources, but these two books are the most widely recognized.

THE PAST

Men and Their Drugs

Many drugs have been administered intravenously for the purpose of anesthesia (Table 1–1), and of these substances, only a few are still used in clinical practice. Nevertheless, it is worthwhile to mention some of the most notable men in this field and the drugs they used for intravenous anesthesia. It is obvious from a review of Table 1–1 that most drugs have not survived the test of time; in fact, David Davis aptly stated, "Many intravenous agents have collapsed. Few have been resuscitated."[7]

Christopher Wren, the prominent English architect, was apparently the first investigator to record the anesthetic effects of a drug. In *Philosophical Transactions* (1665), Wren reported that he could "easily contrive a way to convey any liquid thing immediately into the mass of blood; thus, in pretty big and lean dogs by making ligatures on the veins then opening them on the side of the ligature towards the heart; and by putting into them slender syringes or quills, fastened to bladders containing the matter to be injected."[1] His recognition of a method for administering drugs into the central circulation led him to further experiments, with the encouragement of Robert Boyle.[8] Wren then reported, "The opium, being soon circulated into the brain, did within a short time stupify, though not kill the dog."[1] These reports are generally regarded as the first account of successful anesthetic effects of opium in an animal; but no clinical advantage was taken from these reports.

It is well known that ether delivered by insufflation was developed as a method of inducing anesthesia by Crawford Long in Georgia and William Morton in Boston in the early 1840s. Aware of this significant development in inhalational anesthesia, a Russian surgeon, Pirogoff, in 1846 first tried to produce general anesthesia by the intravenous infusion of ether.[9] These trials were unsuccessful but represented an important step in man's attempt to induce general anesthesia by the intravenous route. Success came soon. A remarkable French scientist, Pierre-Cyprien Ore, was the first physician to administer an intravenous drug for the purpose of providing anesthesia for a surgical procedure. Ore achieved this end while working at the St. André Hospital in Bordeaux in February 1874; his first clinical report regarding anesthesia and surgery was published in 1875.[10] Ore had previously conducted experiments during which he administered chloral hydrate to animals. Then on December 6, 1872, Ore administered 30 mg of chloral hydrate intravenously to a 26-year-old man for treatment of post-traumatic tetanus, and observed that the drug produced a level of unconsciousness sufficient for surgery.[11] The first actual intravenous anesthetic delivered for use in a surgical setting occurred on February 9, 1874, when Ore, again treating a patient with tetanus, administered chloral hydrate so that he was able to "explore the crushed finger at his ease." Because Ore was so enthusiastic about his discovery, he challenged the conventional wisdom and stated that chloral hydrate was superior to chloroform as an anesthetic. His pioneering zeal was "rewarded" by two official reprimands from the Academy of Surgery and dismissal from his duties as surgeon at the hospital on December 31, 1874.[12]

Table 1–1.   Contributions to Intravenous Anesthesia Practice*

Investigators	Intravenous Drugs	Year
Wren	Opium to dogs	1657
Pirogoff	Ether to man	1847
Ore	Chloral hydrate	Feb. 9, 1874†
Krawkow	Hedonal	1905
Babcock	Morphine and scopolamine	1905
Burkhardt	Chloroform and ether	1909
Noel and Southart	Paraldehyde	1913
Graef	Ether and Isopral	1913
Peck and Meltzer	Magnesium sulfate	1916
Naragawa	Ethyl alcohol	1921
Bardet	Somnifen	1921
Keller	Alurate	1927
Bumm	Pernoston	1927
Kirschner	Avertin	1929
Weiss	Phenobarbital	1929
Zerfas	Sodium amytal	1929
Lundy	Pentobarbital	1931
Weese and Scharpff	Epival	1932
Doring	Eunarcon	1933
Desplas and Chevillen	Soneryl	1934
Lundy; Waters	Thiopental	1934
Carrington and Raventos	Thialbarbitone	1946
Laborit and Huguenard	Thorazine, barbiturate, opioid	1950
Dornette	Thiamylol	1954
Stoelting	Methohexital	1957
Frey and Hermann; Thuillier, Domenjog	Propanidid	1957
DeCastro and Mundeleer	Droperidol and fentanyl	1959
Corssen and Domino	Ketamine	1966
Urban et al.; McClish; Stovner Campbell et al.; Clark et al.	Diazepam	1966
Lowenstein et al.	Morphine (high dose)	1969
	Althesin	1971
Doenicke	Etomidate	1973
Kay and Rolly	Diprivan	1977
Brown et al.; Conner et al. Reves et al.	Midazolam	1978
Stanley and Webster	Fentanyl (high dose)	1978
Rolly et al.	Sufentanil	1979
Kay and Pleuvry	Alfentanil	1980

*Compiled from Adams, C.: Intravenous Anesthesia. New York, Paul B. Hoeber, Inc., 1944; Dundee, J.W., and Wyant, G.M.: Intravenous Anaesthesia. Edinburgh, Churchill Livingstone, 1974; and Vandam, L.D.: Intravenous anesthesia—history, currency, prospects. Mt. Sinai J. Med. (N.Y.), 50:316, 1983.
†First successful clinical anesthetic.

At the end of the 1800s and the early 1900s, many clinicians were using morphine and scopolamine intravenously in surgical practice, but this method fell into disfavor because of several deaths reported in 1905.[8,12,13] Concurrent with the abandonment of morphine and scopolamine, however, was the beginning of what can be called the current era of intravenous anesthesia, in St. Petersburg, Russia. There, Krawkow began experiments with the clinical use of hedonal (methyl propyl-carbonol-urethane); its popularity spread in Russia and other parts of Europe.[14] Thus began the use of intravenous compounds for the induction and maintenance of anesthesia that has continued to the present.

The next major experimental steps were made by Noel and Southart in 1913 using paraldehyde, but this method of intravenous anesthesia met with only slight success and limited popularity.[15] In 1916, Peck and Meltzer tried an entirely different type of drug, magnesium sulfate, but like paraldehyde, magnesium sulfate never gained universal popularity.[16] In 1921, Naragawa used ethyl alcohol intravenously for the induction of anesthesia.[17] There probably were many earlier trials with wine and beer, even Wren is thought to have used spirits intravenously, but alcohol was not widely accepted until Marin reported extensive experience with this method of anesthesia in 1929.[18] Ethyl alcohol was not widely used for anesthesia, but its sporadic use continues today.

Although Fischer and von Mering first synthesized a barbiturate, barbital (diethylbarbituric acid) in 1903, it was not until 1921 that Bardet gave Somnifen (diethyl-dielo-barbiturate of diethylamine) to patients.[19] This drug became popular in Europe, especially France and Germany. Somnifen was the beginning of a long line of barbiturate derivatives that were tried in the 1920s and 1930s. Although some of these barbiturates have achieved some popularity in clinical use, it was in 1934 that thiopental, the enduring barbiturate, was first used clinically. Thiopental is still widely used and its development and introduction into clinical use mark the start of the present era.

Some controversy exists over who first actually administered thiopental to a patient. Certainly, both Drs. John Lundy at the Mayo Clinic and Ralph Waters at the University of Wisconsin were pioneers in the early use of this drug. Waters administered thiopental on March 8, 1934, for a short surgical procedure on the tongue (Fig. 1–1); this event appears to be the first clinical use of thiopental.[6] Lundy, however, published the first report of the clinical use of the drug; he first administered thiopental in June of 1934.[5,20] The initial large clinical series was reported by Lundy in 1935.[21] From the beginning of its use, thiopental proved to be effective and grew immensely in popularity. The only time in the 50-year history of its clinical use that thiopental was severely criticized was during World War II, when the drug fell into the hands of unskilled anesthetists, and its administration to casualties at Pearl Harbor resulted in many deaths. In fact, Halford, a surgeon, stated that intravenous anesthesia with thiopental was "an ideal method of euthanasia."[22] The report by Halford was accompanied by an editorial that presented a more moderate position regarding the use of intravenous thiopental in traumatic cases.[23] To this day, that moderate position involving cautious use of thiopental under hypovolemic conditions is maintained. One noteworthy barbiturate derivative is methohexital (1-methyl-5-allyl-5-(*l*-methyl-2 pentynyl) barbituric acid, which was first described by Stoelting in 1957.[24] Methohexital has a greater clearance rate than thiopental, which has assured its continued use in patients in whom rapid clearance is desired. Although many barbiturate derivatives have been introduced since the emergence of thiopental, none have surpassed its widespread use.

Beginning in the 1950s until today, interest in non-barbiturate intravenous anesthetic agents has been extensive. Although many compounds have been introduced into clinical practice, only a few have made significant contributions to the practice of anesthesia. DeCastro and Mundeleer reported the administration

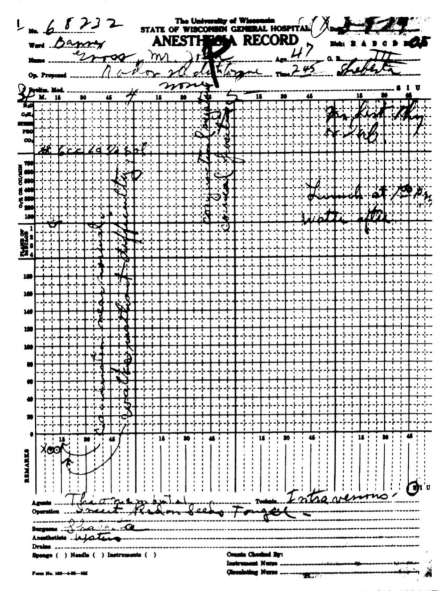

Fig. 1–1. Reproduction of the first administration of thiopental by Waters on March 8, 1934. (From Dundee, J.W., and Wyant, G.M.: Intravenous Anaesthesia. Edinburgh, Churchill Livingstone, 1974, with permission.)

of haloperidol and a potent narcotic, phenoperidine, in 1959.[25] From their work came the drug combination of Innovar (droperidol and fentanyl). The efficacy and safety of this fixed mixture has been questioned by some individuals because of the disparate duration of action of the two constituent compounds. In fact, Vandam stated, "failure to realize the potential for harm of either drug in this mixture has led to serious morbidity and mortality in the hands of the unwary."[8]

In 1966, Corssen and Domino reported the first clinical trials conducted with ketamine.[26] This drug was then, and remains, a unique addition to the field of intravenous anesthesia. Ketamine, a phencyclidine derivative, does not produce the generalized central nervous system depression experienced with barbiturates and most other anesthetics. Ketamine has been termed a "dissociative anesthetic," because "behavioral observations along with electrophysiologic dissociation of the thalamo-neocortical and lymbic symptoms occurred" after its administration. This drug also preserved the cardiovascular reflexes and was less of a depressant of the respiratory tract than are other intravenous anesthetic compounds. Ketamine remains the only phencyclidine derivative available for clinical practice. Another unique compound recently introduced is etomidate, which was studied and described by Doenicke and co-workers in 1973.[27] Etomidate enjoys a certain measure of popularity, particularly in high-risk patients, because of its minimal effects on the cardiovascular system and its relatively short duration of action. The development of the benzodiazepine midazolam, first used clinically in 1978, is remarkable in that this compound is water soluble in vitro yet is highly lipid soluble in vivo, and it has high plasma clearance.[28–30] The other benzodiazepines, even in their earliest clinical trials as anesthetics, were found to be poor intravenous anesthetic induction drugs because of the slow and unpredictable onset of hypnotic effects after their use, as well as their prolonged duration of action.[31]

Men and Their Concepts

Along with the development of new drugs, there has been an equally important evolution in concepts concerning the use of intravenous drugs in the practice of anesthesia. Initially, as with inhalation agents, one drug was expected to do all things: that is, to produce sleep, provide amnesia, and provide sufficient analgesia for the performance of a surgical procedure. Such usage was dangerous, because large doses were required to provide adequate anesthesia, and these doses usually produced depression of vital respiratory and cardiovascular systems. Several investigators, however, realized that intravenous drugs could be used in conjunction with other intravenous anesthetics, as well as with nitrous oxide and even potent inhalation agents, with less risk than that attendant on the use of each drug independently at high doses. This concept was probably first advanced by George W. Crile, who proposed that more than one form of anesthetic could be administered simultaneously to produce the ideal anesthetized state.[32] For example, nerve blocks combined with general anesthetic agents or opioids were preferable to either technique alone. His concept was termed anoci-association, and was the forerunner of what others have termed balanced anesthesia. Laborit and Huguenard proposed that the combination of a major tranquilizer (chlorpromazine), a short-acting barbiturate, and an opioid would induce a state they termed artificial hibernation.[33] This combination of very different compounds was striking and was a completely novel approach to intravenous anesthesia. The recommendation by DeCastro and Mundeleer (1959) that "neurolept anesthesia" could be induced with a butyrophenone, opioid, and nitrous oxide is an extension of the concept of Laborit and Huguenard regarding the use of drugs of diverse, yet specific, actions to produce anesthesia.[25] The butyrophenone produces hypnosis, the opioid provides analgesia, and nitrous oxide contributes weakly to both effects.

The current practice of mixing multiple intravenous drugs and inhalation drugs is called balanced anesthesia. This term was coined by Lundy in 1926 when he described a logical choice of a combination of various anesthetic agents used "in a small enough amount so that it would produce no unsatisfactory effect."[34] He, like Crile, argued that various drugs, such as thiopental, could be used to supplement regional blocks and to produce the balanced anesthetic state, much as one would try to balance one's dietary state. The concept of balanced anesthesia was further advanced in 1954 by Little and Stephen in an eloquent description of the reasons for combining various intravenous drugs to accomplish specific goals in the overall management of anesthesia.[35] They state, "It would be a sin of purgatorial level to administer highly toxic and potentially lethal drugs carelessly and light-heartedly, with no consideration as to their pharmacologic effects, or even as to whether such pharmacologic effects were either desirable or necessary. That drug or those drugs, which are necessary to achieve the purposes of anesthesia for the job at hand, are administered—no more and for a certainty, no less. Clinical pharmacology can only be practiced by employing each drug for a specific effect, in the quantity necessary to achieve that effect." Thus, the concept of using a single intravenous anesthetic drug seemed dead. Further amplification of the principles of intravenous anesthesia was provided by Woodbridge in 1957 in his report on the concepts of depth of anesthesia during balanced anesthesia.[36] Although the word (nothoria) that he introduced to refer to the combinations of various anesthetic levels required during anesthesia did not replace the term anesthesia as he had hoped, he did demonstrate that the classic stages of general anesthesia based on ether anesthesia could no longer be used in modern balanced anesthesia. Thus, the classic stages of anesthesia have been lost in the practice of balanced anesthesia, in which patients either are awake or are in light or deep anesthesia.

Despite the firm establishment of the concept of multiple intravenous anesthetics being an integral part of balanced anesthesia, some investigators recently proposed that, in critically ill patients and in those persons having long-lasting operations, high-dose opioids used alone are the superior anesthetic. This concept is at variance with that of balanced anesthesia, but it is popular among anesthesiologists who practice cardiac anesthesia. Lowenstein and co-workers in 1969, followed by Stanley and Webster in 1979, have argued the safety and usefulness of high-dose opioid anesthesia in major operations.[37–39] The development of many synthetic opioids, primarily from Janssen Laboratories (Fig. 1–2), has resulted in the availability of many drugs for administration with oxygen and a relaxant, in sufficiently high doses to produce anesthesia. Awareness can occur, however, chest wall rigidity during induction is a common problem, and postoperative respiratory depression is highly probable with this technique. Because the use of opioids in high doses causes respiratory depression, it is unlikely that the concept of using opioids as sole anesthetics will be appropriate in situations other than when ventilatory assistance postoperatively is acceptable. The practice of balanced anesthesia with the use of different intravenous drugs to produce sleep, amnesia, and analgesia in small enough quantities to avoid cardiopulmonary depression and to provide rapid emergence will be the enduring concept unless a short-lasting, complete anesthetic drug is developed.

THE PRESENT

Currently, intravenous anesthesia is widely practiced, the obvious reason being that it is a rapid, safe, and effective method of bringing a conscious patient into the anesthetized state. Intravenous anesthesia, however, has not always been as popular as it is today (Fig. 1–3). In Figure 1–3, note the steady increase in percentage of the use of intravenous anesthetics in hospitals in both the United

Dextromoramide	R 875	1956 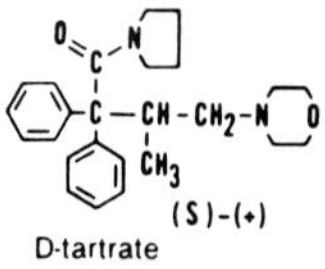
Phenoperidine	R 1406	1957 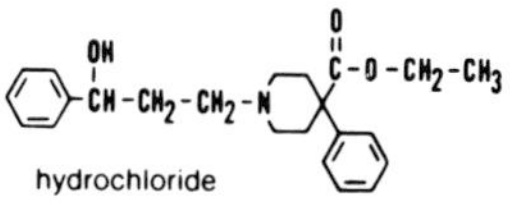
Piritramide	R 3365	1960 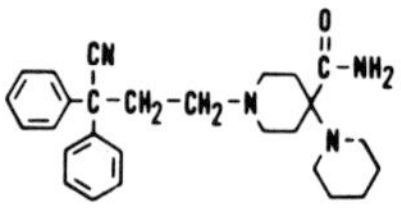
Fentanyl	R 4263	1960 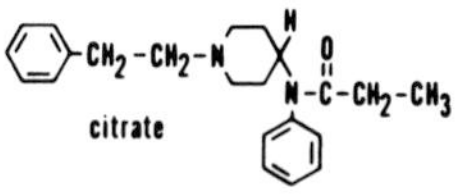
Bezitramide	R 4845	1961 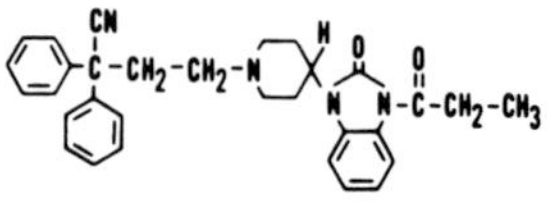
Carfentanil	R 33799	1974 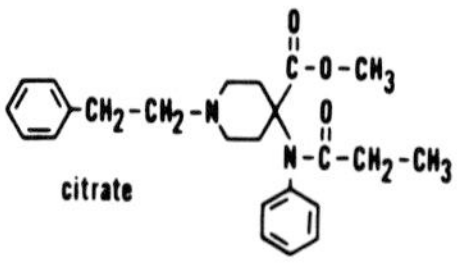
Sufentanil	R 33800	1974 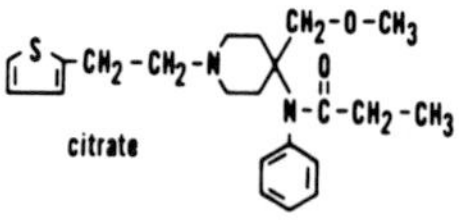
Lefentanil	R 34995	1975 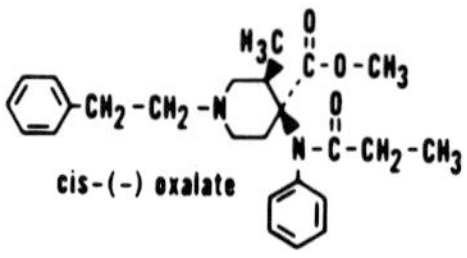
Alfentanil	R 39209	1976 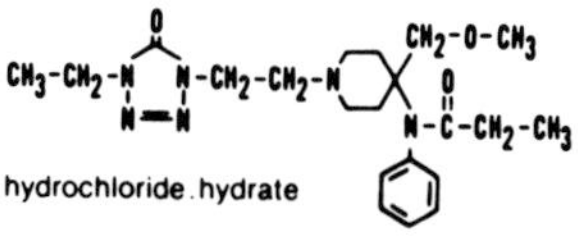

Fig. 1–2. Long line of synthetic opioids produced by the chemist in Janssen Laboratories for use in anesthesia. (From Janssen, P.A.J.: Potent, new analgesics, tailor-made for different purposes. Acta Anaesthesiol. Scand., 26:262, 1982, with permission.)

Kingdom and the United States.[6] If this graph were continued to the present, it undoubtedly would show that well over 90% of hospital staffs use intravenous anesthetics.

Most intravenous anesthetics are used for induction of anesthesia, but these drugs are also now used widely for the maintenance of anesthesia in combination with nitrous oxide and potent inhalation agents. Reasons for the increased use

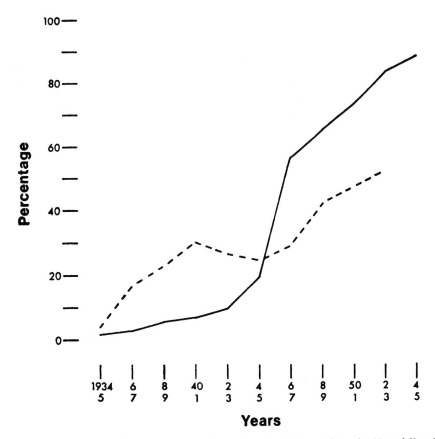

Fig. 1–3. Percentage use of intravenous anesthetics in selected hospitals in the United Kingdom and the United States from 1934 to 1954. (From Dundee, J.W., and Wyant, G.M.: Intravenous Anaesthesia. Edinburgh, Churchill Livingstone, 1974, with permission.)

are the number of specific compounds available to produce the desired results, their safety, the ease of administration, high rate of patient acceptance, and satisfactory emergence from general anesthesia. Of course, these drugs are usually administered by highly trained and skilled individuals whose practice of anesthesiology is firmly based in the knowledge of clinical pharmacology. The physicians and nurses who administer these drugs are familiar with the pharmacokinetic and pharmacodynamic characteristics of intravenous anesthetics so that predictable responses are achieved with selected intravenous anesthetic drugs.

In other chapters of this book, the various intravenous anesthetic drugs that are available for current practice are detailed. Some mention of present anesthetic practice should accompany consideration of the past and future, however. Intravenous drugs can be categorized according to their pharmacologic class (Table 1–2). Within each class, the drugs have certain dependable characteristics on which the clinician can rely and can use. The barbiturates are superb hypnotics, but they lack analgesic properties and provide short and unpredictable amnesia. The opioids are excellent analgesics, but they are poor hypnotics and have unreliable amnestic properties. The benzodiazepines provide excellent amnesia but are unpredictable hypnotics and lack analgesic properties. The phencyclidine ketamine is an excellent analgesic and good hypnotic, but it is associated with emergence hallucinations. The imidazole etomidate is an excellent hypnotic but lacks analgesic properties and provides undependable amnesia. Clinicians make use of the desirable characteristics of a drug, minimizing the undesirable property or properties when formulating an anesthetic management plan. Thus, the combination of a drug that produces good hypnosis (a barbiturate) with a drug that is an excellent analgesic (an opioid) is a rational plan for clinical use—indeed, it is the current practice of balanced anesthesia (vida supra).

THE FUTURE

If the past and present are any indication of the future (and few persons doubt that this is so), we can look with confidence that there will be new intravenous drugs and techniques for clinical use. The ideal intravenous drug has not yet been developed. There are many definitions as to what constitutes the ideal intravenous anesthetic, but it is believed that this ideal anesthetic drug would be one that provides rapid hypnotic, analgesic, and amnestic effects; that is water soluble and does not produce venous or organ damage; that does not depress respiratory or cardiovascular systems; whose effects can be reversed by a specific antagonist; with rapid metabolism, so that termination of administration would result in rapid termination of effect; that has predictable pharmacokinetic actions independent of organ dysfunction (e.g., liver); and, that is easily administered and has a stable shelf-life. Specific central nervous system receptor agonist compounds and even some endogenous biogenic amines could be developed that could satisfy some of these criteria. The perfect drug is still being sought; before it is found, many drugs will be developed that should be an improvement over existing ones.

As the pharmaceutical chemists make progress, so too do the bioengineers. Many intravenous drugs that are now a part of conventional anesthesia delivery will be administered by automated continuous infusion systems. The systems will be driven either by a pharmacokinetic model first reported by Schwilden and further developed by Alvis and co-workers, or by closed-loop devices that have as feedback signals either the processed EEG, on-line drug levels, or some other monitor of anesthetic drug level and depth.[41,42] This system is not science fiction, but probably will be a reality by the turn of the century. Even today, using an automated system, blood levels of fentanyl can be increased and decreased to provide a satisfactory depth of anesthesia by the anesthesiologist, much as he

Table 1–2. Classes and Pharmacodynamic Characteristics of Drugs

Class	Characteristics
Barbiturates	Excellent hypnosis, no analgesia, and poor amnesia
Opioids	Excellent analgesia, no amnesia, poor hypnosis
Benzodiazepines	Excellent amnesia, no analgesia, unpredictable hypnosis
Phencyclidine	Excellent analgesia, good hypnosis and amnesia, produces hallucinations
Imidazole (etomidate)	Excellent hypnosis, lacks analgesia, poor amnesia

increases and decreases the dial of his inhalation anesthetic vaporizer (Fig. 1–4).[43] When these systems are miniaturized, they will become an essential component of anesthesia delivery systems, for they will permit the practice of a quantitative form of intravenous anesthesia. Knowledge of blood levels of intravenous anesthetics will permit anesthesiologists to determine when to stop continuous infusion of the drug. The continuous infusion of anesthesia will avoid the peaks and valleys that occur with intermittent drug administration, and will prevent drug accumulation that can occur without knowledge of the blood-drug levels.[43]

Finally, the ED-50 (MAC concept) or MIC (minimum intravenous concentration) of intravenous anesthetic drugs and drug combinations will become clear. Much of the guess work that currently exists in the practice of intravenous drug administration will be removed through careful systematic investigation of the various intravenous drugs and the drug plasma levels required to achieve satisfactory anesthesia. The task of generating this knowledge will be arduous and long because of the multitude of drugs and the wide variety of drug combinations, but the ability to introduce drugs by continuous infusion will assist in this essential research.

The future of intravenous anesthesia is assured a major place in the practice of anesthesiology. Although we do not dare predict that inhalation agents will be a relic of the past, we are confident that intravenous anesthetics will play an

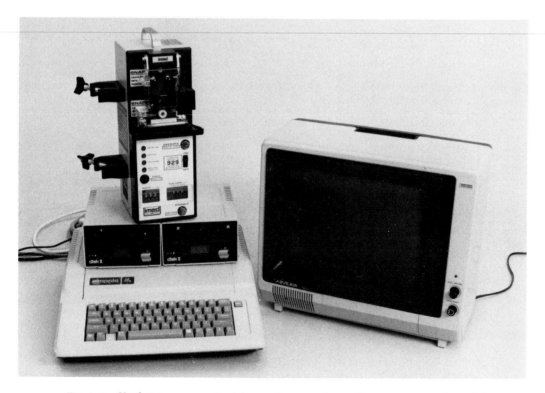

Fig. 1–4. Hardware components of the continuous automated intravenous anesthesia delivery system. The microprocessor (an Apple IIE), with pharmacokinetic data, patient characteristics, and drug concentration automatically infuses and keeps a constant blood level of intravenous anesthetics. (See Alvis, M.J., Reves, J.G., Govier, A.V., Menkhaus, P.G., Henling, C.E., Spain, J.A., and Bradley, E.: Computer-assisted continuous infusion of fentanyl during cardiac anesthesia: Comparison with a manual method. Anesthesiology, 63:41, 1985.).

important role in anesthetic management and will be essential to the care of patients requiring anesthesia for surgical procedures.

REFERENCES

1. Wren, P.C.: *In* Philosophical Transactions. Vol. I for Anno 1665 and 1666. London, T.N. for John Martyn at the Bell.
2. Rynd, F.: Injection of nerves. Dublin Med. Press, *13*:167, 1845.
3. Wood, A.: New method of treating neuralgia by the direct application of opiates to the painful points. Edinb. Med. Surg. J., *82*:265, 1855.
4. Pravaz, C.G.: Sur un noveau moyen d'operer la coagulation du sang dans les arteres, applicable a la guerison des aneurismes. C.R. Seances, Acad. Sci. (III), *36*:88, 1853.
5. Adams, C.: Intravenous Anesthesia. New York, Paul B. Hoeber, Inc., 1944.
6. Dundee, J.W., and Wyant, G.M.: Intravenous Anaesthesia. Edinburgh, Churchill Livingstone, 1974.
7. Davis, D.A.: The collapse and resuscitation of intravenous anesthesia. Clinical Anesthesia. Edited by J.F. Artusio, Jr. Philadelphia, F.A. Davis, 1968, p. 78.
8. Vandam, L.D.: Intravenous anesthesia—history, currency, prospects. Mt. Sinai J. Med., *50*:316, 1983.
9. Henschel, W.F., and Kljucar, S.: Intravenous anesthesia: its development towards its position in today's anesthesia. Acta Anaesthesiol. Belg., *3*:195, 1980.
10. Ore, P.C.: Etudes cliniques sur l'anesthesie chirurgicale par la methode des injections de chloral dans les veines. Paris, J.B. Bailliere et Fils, 1875.
11. Sabathie, M., and Delperier, A.: The first intravenous general anesthesia in the world. Acta Anaesthesiol. Belg., *3*:303, 1974.
12. Babcock, W.W.: A new method of surgical anesthesia. Proc. Phila. County Med. Soc., 26:347, 1905.
13. Van Hoosen, B.: Scopolamine-morphine anesthesia. Chicago, House of Manz, 1915, pp. 15–18.
14. Krawkow, N.F.: Ueber die hedonal-chloroform-narkose. Arch. Exp. Pathol. Pharmakol. Suppl., 317, 1908.
15. Noel, H., and Southart, H.S.: The anaesthetic effects of the intravenous injection of paraldehyde. Ann. Surg., 57:64, 1913.
16. Peck, C.H., and Meltzer, S.J.: Anesthesia in human beings by intravenous injection of magnesium sulphate. JAMA, 67:1131, 1916.
17. Naragawa, K.: Experimentelle studien uber die intravenose infusionsnarkose mittels alkohols. (Mitteilung der Ergebnisse der Tierversuche) J. Exp. Med., 2:81, 1921.
18. Marin, M.G.: Application des alkohol ethilico come anesthetico general per via endovenosa. Mexico, F. Mesones, 1929.
19. Fischer, E., and von Mering, J.: Ueber eine neue Classe von Schlafmitteln. Therap. Gegenw., 5:97, 1903.
20. Lundy, J.S., and Tovell, R.M.: Some of the newer local and general anaesthetic agents. Methods of their administration. Northwest Med., *33*:308, 1934.
21. Lundy, J.S.: Intravenous anesthesia: preliminary report of the use of two new thiobarbiturates. Mayo Clin. Proc., *10*:534, 1935.
22. Halford, F.J.: A critique of intravenous anesthesia in war surgery. Anesthesiology, 4:67, 1943.
23. Editorial: Question of intravenous anesthesia in war surgery. Anesthesiology, 4:74, 1943.
24. Stoelting, V.K.: The use of a new intravenous oxygen barbiturate 25398 for intravenous anesthesia (a preliminary report). Anesth. Analg., 36:49, 1957.
25. DeCastro, J., and Mundeleer, R.: Anesthesie sans barbituriques: la neurolept analgesie. Anesth. Analg., *16*:1022, 1959.
26. Corssen, G., and Domino, E.F.: Dissociative anesthesia: further pharmacologic studies and first clinical experience with phencyclidine derivative CI 581. Anesth. Analg., *45*:29, 1966.
27. Doenicke, A., Kugler, J., Penzel, G., Laub, M., Kalmar, L., Killian, I., and Bezecny, H.: Hirn-funktion und Toleranzbreite nach Etomidate, einem neuen barbituratfreien i.v. applizierbaren hypnoticum. Anaesthesist, 22:357, 1973.
28. Brown, C.R., Sarnquist, F.H., Canup, C.A., and Pedley, T.A.: Clinical, electroencephalographic and pharmacokinetic studies of a water-soluble benzodiazepine, midazolam maleate. Anesthesiology, 50:476, 1979.
29. Conner, J.T., Katz, R.L., Pagano, R.R., and Graham, C.W.: RO 21-3981 for intravenous surgical premedication and induction of anesthesia. Anesth. Analg., 57:1, 1978.
30. Reves, J.G., Corssen, G., and Holcomb, C.: Comparison of two benzodiazepines for anaesthesia induction: midazolam and diazepam. Can. Anaesth. Soc. J., 25:211, 1978.
31. Urban, B.J., Amaha, K., and Steen, S.N.: Investigation of 1-4-benzodiazepine derivatives as basal anesthetic agents. Anesth. Analg., *45*:733, 1966.

32. Crile, G.W.: An experimental and clinical research into certain problems relating to surgical operations. Philadelphia, J.B. Lippincott, 1901.
33. Laborit, H., and Huguenard, P.: Pratique de l'hibernotherapie, en chirurgie et en medicine. Paris, Masson, 1954.
34. Lundy, J.S.: Balanced anesthesia. Minn. Med., 9:399, 1926.
35. Little, D.M., Jr., and Stephen, C.R.: Modern balanced anesthesia: A concept. Anesthesiology, 15:246, 1954.
36. Woodbridge, P.D.: Changing concepts concerning depth of anesthesia. Anesthesiology, 18:536, 1957.
37. Lowenstein, E., Hallowell, P., Levine, F.H., Dagget, W.M., Austen, W.G., and Lever, M.G.: Cardiovascular response to large doses of intravenous morphine in man. N. Engl. J. Med., 281:1389, 1969.
38. Stanley, T.H., and Webster, L.R.: Anesthetic requirements and cardiovascular effects of fentanyl-oxygen and fentanyl-diazepam-oxygen anesthesia in man. Anesth. Analg., 57:411, 1978.
39. Stanley, T.H.: Narcotics as complete anesthetics. *In* Trends in Intravenous Anesthesia. Edited by J.A. Aldrete, Year Book, 1980, p. 367.
40. Janssen, P.A.J.: Potent, new analgesics, tailor-made for different purposes. Acta Anaesthesiol. Scand., 26:262, 1982.
41. Schwilden, H.: A general method for calculating the dosage scheme in linear pharmacokinetics. Eur. J. Clin. Pharmacol., 20:379, 1981.
42. Alvis, M.J., Reves, J.G., Govier, A.V., Menkhaus, P.G., Henling, C.E., Spain, J.A., and Bradley, E.: Computer-assisted continuous infusion of fentanyl during cardiac anesthesia: comparison with a manual method. Anesthesiology, 63:41, 1985.
43. Reves, J.G., Greene, E.R., Jr., and Mackrell, T.N.: Continuous infusion of intravenous anesthetics: automated IV anesthesia, a rational method of drug administration. *In* New Anesthetic Agents, Devices and Monitoring Techniques. Edited by T.H. Stanley. Hingham, MA, Martinus Nijhoff, 1983, pp. 196.

Chapter 2

HISTORY OF NARCOTICS IN ANESTHESIOLOGY

Narcotic analgesics, narcotic anesthetics, and opioids are three terms used to describe a group of drugs that possess morphine or opium-like properties. These properties include varying degrees of analgesia, sedation, respiratory depression, cough suppression, euphoria/dysphoria, muscular rigidity, histamine release, pruritus, meiosis, nausea and vomiting, constipation, biliary colic, urinary retention, and drug dependence. Opium is obtained from the juice of the poppy plant, *Papaver somniferum,* and comprises over 20 alkaloids, of which morphine is the most common (10%) and the best known. The term narcotic, derived from the Greek word for stupor, has been used loosely to describe sleep-inducing agents. More recently, in the legal context, it refers to any substance causing dependence. In this section, the terms opioid, narcotic analgesic, or narcotic anesthetic are used to describe drugs that specifically bind to any of several subspecies of opioid receptors and produce some opioid agonist effects.

EARLY HISTORY

Opioids have been administered by a variety of techniques for thousands of years to allay anxiety and to reduce pain associated with surgery.[1–4] The history of the use of opioids as intravenous anesthetics or analgesic supplements began in 1665 when Johann Sigismund Elsholtz injected crude opium into a dog's vein, producing a degree of analgesia-anesthesia from which the dog later recovered.[5] Despite this promising start, further experiments with intravenous opium languished for more than 2 centuries. In 1806, Serturner isolated morphine and suggested it was the most important of the opium alkaloids for producing either or both analgesia and insensibility.[6] Pravaz described the syringe (which may have first been invented by Rynd in 1845) and Wood the hollow needle in 1854.[4,5,7,8] The isolation of morphine and the invention of the hollow needle and syringe allowed physicians to administer measured amounts of morphine accurately for the first time. As a result, Lorenzo Burno of Turin, Italy, began injecting morphine intramuscularly 1 hour before surgery to lessen preoperative psychic trauma in the late 1850s—the first use of anesthetic premedication.

A technique entitled "mixed anesthesia" evolved over the next decade or two and consisted of the administration of morphine and atropine, intravenously and intramuscularly, in addition to the use of an inhalation agent, usually nitrous oxide or ether.[9,10] This technique was not popular because of the enthusiasm for the use of inhalation agents, diethyl ether and chloroform (without intravenous supplementation), and the awakening interest in the use of pure intravenous anesthesia after the introduction of chloral hydrate in 1872.[5] The concept of mixed anesthesia, however, helped to promote morphine, and probably atropine and scopolamine as well, as premedication drugs, which when given before and sometimes during surgery would decrease requirements for inhalation anesthetics and therefore enable deep levels of anesthesia to be attained with less depression of the major organ systems.[11]

Late in the nineteenth century, a technique evolved in which large amounts of morphine (1 to 2 mg/kg) were used with scopolamine (1 to 3 mg/70 kg) intramuscularly and intravenously as the sole anesthetic agents.[12–17] This type of anesthesia was used in all types of operations as well as for obstetric patients, and stimulated the publication of many articles and books from 1900 to 1912. Although patients would occasionally move and therefore had to be restrained during certain operations, pre- and postoperative excitement and memory of the operation itself were rare. Unfortunately, initial enthusiasm for morphine-scopolamine anesthesia soon waned because of an alarming increase in operative mortality.[17] Although the exact cause of this increase in mortality is not clear, it may well have been related to inadequate intra- and postoperative respiratory support; devices for mechanical ventilation of patients and awareness of the need for such support were both lacking at that time.

For some time thereafter, interest in opiates for surgical patients focused on their use for preoperative medication or postoperative analgesia. Thus, when hydrocodone bitartrate (Dicodid) and hydromorphone hydrochloride (Dilaudid) were first introduced in 1923 and 1926, respectively, they were used almost exclusively before or after surgery rather than intraoperatively.[2] Opiates used during surgery were intended to supplement waning local or regional anesthesia or to provide additional analgesia during inhalation (nitrous oxide and ether) or intravenous (chloral hydrate and urethane) anesthesia for brief examinations, such as cystoscopy, gastroscopy, or endoscopy.[2,18]

The introduction of sodium thiopental in 1934 was greeted with enthusiasm because of the speed and ease of induction of anesthesia.[5,18,19] It soon became apparent, however, that enormous doses were required for long-lasting analgesia when this drug was used alone.[1,18] Such doses also produced significant intraoperative cardiovascular and respiratory depression and a long postoperative recovery period. Nevertheless, the discovery of thiopental did stimulate interest in the barbiturates and other intravenous agents.[5,19]

Initial attempts to synthesize a new atropine-like spasmolytic agent resulted in the synthesis of meperidine (pethidine and Demerol), the first entirely synthetic narcotic, in 1938.[20] This discovery enabled the introduction of nitrous oxide-meperidine anesthesia by Neff, Mayer, and Perales in 1947,[21] a technique in which nitrous oxide was supplemented with intravenous increments of meperidine, together with d-tubocurarine, sodium thiopental, or both, as well as other thiobarbiturates as needed. This report was an important stimulus for the return of narcotic compounds to the operating theater; shortly thereafter, morphine, alphaprodine, and other opioids began to appear as alternative constituents of the basic nitrous oxide-narcotic technique.[18,22–24] The original hope that meperidine and its congeners (e.g., alphaprodine) would provide analgesia with less (or no) addiction liability and respiratory depression than occurs with morphine use unfortunately proved false.[24] This idea, however, subsequently resulted in efforts to synthesize narcotic antagonists (see subsequent discussion).[25–28]

In the early 1950s, numerous attempts were made to improve the potency and usefulness of narcotics as anesthetics (P. Janssen, personal communication). In France, attempts were made to produce sedation with intense analgesia, termed twilight sleep or artificial hibernation. These techniques were popularized with the use of mixtures of tranquilizers (phenothiazines) and narcotics called lytic cocktails.[29] Early investigations in which these compounds were used focused attention on the need for more potent narcotic analgesics with fewer side-effects and a higher safety margin. The result was the synthesis of dextromoramide, phenoperidine, piritramide, and finally, fentanyl.[30-34] Fentanyl was most impressive because of its greater potency (150 times that of morphine), higher therapeutic index (LD_{50}/ED_{50}) (400 versus 4.8 for meperidine and 70 for morphine) and the *absence of side-effects*. The studies that led to the synthesis of fentanyl laid the foundation for better understanding the structure-activity relationships of narcotic analgesics, and stimulated interest in developing compounds with even greater potency and safety margins.[33,35,36]

MODERN DRUGS

DeCastro and co-workers developed the concept of neuroleptanalgesia, which combines the use of a major tranquilizer, most frequently the butyrophenone droperidol, and a potent opioid analgesic, fentanyl or phenoperidine.[37] Neuroleptanalgesia is characterized by analgesia, amnesia, absence of overt motor activity, suppression of autonomic reflexes, and maintenance of cardiovascular stability. The use of droperidol and fentanyl, available in the United States as a 50:1 mixture of 2.5 mg and 50 μg, respectively (manufactured as Innovar), gained popularity in both the United States and Europe. The combination is now usually used as a component of a balanced anesthestic technique with nitrous oxide (50 to 70%) in oxygen.

The most important recent development in the evolution of the opioids occurred in 1969, when Lowenstein and colleagues reintroduced the concept that opioids in sufficient doses can be anesthetics.[38] The beginnings of open-heart surgery featured importantly in this event because clinicians were attempting to anesthetize and to operate on patients with markedly impaired cardiovascular and pulmonary function and in whom even small degrees of myocardial depression could be catastrophic. Thus, the discovery that morphine (1 to 3 mg/kg) with oxygen (100%) produced anesthesia without myocardial depression, and often with increased cardiac output, was initially widely acclaimed.[39-43] Significant disadvantages soon became apparent, however, including incomplete amnesia, occasional histamine-related reactions (cutaneous flushing, hypotension, and bronchoconstriction), marked increases in intraoperative and postoperative blood and fluid requirements, and especially prolonged postoperative respiratory depression.[39-44] In addition, cardiovascular stability was not always complete: bradycardia, hypotension, or hypertension occurred frequently and the addition of nitrous oxide caused cardiovascular depression.[24,39] Difficulties with morphine anesthesia were most evident in patients undergoing coronary artery surgery, particularly those lacking a history of heart failure.[39,43,44]

Because of these problems with morphine-oxygen anesthesia, a suitable alternative was sought among existing opioids. Meperidine was the first substitute studied. Unfortunately, results of initial investigations in the dog and in man showed that, even after low doses (2 to 2.5 mg/kg) were delivered intravenously, meperidine caused significant cardiovascular depression and tachycardia.[45–48] Anesthetic doses (10 mg/kg) produced a marked decrease in cardiac output and even cardiac arrest.[45] Meperidine was found to be 20 times more depressant to the contractile element of the isolated cat papillary muscle than equianalgesic doses of morphine.[49] In patients given meperidine (2 to 3 mg/kg) and nitrous oxide for major orthopedic surgery, cardiac output was reduced 50%, together with appreciable decreases in stroke volume and arterial blood pressure.[48] After about 1 year, it was concluded that meperidine was not a suitable alternative to morphine as an anesthetic in patients with serious cardiovascular disease. Additional studies demonstrated that alphaprodine and piritramide were not appreciably different from meperidine.[49,50]

Investigators interested in opioid anesthesia then began to study fentanyl.[51–54] In animals anesthetized with other anesthetics, fentanyl caused only minor changes in cardiovascular function, e.g., small decreases in blood pressure and minimal or no change in ventricular performance.[51,53] Huge doses of fentanyl, up to 3 mg/kg, given to dogs under basal anesthesia with barbiturates were found to produce a dose-dependent decrease in heart rate; only small reductions in cardiac output, peripheral resistance, and arterial pressure; and an increase in stroke volume.[54] These findings suggested that fentanyl might be a useful "anesthetic" in man.

Fentanyl (50 to 100 μg/kg) with oxygen (100%) was then evaluated as an anesthetic in patients undergoing mitral valve and coronary artery surgery.[55,56] Changes in cardiovascular dynamics with induction doses ranging from 8 to 30 μg/kg consisted of small decreases in heart rate and arterial blood pressure. All other cardiovascular variables studied, including cardiac output, remained unchanged, even with additional doses up to 100 μg/kg.

Fentanyl is currently popular for use as a narcotic anesthetic, despite its potential for cardiovascular depression and stimulation, respiratory depression, muscle rigidity, and, occasionally, incomplete anesthesia.[57–60] Its success, particularly in higher doses, portends changes in anesthetic practice of the future, especially with newer, more potent analgesics with higher therapeutic indices and other desirable pharmacokinetic characteristics (see Chapter 3).

Sufentanil is a new synthetic opioid that is approximately 5 to 10 times more potent than fentanyl and has a therapeutic index (LD_{50}/ED_{50}) approximately 100 times greater than that of fentanyl (25,000 versus 277) in rats. Sufentanil was approved for clinical use by the United States Food and Drug Administration in 1984 as an anesthetic supplement and complete anesthetic.[61] The cardiovascular actions of this opioid are similar to those of fentanyl; however, sufentanil may be more effective in blocking sympathetic activation during surgical stimulation, especially in patients prone to intraoperative hypertension.

Alfentanil is another new narcotic analgesic that may soon be available in the United States. Alfentanil is one fourth as potent as and is shorter acting than fentanyl.[62] Its therapeutic index is also high (1080) in rats.[47] These actions have indicated that the drug may be of use as an anesthetic induction agent or analgesic supplement, especially in patients undergoing short operative procedures.

AGONIST-ANTAGONISTS

A highlight in the history of narcotics in anesthesiology has been the search for a potent analgesic that results in minimal or no depression of respiration. An alternative goal would be to develop a safe and potent antagonist of the respiratory side-effects of narcotic analgesics. The first opioid antagonist, *N*-allylnorcodeine, was synthesized by Pohl in 1914 in an attempt to improve the analgesic properties of codeine.[63] The discovery that this compound mildly antagonized the respiratory depression and sleep produced by morphine remained unnoticed for 24 years until McCawley et al. attempted to prepare *N*-allylnormorphine (nalorphine) as a strong analgesic with "built-in" antagonistic action.[64] Successfully synthesized later by Weijland and Erickson in 1942, the compound was found to be strongly antagonistic to most of the effects of morphine.[65–67] In larger doses, nalorphine is a potent analgesic in man and in animals.[68–70] Unfortunately, these doses of nalorphine produce severe psychotomimetic effects, rendering the drug unsuitable as an analgesic, although in lower dosage it is an effective opioid antagonist.

The discovery of nalorphine stimulated a search for other agonist-antagonist drugs, mostly with only minor molecular modification of existing opioids.[71] The next such agonist-antagonist used widely in man was pentazocine, the *N*-dimethylallyl derivative of phenazocaine.[72,73] Pentazocine has one-third to one-fifth the analgesic properties of morphine, but in equipotent doses it produces similar degrees of respiratory depression.[74,75]

More recently, two totally different synthetic agonist-antagonist analgesics, butorphanol and nalbuphine, have become available. The synthesis of butorphanol (BC-2627) was reported in 1972.[76] In man, its analgesic potency is 508 times that of morphine, and its duration of action is similar to that of morphine.[77–80] Although respiratory depression produced by butorphanol (2 mg) is equivalent to that of morphine (10 mg), respiratory depression does not increase in a dose-related fashion with increasing doses of butorphanol as it does with morphine.[81]

Nalbuphine is structurally related to the opioid, oxymorphone, and to the opioid antagonist, naloxone. Its analgesic potency and duration are similar to those of morphine and have been attributed to an action at kappa opioid receptors.[82] Nalbuphine also binds to, but only produces a minimal agonist effect on, the classic pure agonist mu receptors, which are thought to mediate analgesia and respiratory depression produced by morphine and other opioids.[83,84] Competitive interaction between nalbuphine and agonist opioids at those receptors may explain the opioid-antagonistic activity of nalbuphine. The future role of the agonist-antagonists in clinical anesthesia is uncertain but is potentially exciting.

REFERENCES

1. Theophrastus: *C.f.,* Wooton, A.C.: Chronicles of Pharmacy. London, Macmillan, 1910.
2. Foldes, F.F., Swerdlow, M., and Siker, E.S.: Narcotics and Narcotic Antagonists. Springfield, Charles C Thomas, 1964, pp. 1–7.
3. de Chaulica, G., and La Wall, C.F.: 4000 Years of Pharmacy. Philadelphia, Lippincott, 1927.
4. Gwathmey, J.T.: Anesthesia. New York, Macmillan, 1925.
5. Adams, R.C.: Intravenous Anesthesia. New York, Hoeber, 1944.
6. Serturner, F.W.A.: Darstellung der reinen Mohnsäure nebst einer chemischen Untersuchung des Opiums mit vorzüglicher Hinsicht auf einen darin neu entdeckten Stoff und die dahin gehörigen Beherkungen. J. Pharm. Aerzte Apoth. Chem., *14*:47, 1806.
7. Pravaz, C.G.: Sur un nouveau moyen d'opérér la coagulation du sang dans les arteries. Applicable à la guérison des aneurismes. C. R. Seances Acad. Sci. [III], *36*:88, 1853.
8. Wood, A.: New method of treating neuralgia by the direct application of opiates to the painful joints. Edinb. Med. J., 82:265, 1855.
9. Kane, H.H.: The Hypodermic Injection of Morphia. New York, Chas. L. Bermingham, 1880.
10. Dogliotti, A.M.: Anesthesia: Narcosis, Local, Regional, Spinal. Chicago, S.B. Debour, 1939.
11. Bernard, C.: Lecons sur des Anesthesiques et sur l'Asphyxie. Paris, Masson, 1875.
12. Schneiderlin, H.D.: Eine neue Narkose. Aerztl Mitt a Baden, *54*:101, 1900.

13. Babcock, W.W.: A new method of surgical anesthesia. Proc. Phila. County Med. Soc., 26:347, 1905.
14. Smith, R.R.: Scopolamine-morphine anesthesia, with report of two hundred and twenty-nine cases. Surg. Gynecol. Obstet., 8:414, 1908 (Abstr.).
15. Holt, W.L.: Scopolamine-morphine in obstetrics. Am. J. Clin. Med., 14:565, 1907.
16. Van Hoosen, M.A.: Scopolamine-Morphine Anesthesia. Chicago, House of Manz, 1915.
17. Boit, H.: Die kombination vol skopolamin-dilaudid mit ortlicher betaubung und mit evipanzu-satznarkose bei mittleren und grossen operationen. Zentralbl. Chir., 61:1662, 1934.
18. Foldes, F.F., Swerdlow, M., and Siker, E.S.: Narcotics and Narcotic Antagonists. Springfield, Charles C Thomas, 1964, pp. 7–9.
19. Lundy, J.S.: Intravenous and regional anesthesia. Ann. Surg., 110:878, 1939.
20. Eisleb, O., and Schaumann, O.: Dolantin, ein neuartiges spasmolytikum und analgeticum. Dtsch. Med. Wochenschr., 65:967, 1939.
21. Neff, W., Mayer, E.C., and de la Luz Perales, M.: Nitrous oxide and oxygen anesthesia with curare relaxation. Calif. Med., 66:67, 1947.
22. Foldes, F.F., Swerdlow, M., Lipschitz, E., Weber, G., and Pick, L.A.: The combined use of nisentil hydrochloride and levallorphan tartrate for the supplementation of nitrous oxide-oxygen anesthesia. Can. Anaesth. Soc. J., 2:362, 1955.
23. Siker, E.S., Foldes, F.F., Pahk, N.M., and Swerdlow, M.: Nisentil (1,3,dimethyl-4-phenyl-4 pro-pionoxy piperidine): a new supplement for nitrous oxide-oxygen, thiopentone (pentothal sodium) anesthesia. Br. J. Anaesth., 26:405, 1954.
24. Eddy, N.B., Halbach, H., and Braenden, O.J.: Synthetic substances with morphine-like effect. Clinical experience: potency, side-effects, addiction liability. Bull. WHO, 17:569, 1957.
25. Eckenhoff, J.E., Elder, J.D., and King, B.D.: The effect of N-allyl normorphine in treatment of opiate overdose. Am. J. Med. Sci., 222:115, 1951.
26. Hamilton, W.K., and Cullen, S.C.: Effect of levallorphan tartrate upon opiate-induced respiratory depression. Anesthesiology, 14:550, 1953.
27. Schnider, O., and Hellerbach, J.: Synthese von morphinanen (2. Mitterkung). Helv. Chir. Acta, 33:1437, 1950.
28. Lunn, J.N., Foldes, F.F., More, J., and Brown, I.M.: The influence of N-allyloxymorphone on the respiratory effects of oxymorphone in anesthetized man. Pharmacologist, 3:66, 1961.
29. Laborit, H., and Huguenard, P.: Practique, de l'hibernotherapie in chirurgie et en medicine. Paris, Masson et cie, 1954.
30. Janssen, P.A.J., and Jageneau, A.H.: A new series of potent analgesics. J. Pharm. Pharmacol., 10:14, 1958.
31. Janssen, P.A.J., and Eddy, N.B.: Compounds related to pethidine-IV: new general chemical methods of increasing the analgesic activity of pethidine. J. Med. Chem., 2:32, 1960.
32. Janssen, P.A.J.: Pirinitramide (R 3365), a potent analgesic with unusual chemical structure. J. Pharm. Pharmacol., 13:513, 1961.
33. Janssen, P.A.J.: A review of the chemical features associated with strong morphine-like activity. Br. J. Anaesth., 34:260, 1962.
34. Janssen, P.A.J.: The inhibitory effect of fentanyl and other morphine-like analgesics on the warm water-induced tail withdrawal reflex in rats. Drug. Res., 13:502, 1963.
35. Van Bever, W.F.M., Niemegeers, C.J.E., Schellekens, K.H.L., and Janssen, P.A.J.: N-4-substi-tuted 1-(2-arylethyl)-4-piperidinyl-N-phenylpropanamides, a novel series of extremely potent an-algesics with unusually high safety margin. Drug Res., 26:1548, 1976.
36. Niemegeers, C.J.E., Schellekens, K.H.L., Van Bever, W.F.M., and Janssen, P.A.J.: Sufentanil, a very potent and extremely safe intravenous morphine-like compound in mice, rats and dogs. Drug Res., 26:1551, 1976.
37. DeCastro, J., and Mundeleer, R.: Anesthesie sans barbituratiques: la neuroleptanalgesie. Anesth. Analg., 16:1022, 1959.
38. Lowenstein, E., Hallowell, P., Levine, F.H., Daggett, W.M., Austin, G., and Laver, M.B.: Cardiovascular response to large doses of intravenous morphine in man. N. Engl. J. Med., 281:1389, 1969.
39. Stoelting, R.K., and Gibbs, P.S.: Hemodynamic effects of morphine and morphine-nitrous oxide in valvular heart disease and coronary artery disease. Anesthesiology, 38:42, 1973.
40. Stanley, T.H., Gray, N.H., Stanford, W., and Armstrong, R.: The effects of high-dose morphine in fluid and blood requirements in open-heart procedures. Anesthesiology, 38:536, 1973.
41. Hasbrouk, J.D.: Morphine anesthesia for open-heart surgery. Ann. Thorac. Surg., 10:364, 1970.
42. McDermott, R.W., and Stanley, T.H.: The cardiovascular effects of low concentrations of nitrous oxide during morphine anesthesia. Anesthesiology, 41:89, 1974.
43. Arens, J.F., Benbow, B.P., Ochsner, J.L., and Theard, R.: Morphine anesthesia for aorto-coronary bypass procedures. Anesth. Analg., 51:901, 1972.
44. Lowenstein, E.: Morphine "anesthesia"—a perspective. Anesthesiology, 35:563, 1971.

45. Freye, E.: Cardiovascular effects of high dosages of fentanyl, meperidine and naloxone in dogs. Anesth. Analg., *53*:40, 1974.

46. Stanley, T.H., Bidwai, A.V., Lunn, J.K., and Hodges, M.R.: Cardiovascular effects of nitrous oxide during meperidine infusion in the dog. Anesth. Analg., *56*:836, 1977.

47. de Castro, J., Van de Water, A., Wouters, L., Xhonneux, R., Reneman, R., and Kay, B.: Comparative study of cardiovascular, neurological and metabolic side effects of eight narcotics in dogs. Parts I, II, and III. Acta Anaesthesiol. Belg., *30*:5, 1979.

48. Stanley, T.H., and Liu, W.S.: Cardiovascular effects of nitrous oxide-meperidine anesthesia before and after pancuronium. Anesth. Analg., *56*:669, 1977.

49. Strauer, B.: Contractile responses to morphine, piritramide, meperidine and fentanyl: A comparative study of effects on the isolated ventricular myocardium. Anesthesiology, *37*:304, 1972.

50. Reddy, P., Liu, W.S., Port, D., Gillmor, S., and Stanley, T.H.: Comparison of haemodynamic effects of anaesthetic doses of alphaprodine and sufentanil in the dog. Can. Anaesth. Soc. J., *27*:345, 1980.

51. Patschke, D., Gethmann, J.W., Hess, W., Tajrrow, J., and Waibel, H.: Hemodynamic koronardruchblutung und myocardialer sauerstoffverbrauch unter hohen fentanyl und piritramidosen. Anaesthesist, *25*:309, 1976.

52. Freye, E.: Effects of high doses of fentanyl on myocardial infarction and cardiogenic shock in the dog. Resuscitation, *3*:105, 1974.

53. Eisele, J.H., Reitan, J.A., Torten, M., and Miller, C.H.: Myocardial sparing effect of fentanyl during halothane anesthesia in dogs. Br. J. Anaesth., *47*:937, 1975.

54. Liu, W.S., Bidwai, A.V., Stanley, T.H., and Loeser, E.A.: Cardiovascular dynamics after large doses of fentanyl and fentanyl plus N_2O in the dog. Anesth. Analg., *55*:168, 1976.

55. Stanley, T.H., and Webster, L.R.: Anesthetic requirements and cardiovascular effects of fentanyl-oxygen and fentanyl-diazepam-oxygen anesthesia in man. Anesth. Analg., *57*:411, 1978.

56. Lunn, J.K., Webster, L.R., Stanley, T.H., and Woodward, A.: High dose fentanyl anesthesia for coronary artery surgery: Plasma fentanyl concentration and influence of nitrous oxide on cardiovascular responses. Anesth. Analg., *58*:390, 1979.

57. Stanley, T.H., Berman, L., Green, O., and Robertson, D.: Plasma catecholamine and cortisol responses to fentanyl-oxygen anesthesia for coronary artery operations. Anesthesiology, *53*:250, 1980.

58. Stanley, T.H.: The pharmacology of intravenous narcotic anesthetics. *In* Anesthesia. Edited by R.D. Miller, New York, Churchill Livingstone, 1981, pp. 425–449.

59. Robinson, S., and Gregory, G.A.: Fentanyl-air-oxygen anesthesia for ligation of patent ductus arteriosus in preterm infants. Anesth. Analg., *60*:331, 1981.

60. Sebel, P.S., Bovill, J.G., Wauquier, A., and Rog, P.: Effects of high dose fentanyl anesthesia on the electroencephalogram. Anesthesiology, *55*:203, 1981.

61. de Lange, S., Boscoe, M., Stanley, T.H., and Pace, N.: Comparison of sufentanil-O_2 and fentanyl-O_2 for coronary artery surgery. Anesthesiology, *56*:112, 1982.

62. Nauta, J., de Lange, S., Koopman, D., Spierdijk, J., and Stanley, T.H.: Anesthetic induction with alfentanil: a new short-acting narcotic analgesic. Anesth. Analg., *61*:267, 1982.

63. Pohl, J.: Uber das *N*-allylnorcodeine, einen antagonisten des morphins. J. Exp. Path. Ther., *17*:370, 1915.

64. McCawley, W.L., Hart, E.R., and Marsh, D.F.: The preparation of *N*-allylnormorphine. J. Am. Chem. Soc., *63*:314, 1941.

65. Weijland, J., and Erickson, A.E.: *N*-allylnormorphine. J. Am. Chem. Soc., *64*:869, 1942.

66. Unna, K.: Antagonist effect of *N*-allylnormorphine upon morphine. J. Pharmacol. Exp. Ther., *79*:27, 1943.

67. Hart, E.R., and McCawley, W.L.: The pharmacology of *N*-allylnormorphine as compared with morphine. J. Pharmacol. Exp. Ther., *82*:339, 1944.

68. Schnider, O., and Hellerback, J.: Synthese von morphinan. Helv. Chim. Acta, *33*:1437, 1950.

69. Pearl, J., Stander, H., and McKean, D.B.: Effects of analgesics and other drugs on mice in phenylquinone and rotarod test. J. Pharmacol. Exp. Ther., *167*:9, 1969.

70. Perrine, T.D., Atwell, L., Tice, I.B., Jacobson, A.E., and May, E.L.: Analgesic activity as determined by the Nilsen method. J. Pharm. Sci., *61*:86, 1972.

71. Clark, R.L., Pessolano, A.A., and Weijland, J.: *N*-substituted eponymorphinans. J. Am. Chem. Soc., *75*:4974, 1953.

72. Jasinski, D.R., Martin, W.R., and Hoeldtke, R.D.: Effects of short and long-term administration of pentazocine in man. Clin. Pharmacol. Ther., *11*:385, 1970.

73. Fraser, H.R., and Rosenberg, D.E.: Studies on the human addiction liability of 2-hydroxy-5,9-dimethyl-2-(3,3-dimethylallyl)-6,7-benzomorphan (Win 20,228): a weak narcotic antagonist. J. Pharmacol. Exp. Ther., *143*:149, 1964.

74. Leaman, D.M., Nellis, S.H., Zelis, R., and Field, J.M.: Effects of morphine sulfate on human coronary blood flow. Am. J. Cardiol., *41*:324, 1978.

75. Lee, G., De Maria, A.N., Amsterdam, E.A., Realyvasquez, F., Angel, J., Morrison, S., and Mason,

D.T.: Meperidine and pentazocine on cardiocirculatory dynamics in patients with acute my-ocardial infarction. Am. J. Med., *60*:949, 1976.

76. Monkovic, I., Conway, T.T., Wang, H., Perron, Y.G., Patcher, I.J., and Belleau, B.: Total synthesis and pharmacological activities of N-substituted 3,14 dihydroxymorphinans. J. Am. Chem. Soc., *95*:7910, 1973.
77. Dobkin, A.B., Eamkaow, S., Zak, S., and Caruso, F.S.: Butorphanol: a double-blind evaluation in postoperative patients with moderate or severe pain. Can. Anaesth. Soc. J., *21*:600, 1974.
78. Tavakoli, M., Corssen, G., and Caruso, F.S.: Butorphanol and morphine: a double-blind comparison of their parenteral analgesic activity. Anesth. Analg., *55*:394, 1976.
79. Del Pizzo, A.: Butorphanol: a double-blind intramuscular analgesic comparison with morphine sulfate in postoperative patients with moderate or severe pain. Curr. Ther. Res., *20*:221, 1976.
80. Gilbert, M.S., Hanover, R.M., Moylan, D.S., and Caruso, F.S.: Intramuscular butorphanol and meperidine in postoperative pain. Clin. Pharmacol. Ther., *20*:359, 1976.
81. Nagashima, H., Karamanian, A., Malovany, R., Radnay, P., Ang, M., Koerner, S., and Foldes, F.F.: Effects of intravenous butorphanol and morphine. Clin. Pharmacol. Ther., *19*:738, 1976.
82. Beaver, W.T., and Feise, G.A.: A comparison of the analgesic effect of intramuscular nalbuphine and morphine in patients with postoperative pain. J. Pharmacol. Exp. Ther., *204*:487, 1978.
83. De Fazio, C.A., Moscicki, J.C., and Magruder, M.R.: Anesthetic potency of nalbuphine and interaction with morphine in rats. Anesth. Analg., *60*:629, 1981.
84. Gilbert, P.E., and Martin, W.R.: The effects of morphine and nalorphine-like drugs in the non-dependent, morphine-dependent and cyclazocine-dependent chronic spinal dog. J. Pharmacol. Exp. Ther., *198*:66, 1976.

Chapter 3

CHEMISTRY OF NARCOTIC COMPOUNDS

CLASSIFICATION

Narcotic-analgesic compounds have long been classified as naturally occurring, semisynthetic, and synthetic (Table 3–1).[1,2] Although an increased understanding of the structure-activity relationships of these compounds has suggested that classification by chemical structure may be more rational, the unknowns in opioid structure-activity relationships still are sufficient to defend the use of the older classification in this chapter.

The naturally occurring narcotics are obtained from the poppy plant, *Papaver somniferum,* the source of more than 20 pharmacologically active alkaloids that constitute opium. The only useful members of this group can be divided into 2 chemical classes, phenanthrenes (morphine and codeine) and benzylisoquinoline derivatives (papaverine). Only morphine (Fig. 3–1) is important as an intravenous anesthetic or analgesic.

The semisynthetic narcotics are derivatives of morphine in which any one of several changes has been made, e.g., etherification of one hydroxyl group (codeine), esterification of both hydroxyl groups (heroin), oxidation of the alcoholic hydroxyl to a ketone, or saturation of a double bond on the benzene ring (hydromorphone hydrochloride [Dilaudid]).

The synthetic compounds may be divided into four groups, of which the first three resemble morphine: the morphinan derivatives (levorphanol), the diphenyl

Table 3–1. Classification of Narcotic Compounds

Naturally occurring
    Morphine
    Codeine
    Papaverine

Semisynthetic
    Heroin
    Dilaudid

Synthetic
    Morphine derivatives (levorphanol)
    Methadone derivatives (methadone)
    Benzomorphan derivatives (pentazocine)
    Phenylpiperidine derivatives (meperidine, fentanyl, sufentanil, and alfentanil)

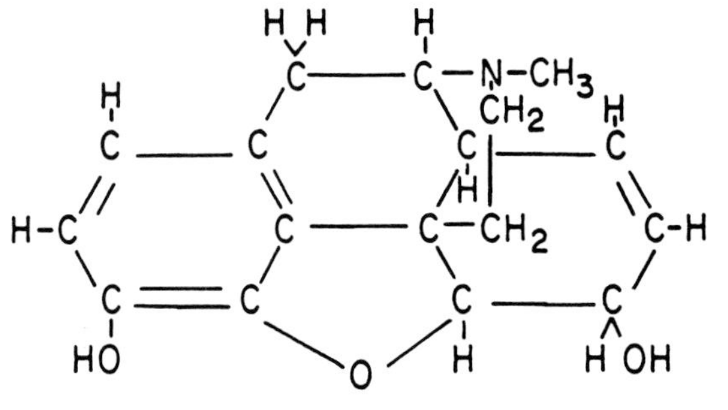

Fig. 3–1. Structural formulas of morphine and its antagonist, naloxone.

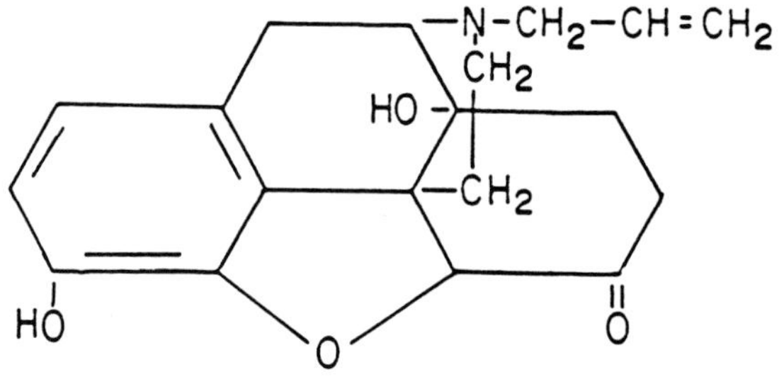

or methadone derivatives (methadone and *d*-propoxyphene), the benzomorphans (phenazocine and pentazocine), and the phenylpiperidine derivatives (meperidine and fentanyl). Although many of these compounds have been suggested for intravenous analgesia or anesthesia, only the phenylpiperidines are in current use during surgery. Pentazocine and methadone are, however, frequently used to provide postoperative analgesia.

MODE OF ACTION

The mode of action of narcotic compounds can be explained in terms of receptor sites in the central nervous system (CNS) and elsewhere, their interaction with central and peripheral nervous system transmitters, and their chemical structure.

SITE OF ACTION

The existence of specific narcotic (opiate) receptors in the CNS has long been postulated. Determination of their precise location and identification was not feasible until recently because narcotics bind to most biologic membranes, including opiate receptors.[3-5] Non-binding can be excluded from binding receptors by measuring total membrane binding with stereospecific radioactive opiates and measuring nonspecific binding with compounds chemically similar to opiates but lacking narcotic activity (e.g., dextromoramide). Stereospecific binding is determined by the difference between the results of the two determinations.[3-5]

The initial discovery suggested that opiate receptors were found only in certain areas of the CNS.[6,7] Subsequently, numerous classes of opiate receptors were found widely distributed throughout the brain, spinal cord, and other major organ systems, including the liver, lungs, heart, uterus, and certain white blood cells.[5,8–13] Distribution of the mu or classic morphine receptor in the CNS is not uniform. The highest mu receptor densities are found in a small part of the ventral mesencephalon (mammary bodies), in the mesolimbic area (nucleus accumbens and tuberculum olfactorium), the thalamus, striatum, amygdala, hypothalamus, and periaqueductal gray and mid-brain raphe.[5,13] These regions are thought to be involved with pain perception and integration, as well as with emotional responses to pain; in all these areas, microinjections of morphine or direct electric stimulation produce analgesia that is reversible by naloxone.[6,7] The cortex, especially the frontal cortex, also contains mu receptors, at least in rats.[5] Interestingly, mu opioid receptors are present in both ventral and dorsal portions of the spinal cord, slightly more in the dorsal than the ventral regions and more in the thoracic than the lumbar region.[5]

In addition to analgesia and alterations in emotional responses to pain, opiates produce other effects, such as reducing spontaneous ventilation and ventilatory responses to carbon dioxide, decreasing tension in vascular smooth muscle, and increasing smooth muscle tone in other organs (e.g., urethral sphincter and biliary tract). All these effects are attributable to stimulation of one or more of the abovementioned opiate receptors.[13] There are clearly at least three to six populations of opiate receptors of varying sensitivity to different opiates and congeners, but their tonic or phasic interactions and purpose are unclear.

ENDOGENOUS OPIATE-LIKE PEPTIDES

The long-recognized specificity of CNS receptors for morphine and other narcotics was suggestive of the possible existence of an endogenous, narcotic-like compound involved in pain perception.[9–13] In 1975, two pentapeptides with significant opiate-like activity were found in the brain and were called enkephalins.[14–16] These pentapeptides are present throughout the brain and spinal cord, with highest density in regions that are rich in opiate receptors.[14,15] In addition to the CNS, the enkephalins appear only in the gastrointestinal tract.[7] Their striking restriction to the CNS and one or more other organs suggests that they may act as neurohormones.

Enkephalins, however, are not the only opioid peptides in the CNS. Larger peptides containing the intact sequence of amino acids found in the enkephalins have been found in the pituitary gland. Called endorphins, these compounds bind to opiate receptors and have marked narcotic activity. They in turn are part of an even larger pituitary extract, lipotropin (Fig. 3–2).[17]

The exact relationship of enkephalins to endorphins and the purpose of both in the CNS are not clear. In assays of opiate binding in synaptosomes, the activity of these peptides is indistinguishable from that of morphine. On a molar basis, the enkephalins and most of the endorphins are about as active as morphine. In contrast, β-endorphin is 5 to 10 times more potent than morphine. Because enkephalins are rapidly metabolized when injected intravenously or directly into the cerebral ventricles, their analgesic actions are difficult to evaluate in vivo, although they do produce significant analgesia for 15 to 60 minutes. Remarkably, some endorphins appear to produce analgesia in specific body areas, e.g., the face and neck. In contrast, β-endorphin produces analgesia of the entire body. Endorphins also affect temperature, mood, and the secretion of other neurohor-

```
H-GLU-LEU-THR-GLY-GLU-ARG-LEU-GLU-GLN-ALA-ARG-
  1
GLY-PRO-GLU-ALA-GLN-ALA-GLU-SER-ALA-ALA-ALA-

ARG-ALA-GLU-LEU-GLU-TYR-GLY-LEU-VAL-ALA-GLU-ALA-

GLU-ALA-ALA-GLU-LYS-LYS-ASP-SER-GLY-PRO-TYR-LYS-

MET-GLU-HIS-PHE-ARG-TRP-GLY-SER-PRO-PRO-LYS-ASP-

LYS-ARG-TYR-GLY-GLY-PHE-MET-THR-SER-GLU-LYS-SER-
            61                65
GLN-THR-PRO-LEU-VSL-THR-LEU-PHE-LYS-ASN-ALA-ILE-
                          76  77
ILE-LYS-ASN-ALA-HIS-LYS-LYS-GLY-GLN-OH
            87                    91
```

Fig. 3–2. Beta-lipotropin (β-LPH), a 91 amino acid pituitary hormone, contains some endorphins and enkephalins within its structure. Met-enkephalin corresponds to the 61-65 amino acid sequence of this hormone. Alpha-, beta-, gamma-, and delta-endorphin correspond to the 61-76, 61-91, 61-77, and 61-87 amino acid sequences of beta-lipotropin, respectively.

mones.[16] Conceivably, manipulation of these peptides in the CNS or administration of similar synthetic compounds might produce desirable analgesic or anesthetic effects in surgical patients.

What is the role of the endogenous opiates in man? These peptides may influence both normal and abnormal behavior and even drug addiction and withdrawal. They may also play an important, if imprecisely defined, part in the physiologic response to metabolic and psychologic stress, immunologic reactions, and circulatory responses during certain disease processes, e.g., sepsis and hypovolemic shock.[13,15–21]

The endogenous opiates exist in virtually all vertebrate species and in many invertebrates as well. Highest concentrations of β-endorphin occur in the pituitary gland (anterior and intermediate lobes greater than posterior lobe) and in the medial basal and arcuate regions of the hypothalamus. Some long-axoned endorphin-releasing neurons synapse at upper brain stem locations, including diencephalic, telencephalic, medullary, and spinal cord nuclei. β-Endorphin also exists outside the CNS in the small intestine, placenta, and plasma. The enkephalins are widely distributed in many areas of the CNS (amygdala, globus pallidus, striatum, hypothalamus, thalamus, brain stem, and spinal cord dorsal horn laminae I and II) and in the peripheral nervous system (peripheral ganglia, autonomic nervous system, adrenal medulla, gastrointestinal tract, and plasma).

STRUCTURE-ACTIVITY RELATIONSHIPS

Pure Agonist (Mu) Receptor-Stimulating Narcotics

Structurally, narcotics are complex, three-dimensional compounds existing as two stereoisomers,[7] of which usually only one isomer is able to produce analgesia. Indeed, the presence or absence of analgesic activity is intimately related to its stereochemical structure in keeping with the "lock-and-key" hypothesis of narcotic action.[2,5,22–25] Hence, relatively minor changes in conformation of a narcotic molecule significantly alter pharmacologic activity. This concept and dissatisfaction with available opioids, especially morphine and meperidine, as less than optimal molecules to reach and stimulate the opioid (mu) receptor have been two major forces in the design and development of better compounds.

Lipid solubility has long been recognized as a key factor in the passage of drugs across the blood-brain barrier. Because meperidine is almost 30 to 35 times more lipid soluble than morphine (octanol pH 7.4 buffer partition coefficient = 38.8 to 1.42), chemists began experimenting with congeners of meperidine.[26] Because benzene rings are known to enhance lipid solubility, a phenyl group replaced 1 hydrogen of the methyl group attached to the nitrogen in meperidine in one of the earliest compounds studied (Fig. 3–3) (P. Janssen, personal communication). The result was enhanced analgesic activity, although the spatial arrangements of those elements of the molecule chiefly responsible for interacting with the receptor were still less than ideal. It was subsequently found that, by separating the phenyl group linking the nitrogen on meperidine by 3 carbons instead of 1 and then adding a hydroxyl group to the third carbon, a compound, later called phenoperidine, could be created (Fig. 3–3). This compound was 20 times more potent than morphine and approximately 200 times more potent than meperidine.[22]

Continuing attempts to optimize molecular configuration eventuated in fentanyl (Fig. 3–4), a compound with 100 to 300 times the potency of morphine (depending on the species evaluated).[22–24] Note that the distance between the piperidine nitrogen and the benzene ring is reduced from 3 to 2 carbon atoms, the ester on the right side of the molecule is reversed, and one of its oxygen molecules is replaced with a nitrogen.

In addition to increased potency, fentanyl possesses an analgesic therapeutic index approximately 4 times that of morphine (277 versus 70) and more than 50 times that of meperidine (277 versus 5). By attaching a small C-O-C tail (Fig. 3–4), fentanyl is converted to a new variant called carfentanil. This molecule has a potency of approximately 10,000 times that of morphine and a therapeutic index of about 8500 in (non-ventilated) rats.[27] A derivative of carfentanil, called sufen-

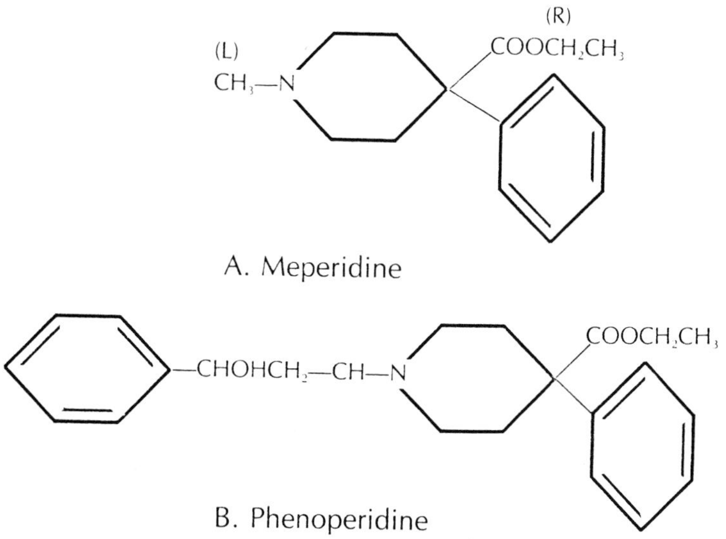

A. Meperidine

B. Phenoperidine

Fig. 3–3. Structural formulas for meperidine and phenoperidine.

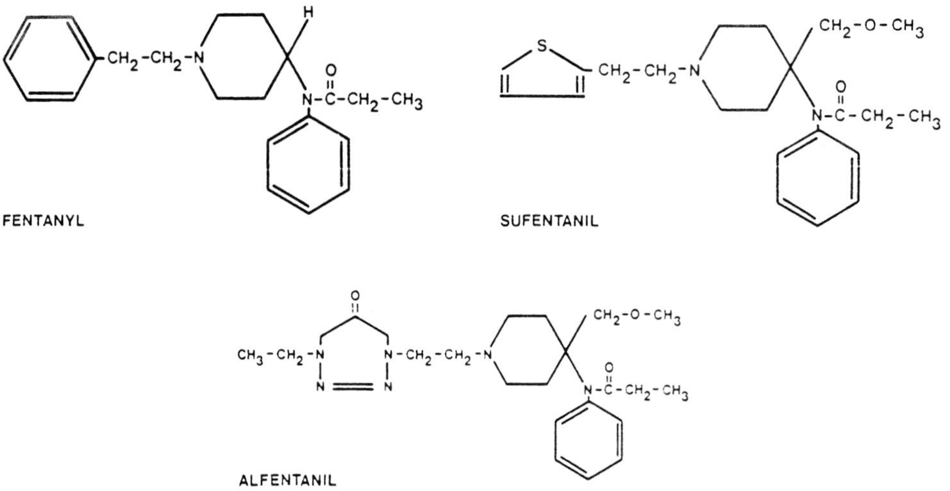

FENTANYL

SUFENTANIL

ALFENTANIL

Fig. 3–4.   Structural formulas for fentanyl, sufentanil, and alfentanil.

tanil (Fig. 3–4), is about 5000 times more potent than morphine and has an even higher analgesic therapeutic index than carfentanil, more than 25,000.[24]

Note that the degree of lipid solubility of sufentanil is about 1000 times that of morphine.[24] An important concept in the search for better narcotics is the hypothesis that increased potency implies increased specificity for the opioid (mu) receptor, including greater lipid solubility. Therefore, fewer molecules are required to cross the blood-brain barrier to reach receptor sites, thus leaving fewer molecules available in the circulation to produce unwanted reactions. The data

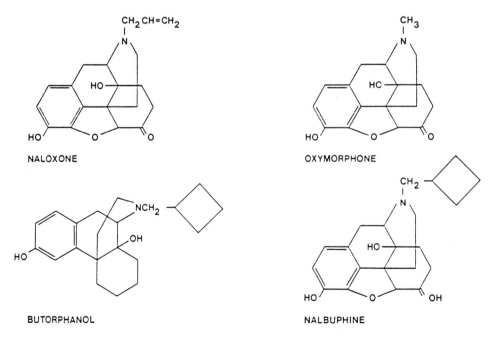

NALOXONE

OXYMORPHONE

BUTORPHANOL

NALBUPHINE

Fig. 3–5.   Structural formulas of opioid antagonists and mixed agonist-antagonists.

indicate that the gain in potency of sufentanil has been achieved, not with increased toxicity but with increased safety.

Agonist-Antagonist Narcotics

The one molecular modification essential to produce a narcotic antagonist is alkylation of the piperidine nitrogen with a three-carbon side chain, such as propyl, allyl, or methallyl (see Fig. 3–1).[28] Other alterations in the molecule have resulted in a variety of compounds with mixed agonist and antagonist activity (Fig. 3–5).[29–33] Although these compounds vary widely in potency, side-effects, and therapeutic indices, none comes even close to the analgesic effectiveness of the newer, potent, pure agonist compounds.

REFERENCES

1. Stanley, T.H.: The pharmacology of intravenous narcotic anesthetics. *In* Anesthesia. Edited by R.D. Miller, New York, Churchill Livingstone, 1981, pp. 425–449.
2. Foldes, F.F., Swerdlow, M., and Siker, E.S.: Chemistry of narcotics and narcotic antagonists. *In* Narcotics and Narcotic Antagonists. Springfield, Charles C Thomas, 1954, pp. 10–26.
3. Leysen, J., and Laduron, P.: Differential distribution of opiate and neuroleptic receptors and dopamine-sensitive adenylate cyclase in rat brain. Life Sci., *20*:281, 1977.
4. Leysen, J., Tollenaere, J.P., Koch, M.H.J., and Laduron, P.: Differentiation of opiate and neuroleptic receptor binding in rat brain. Eur. J. Pharmacol., *43*:253, 1977.
5. Leysen, J., Gommeren, W., and Niemegeers, C.J.E.: ^{3}H-Sufentanil, a superior ligand for μ-opiate receptors; binding properties and regional distribution in rat brain and spinal cord. Eur. J. Pharmacol., *87*:209, 1983.
6. Pert, C.B., Kuhar, M.J., and Snyder, S.H.: Opiate receptor autoradiographic localization in rat brain. Proc. Natl. Acad. Sci. USA, *73*:3729, 1976.
7. Snyder, S.H.: Opiate receptors in the brain. N. Engl. J. Med., *296*:266, 1977.
8. Martin, W.R., Eades, C.G., Thompson, J.A., Huppler, R.E., and Gilbert, P.E.: The effects of morphine- and nalorphine-like drugs in the nondependent and morphine-dependent chronic spinal dog. J. Pharmacol. Exp. Ther., *197*:517, 1976.
9. Lord, J.A.H., Waterfield, A.A., Hughes, J., and Kosterlitz, H.W.: Endogenous opioid peptides: multiple agonists and receptors. Nature, 267:495, 500, 1977.
10. Wuster, M., Schulz, R., and Herz, A.: The direction of opioid agonists towards μ-, δ- and ε-receptors in the vas deferens of the mouse and the rat. Life Sci., *27*:163, 1980.
11. Goodman, R.R., Snyder, S.H., Kuhar, M.J., and Young, W.S., III: Differentiation of delta and mu opiate receptor localizations by light microscopic autoradiography. Proc. Natl. Acad. Sci. USA, 77:6239, 1980.
12. Yaksh, T.L., and Rudy, T.A.: Narcotic analgesics: CNS sites and mechanisms of action as revealed by intracerebral injection techniques. Pain, *4*:299, 1978.
13. Yaksh, T.: Opiate receptors and endorphins. 1982 ASA Refresher Course, October, 1982, pp. 134.
14. Hughes, J., Smith, T.W., and Kosterlitz, H.W.: Identification of two related penta peptides from the brain with potent opiate agonist activity. Nature, *258*:577, 1975.
15. Fredrickson, R.C.A.: Enkephalin pentapeptides—a review of current evidence of a physiological role in vertebrate neurotransmission. Life. Sci., *21*:23, 1977.
16. Goldstein, A.L.: Opioid peptides (endorphins) in pituitary and brain. Science, *193*:1081, 1976.
17. Krieger, D.T., Yamaguchi, H., and Liotta, A.S.: Human plasma ACTH, lipotropin, and endorphin. *In* Neurosecretion and Brain Peptides. Edited by J.B. Martin, S. Reichlin, and K.L. Bick. New York, Raven Press, 1981, pp. 541–556.
18. Lewis, R.V., Stern, A.S., Kimura, S., Rossier, J., Stein, S., and Udenfriend, S.: An about 50,000-dalton protein in adrenal medulla: a common precursor of [Met]- and [Leu]enkephalin. Science, *208*:1459, 1980.
19. Holaday, J.W., and Faden, A.I.: Naloxone reverses the pathophysiology of shock through an antagonism of endorphin systems. *In* Neurosecretion and Brain Peptides. Edited by J.B. Martin, S. Reichlin, and K.L. Bick. New York, Raven Press, 1981, pp 421–434.
20. Peters, W.P., Johnson, M.W., Friedman, P.A., and Mitch, W.E.: Pressor effect on naloxone in septic shock. Lancet, *1*:529, 1981.
21. Sapru, H.N., Willette, R.N., and Krieger, A.J.: Stimulation of pulmonary J receptors by an enkephalin-analog. J. Pharmacol. Exp. Ther., *217*:228, 1981.
22. Beckett, A.H., and Casey, A.F.: Synthetic analgesics, stereochemical considerations. J. Pharm. Pharmacol., *6*:986, 1954.

23. Beckett, A.H.: Analgesics and their antagonists: some steric and chemical considerations. Part I. The dissociation constants of some tertiary amines and synthetic analgesics, the conformations of the methadone-type compounds. J. Pharm. Pharmacol., 8:848, 1956.
24. Cookson, R.F., and Towse, G.D.W.: The search for new analgesics. Clin. Res. Rev., 1:219, 1981.
25. Meuldermans, W.E.G., Hurkmans, R.M.A., and Heykants, J.J.P.: Plasma protein binding and distribution of fentanyl, sufentanil, alfentanil, and lofentanil in blood. Arch. Int. Pharmacodyn. Ther., 257:4, 1982.
26. Cousins, M.J., and Mather, L.E.: Intrathecal and epidural administration of opioids. Anesthesiology, 61:276, 1984.
27. Van Bever, W.F.M., Niemegeers, C.J.E., and Schellekens, K.H.L.: N-4 substituted 1(2-aryl-ethyl)4-piperidenyl-N-phenylpropanamides, a novel series of extremely potent analgesics with unusually high safety margin. Arzneimittelforsch., 26:1548, 1973.
28. Clark, R.L., Pessolano, A.A., and Weijland, J.: N-substituted eponymorphinans. J. Am. Chem. Soc., 75:4974, 1953.
29. Miller, R.R.: Evaluation of nalbuphine hydrochloride. Am. J. Hosp. Pharm., 37:942, 1980.
30. DiFazio, C.A., Moscicki, J.C., and Magruder, M.R.: Anesthetic potency of nalbuphine and interaction with morphine in rats. Anesth. Analg., 60:629, 1981.
31. Monkovic, I., Conway, T.T., Wang, H., Perron, Y.G., Patcher, I.J., and Belleau, B.: Total synthesis and pharmacological activities of N-substituted 3,14 dehydroxymorphinans. J. Am. Chem. Soc., 95:7910, 1973.
32. Lee, G., De Maria, A.N., Amsterdam, E.A., Realyvasquez, F., Angel, J., Morrison, S., and Mason, D.T.: Meperidine and pentazocine on cardiocirculatory dynamics in patients with acute myocardial infarction. Am. J. Med., 60:949, 1976.
33. Jewitt, D.E., Maurer, B.J., Sonnenblick, E.J., and Shillingford, J.P.: Pentazocine: effect on ventricular muscle and hemodynamic changes in ischemic heart disease. Circulation, 44(Suppl. II):118, 1971.

Chapter 4

PHARMACOKINETICS OF NARCOTIC COMPOUNDS

Pharmacokinetics is the quantitative study of the disposition of drugs in the body, and includes the processes of absorption, distribution, biotransformation, and excretion.[1-3] This chapter is a discussion of the pharmacokinetics of the commonly used narcotic analgesics and anesthetics (morphine, meperidine, and fentanyl), along with the newer opioids (alfentanil and sufentanil) (Table 4–1).

It is generally agreed that there is large variability in patient response to narcotic anesthetics. Although poorly understood, this variability is primarily a result of variations in pharmacodynamics, i.e., the effects of a given concentration of a drug on the body, and pharmacokinetics, i.e., the factors determining concentrations of a drug after a given dose, over time. Coupled with the acknowledgment that narcotic anesthesia is different from, and in some respects "lighter" than, potent inhalational anesthesia, the clinician should be aware that pharmacokinetic principles are just that—scientific foundations that are clinically valuable only when coupled with clinical skill, experience, and judgment.

Most clinicians administer inhalational anesthetics "to a desired effect" rather than to any predetermined or "magic" concentration. Likewise, and in spite of recent publications of the pharmacokinetic profiles of numerous narcotic analgesics, it should not be anticipated that mathematic formulas derived from recent

Table 4–1. Averaged Pharmacokinetic Data for Five Opioids*

Pharmacokinetic Parameters	Morphine	Meperidine	Fentanyl	Alfentanil	Sufentanil
pka	8.0	8.5	8.4	6.5	8.0
Percent un-ionized at pH 7.4	23	<10	<10	90	20
Octanol:water partition coefficient (apparent at pH 7.4)	1.4	39	813	145	1778
Percent bound to plasma proteins	30	70	84	92	93
$T_{1/2} \pi$ (min)	0.9–2.4	—	1–3	1–3	0.5–2
$T_{1/2} \alpha$ (min)	10–20	5–15	5–20	5–20	5–15
$T_{1/2} \beta$ (hr)	2–4	3–5	2–4	1–2	2–3
$V_d cc$ (L/kg)	0.1–0.4	1–2	0.5–1.0	0.1–0.3	0.1
$V_d ss$ (L/kg)	3–5	3–5	3–5	0.5–1.0	2.5
Clearance (ml/min)	10–20	8–18	10–20	3–8	10–12

*Data obtained from multiple references (see text).

increased understanding of opioid pharmacology permit empiric delivery of narcotic anesthesia. Rather, titration to a desired clinical effect remains the principle that should govern the use of analgesic or anesthetic doses of opioids.

MORPHINE

Bi- or tri-exponential equations are used to describe the distribution of morphine to one or two peripheral compartments in the body, after intravenous injection. In several reports, investigators have documented a rapid distribution half-life (t½ π) of between 0.9 and 2.4 minutes and a slow distribution half-life (t½ α) of 10 to 20 minutes.[1-7] Thus, free morphine leaves the blood rapidly, and is taken up by the parenchymatous tissues and skeletal muscle. At a pH of 7.4, about 25% of morphine is un-ionized and one third is bound to plasma proteins, mostly serum albumin. Morphine is not lipid soluble; its octanol to water partition coefficient when un-ionized is 6 in contrast to a coefficient of 11,000 for fentanyl. As a result, the penetration of morphine into the central nervous system (CNS) is delayed and does not parallel its disappearance from plasma.[7-9] Exit of the drug from the CNS is also delayed, which is probably the most important explanation for its long duration of action. Despite a much smaller fat to plasma protein partition coefficient (0.8:1) than that of fentanyl (35:1), the volume of distribution of morphine at steady state is large (approximately 4 ± 1.0 L/kg).[1-4] Tissues other than fat, therefore, are responsible for the extensive uptake of morphine.

Clearance of morphine from the body largely depends on hepatic biotransformation (mostly glucuronidation, some N-demethylation, and possibly some oxidation to pseudomorphine or methylation to codeine) and renal excretion. Only 5 to 10% of morphine and its metabolites are excreted in feces.[8-10] The high clearance rate (10 to 20 ml/kg/minute) of morphine is consistent with a high hepatic extraction ratio.[1-7] Thus, the rate of clearance of morphine is dependent on hepatic blood flow. Re-uptake by the blood from peripheral depots is another important limiting factor in the metabolism of morphine. Only about 10% of morphine is excreted unchanged in the urine.[8-10] Although usually inactive, the metabolite, morphine-3-glucuronide, may exercise some opioid effect in certain pathophysiologic states (e.g., renal failure).[11] The elimination half-life (t½ β) of morphine is 2 to 4 hours.[1-6] Physiologic and pathophysiologic factors that influence the pharmacokinetics of morphine, meperidine, and fentanyl are simultaneously discussed in a subsequent section.

MEPERIDINE

The plasma concentration versus time decay curve of meperidine is characterized by a bi-exponential equation with reported distribution half-lives (t½ α) varying from 5 to 15 minutes.[12-16] Meperidine has a plasma protein binding capacity that is greater than that of morphine. About 70% of meperidine is bound to α₁-acid glycoprotein. Meperidine binds only to a minor extent to plasma albumin. Meperidine is even less un-ionized (less than 10%) than morphine at physiologic pH, but it is significantly more lipid soluble. The volume of distribution of meperidine is quite similar to that of morphine (about 4 ± 1 L/kg), as is its clearance (about 8 to 18 ml/kg/minute).[12-16] Like morphine, a high hepatic extraction ratio results in biotransformation that is dependent on hepatic blood flow. Principal metabolic pathways of meperidine include N-demethylation and de-esterification, producing normeperidine, meperidinic acid, and normeperidinic acid as the major metabolites. Normeperidine has some opioid action, and is roughly twice as potent as its parent compound in producing seizures in animals.[17] Seizure activity is a major side-effect of meperidine, which causes its therapeutic index to be more than tenfold lower than that of morphine (5 versus 70). The elimination half-life (t$\frac{1}{2}$ β) for meperidine is approximately 4 ± 1 hours, and excretion of metabolites occurs predominantly through the kidney.[12–16] The elimination half-life of normeperidine is considerably greater than that of meperidine, and cumulative doses, paired with renal and hepatic disease, can easily produce overdosage and toxicity.[18]

FENTANYL

After bolus administration, the plasma concentration of fentanyl declines in a tri-exponential fashion. Like morphine, the rapid distribution half-life (t$\frac{1}{2}$ π) of fentanyl is only 1 to 3 minutes; its slower distribution half-life varies between 5 and 20 minutes.[19–21] Fentanyl is significantly bound (about 80%) to plasma proteins, and less than 10% is un-ionized at physiologic pH. When compared with morphine, penetration of fentanyl into the CNS is greater because of a markedly greater lipid solubility. This characteristic is clearly the most important reason for the rapid onset and shorter duration of action of fentanyl. The volume of distribution of the drug at steady state (about 4 L/kg) is quite similar to that of morphine and meperidine, as is its clearance (10 to 20 ml/kg/minute).[20–22] Clearance of fentanyl is predominantly dependent on hepatic metabolism, although other sites of metabolism do exist (e.g., lung).[23] Less than 10% of fentanyl is excreted unchanged in the urine.[19] Again, hepatic blood flow and peripheral perfusion and re-uptake of fentanyl are important biotransformation rate-limiting factors. Slow re-uptake from fat depots yields an elimination half-life (t$\frac{1}{2}$ β) that is similar to those of meperidine and morphine (about 2$\frac{1}{2}$ to 3$\frac{1}{2}$ hours).[19–22,24,25] The metabolism of fentanyl is complex, although none of the metabolites exerts significant opioid action.[26,27]

PHYSIOLOGIC AND PATHOPHYSIOLOGIC FACTORS AFFECTING OPIOID PHARMACOLOGY

The pharmacokinetic profiles of opioids are easily altered by numerous normal or pathologic processes that ultimately change opioid drug disposition and thus the pharmacodynamics of the compound. Variations in arterial pH can affect drug ionization, plasma protein binding, and drug disposition in a variety of tissues. Morphine, meperidine, and fentanyl are all weak bases. As demonstrated by the Henderson-Hasselbalch equation, $PH = pka + \log \dfrac{\text{Proton acceptor (B)}}{\text{Proton donor (BH}^+)}$, weak bases (ionized as a proton donor) become less ionized as the pH rises. Thus, an increase in arterial pH should increase the penetration of morphine into the brain;[28–30] however, protein binding will also be enhanced and cerebral blood flow will decrease because of respiratory alkalosis, although the sum of effects may not be readily apparent. Interestingly, *respiratory alkalosis* has been shown to be associated with increased levels of fentanyl in the brain.[39] Increased duration of respiratory depression (caused by increased tissue binding and slower CNS removal) has also been associated with respiratory alkalosis.[31] *Respiratory acidosis* should result in opposite effects, i.e., increased plasma ionization, decreased plasma protein binding, and increased cerebral blood flow. Hypercarbia usually results in plasma and brain concentrations of morphine that are higher than those associated with normocarbia.[32] The complex nature of the effects of changes in pH guarantees conflicting reports, as well as difficulties in defining the sum of separate effects and their clinical significance.[33]

Biphasic respiratory depression and secondary peaks in fentanyl plasma concentrations have been described.[34–36] The role that acid-base equilibria and stomach sequestration play in contributing to this phenomenon is uncertain and deserves further detailed study.[37,38]

Age profoundly affects opioid action. In several studies, older patients were found to sustain higher plasma concentrations after opioid administration on the basis of weight.[39,40] A strong positive correlation between age and the incidence of unconsciousness after 30 μg/kg of fentanyl was delivered intravenously has been described.[41] In this study, all patients over 60 years of age, but only one half of those patients less than 40 years of age, lost consciousness, whether or not they were premedicated with diazepam.[41] Unfortunately, changes in the volumes of distribution and clearance do not consistently explain these results. An alternative explanation may be in the number, affinity, or sensitivity of opioid receptors. Whether infants and children have significantly different pharmacokinetics for morphine, meperidine, or any of the other opioids is unclear. Neonates eliminate meperidine more slowly than do adults.[33]

Dose usually does not alter pharmacokinetic variables.[40–42] This fact intimates that biotransformation and excretion mechanisms are not easily saturated by clinical doses of opioids, and that kinetics usually remain first order (drug concentration dependent).

In individuals with acute (hepatitis) and chronic cirrhosis, there is a prolonged elimination half-life and a prolonged clearance rate of meperidine and probably of other opioids as well.[42–45] Interestingly, cirrhosis does not alter hepatic clearance or duration of action of fentanyl. The volume of distribution of meperidine is only slightly increased in the presence of hepatitis and cirrhosis, and protein binding is unaffected by these diseases.[43,44] All of these data suggest that, although initial doses of opioids may have an approximately normal duration of action, subsequent administration of the drug could result in more prolonged effects.

Active metabolites of opioids are usually of clinical importance only during *renal failure*. Although fentanyl has no or few active metabolites, both morphine-3-glucuronide and normeperidine may play a role in the prolonged effect (or toxicity) observed with the administration of morphine or meperidine to patients with renal failure.[11,45] Although acute and chronic renal disease produces changes in protein binding (e.g., decreases with morphine), this fact is probably of no clinical importance.[46]

Cardiopulmonary bypass can markedly alter drug pharmacokinetics. Elimination half-life is prolonged because of a larger volume of distribution and decreased hepatic blood flow.[47–50] Plasma protein binding decreases (due to dilution), and although total plasma drug concentration is reduced, decreases in free concentration are buffered by large peripheral compartment stores. Decreased tissue (skeletal muscle) perfusion during bypass or bypassed tissue (lung) can affect drug kinetics, and decreases in hepatic perfusion and body temperature slow hepatic drug clearance and metabolism. The bypass apparatus also absorbs significant amounts of fentanyl.[46]

SUFENTANIL

Sufentanil is a potent synthetic opioid agonist that is 5 to 10 times more potent than fentanyl. The plasma decay curve of sufentanil fits a three-compartment model, with a rapid (t½ π) distribution half-life of 0.72 minute and a t½ α of 13.7 minutes.[51] Sufentanil is highly protein bound (92.5%), predominantly to α_1-acid glycoprotein; is quite lipophilic; and has a faster onset of action than fentanyl.[51–54] At steady state, the volume of distribution of sufentanil is 2.48 L/kg, somewhat less than that of fentanyl. This determination, coupled with a shorter elimination half-life (t½ β of 148 minutes), may explain the shorter duration of postoperative respiratory depression and shorter time to endotracheal extubation that has been reported.[53] The clearance rate (11.8 ml/kg/minute) and hepatic extraction ratio (0.72) of this synthetic opioid are similar to those of fentanyl. As with fentanyl, the effect of small doses of sufentanil is likely to be terminated by redistribution to the peripheral compartment. With larger doses, plasma concentrations are not rendered subtherapeutic by redistribution because of the relative saturation of the peripheral compartment. In this instance, hepatic biotransformation is responsible for termination of clinical effect.

ALFENTANIL

Alfentanil is another new fentanyl derivative. It is approximately one third to one fifth as potent as fentanyl, but it has a faster onset and shorter duration of action. At doses between 50 and 260 µg/kg, t½ π and t½ α have been reported to be about 2 to 3 minutes and 10 to 20 minutes, respectively.[55,56] Alfentanil is significantly less lipophilic than fentanyl and has a smaller (0.5 to 1.0 L/kg) volume of distribution at steady state. Alfentanil is approximately 10% ionized at pH 7.4, but is highly bound to plasma proteins. Although rapidly metabolized by the liver, alfentanil is found to have a clearance rate that is less than that of fentanyl (4 to 8 versus 10 to 20 ml/kg/minute). The small volume of distribution of alfentanil at steady state, however, results in an elimination half-life (t½ β) that is considerably less than that of fentanyl (1.5 versus 3.5 hours). The markedly different pharmacokinetic profile of the drug explains its more rapid onset of action and shorter duration of effect; it may be most suitably applied by using infusion techniques.

PHARMACOKINETICS AND CLINICAL USE OF INTRAVENOUS NARCOTIC ANESTHETICS

The nature of narcotic anesthesia (i.e., "light anesthesia") and the most popular techniques in the past (i.e., bolus injection producing initially supratherapeutic blood levels and relative, albeit, safe overdose) have often led to prolonged anesthetic effects postoperatively. Investigators interested in minimizing this "side-effect" have searched for ways of more accurately delivering opioids while ensuring that plasma concentrations are "anesthetic." The use of pharmacokinetic principles and the theoretic ability to produce known plasma concentrations of drugs have led to a more scientific approach in the attempt to refine the administration of opioid anesthesia.[57–60]

Alfentanil is relatively more "predictable" than fentanyl in that its elimination is less variable. Its smaller volume of distribution reduces the contribution of redistribution to termination of drug effect, and its lower hepatic clearance rate renders drug clearance less dependent on hepatic blood flow.[59,60] These are modest gains, however, when one considers the gaps in our knowledge of fundamental principles, such as the relationship between pharmacokinetics and dynamics, the importance of receptor kinetics, and factors producing variations in these relationships, that remain largely unanswered.

The role and importance of pharmacokinetics will continue to be defined (e.g., obesity increases the elimination half-life of alfentanil because of decreased clearance,[61] and cardiopulmonary bypass increases the volume of distribution for alfentanil and fentanyl[47]). These investigations will at least provide valuable food for thought. Whether the clinician can then provide a clinically safer and better anesthetic remains to be seen. How much drug administered at what rate to produce what concentration (measured or assumed) to yield certain effects, and what clinical factors must be considered to calculate accurately the anesthetic requirements of patients, are basic questions that now appear overwhelming but may one day be straightforward.

REFERENCES

1. Stanski, D.R., Greenblatt, D.J., and Lowenstein, E.: Kinetics of intravenous and intramuscular morphine. Clin. Pharmacol. Ther., 24:52, 1978.
2. Dahlstrom, B., Bolme, P., Feychting, H., Noack, G., and Paalzow, L.: Morphine kinetics in children. Clin. Pharmacol. Ther., 26:354, 1979.
3. Stanski, D.R., Paalzow, L., and Edlund, P.O.: Morphine pharmacokinetics: GLC assay versus ratio immunoassay. J. Pharm. Sci., 71:314, 1982.
4. Murphy, M.R., and Hug, C.C., Jr.: Pharmacokinetics of intravenous morphine in patients anesthetized with enflurane-nitrous oxide. Anesthesiology, 54:187, 1981.
5. Dahlstrom, B., Tamsen, A., Paalzow, L., and Hartvig, P.: Patient controlled analgesia therapy. IV: Pharmacokinetics and analgesic plasma concentrations of morphine. Clin. Pharmacokinet., 7:266, 1982.
6. Hug, C.C., Jr., Murphy, M.R., Rigel, E.P., and Olson, W.A.: Pharmacokinetics of morphine injected intravenously into the anesthetized dog. Anesthesiology, 54:38, 1981.
7. Way, E.L., and Adler, T.K.: The biological disposition of morphine and its surrogates. 1. Bull. WHO, 25:227, 1961.
8. Wolff, W.A., Riegel, C., and Fry, E.G.: The excretion of morphine by normal and tolerant dogs. J. Pharmacol. Exp. Ther., 47:391, 1933.
9. Yeh, S.Y.: Urinary excretion of morphine and its metabolites in morphine dependent subjects. J. Pharmacol. Exp. Ther., 192:201, 1975.
10. Brunk, S.F., and Della, M.: Morphine metabolism in man. Clin. Pharmacol. Ther., 16:51, 1974.
11. Sasajima, M.: Analgesic effect of morphine-3-glucuronide. Keio Igaka, 47:421, 1970.
12. Mather, L.E., Tucker, G.T., Pflug, A.E., Lindop, M.J., and Wilkerson, C.: Meperidine kinetics in man: intravenous injection in surgical patients and volunteers. Clin. Pharmacol. Ther., 17:21, 1975.
13. Klotz, U., McHorse, T.S., Wilkinson, G.R., and Schenker, S.: The effect of cirrhosis on the disposition and elimination of meperidine in man. Clin. Pharmacol. Ther., 16:667, 1974.
14. Verbeeck, R.K., Branch, R.A., and Wilkinson, G.R.: Meperidine disposition in man: influence of urinary pH and route of administration. Clin. Pharmacol. Ther., 30:619, 1981.
15. Stambaugh, J.E., Wainer, I.W., Sanstead, J.K., and Hemphill, D.M.: The clinical pharmacology of meperidine: comparison of routes of administration. J. Clin. Pharmacol., 16:245, 1976.
16. Austin, K.L., Stapleton, J.V., and Mather, L.E.: Multiple intramuscular injections: a major source of variability in analgesic response to meperidine. Pain, 8:47, 1980.
17. Miller, J.W., and Anderson, H.H.: The effect of N-demethylation on certain pharmacologic actions of morphine, codeine and meperidine in the mouse. J. Pharmacol. Exp. Ther., 112:191, 1954.
18. Szeto, H.H., Inturrisi, C.E., Houde, R., Saal, S., Cheigh, J., and Reidenberg, M.: Accumulation of normeperidine, an active metabolite of meperidine, in patients with renal failure or cancer. Ann. Intern. Med., 86:738, 1977.
19. McClain, D.A., and Hug, C.C., Jr.: Intravenous fentanyl kinetics. Clin. Pharmacol. Ther., 28:106, 1980.
20. Fung, D.L., and Eisele, J.H.: Fentanyl pharmacokinetics in awake volunteers. J. Clin. Pharmacol., 20:652, 1980.
21. Schleimer, R., Benjamini, E., Eisele, J., and Henderson, G.: Pharmacokinetics of fentanyl as determined by radioimmunoassay. Clin. Pharmacol. Ther., 23:188, 1978.
22. Hug, C.C., Jr., Murphy, M.R., Sampson, J.F., Terblanche, J., and Aldrete, J.A.: Biotransformation of morphine and fentanyl in anhepatic dogs. Anesthesiology, 55:A261, 1981.
23. Bower, S., and Hull, C.J.: The comparative pharmacokinetics of fentanyl and alfentanil. Br. J. Anaesth., 54:871, 1982.

24. Koska, A.J., Kramer, W.G., Romagnoli, A., Keats, A.S., and Sabawala, P.B.: Pharmacokinetics of high-dose meperidine in surgical patients. Anesth. Analg., *60*:8, 1981.
25. Hug, C.C., Jr., and Murphy, M.R.: Tissue redistribution of fentanyl and termination of its effects in rats. Anesthesiology, *55*:369, 1981.
26. Goromaru, T., Furuta, T., Baba, S., Yoshimura, N., Miyawaki, T., Sameshima, T., and Miyao, J.: Metabolism of fentanyl in rats and man. Anesthesiology, *55*:A173, 1981.
27. Benson, D.W., Kaufman, J.J., and Koski, W.S.: Theoretic significance of pH dependence of narcotics and narcotic antagonists in clinical anesthesia. Anesth. Analg., *55*:253, 1976.
28. Finck, A.D., Berkowitz, B.A., Hempstead, J., and Ngai, S.H.: Pharmacokinetics of morphine: effects of hypercarbia on serum and brain morphine concentrations in the dog. Anesthesiology, *47*:407, 1977.
29. Nishitateno, K., Ngai, S.H., Finck, A.D., and Berkowitz, B.A.: Pharmacokinetics of morphine: concentrations in the serum and brain of the dog during hyperventilation. Anesthesiology, *50*:520, 1979.
30. Ainslie, S.G., Eisele, J.H., and Corkill, G.: Fentanyl concentrations in brain and serum during respiratory acid-base changes in the dog. Anesthesiology, *51*:293, 1979.
31. Gill, K.J., Cartwright, D.P., Scoggins, A., Gray, A.J., and Prys-Roberts, C.: Ventilatory depression related to plasma fentanyl concentrations during and after anaesthesia. Br. J. Anaesth., *52*:632P, 1980.
32. Chan, K., Vaughan, D.P., and Mitchard, M.: Plasma concentrations and urinary excretion of pethidine and metabolites. Abstracts of the Symposium on the Assessment of Drug Metabolism in Man—Methods and Clinical Applications. University of Dundee, 1974.
33. Cooper, L.V., Stephen, G.W., and Aggett, P.J.A.: Elimination of pethidine and bupivicaine in the newborn. Arch. Dis. Child., *52*:638, 1977.
34. Stoeckel, H., Hengstmann, J.H., and Schuttler, J.: Pharmacokinetics of fentanyl as a possible explanation of recurrence of respiratory depression. Br. J. Anaesth., *51*:741, 1979.
35. Becker, L.D., Paulson, B.A., Miller, R.D., Severinghaus, J.W., and Edmond, I.E.: Biphasic respiratory depression after fentanyl-droperidol or fentanyl alone used to supplement nitrous oxide anesthesia. Anesthesiology, *44*:291, 1976.
36. Stoeckel, H., Schuttler, J., Magnussen, H., and Hengstmann, J.H.: Plasma fentanyl concentrations and occurrence of respiration depression in volunteers. Br. J. Anaesth., *54*:1087, 1982.
37. Trudowski, R.J., and Gessner, T.: Gastric sequestration of meperidine following intravenous administration. Abstracts of Scientific Papers, American Society of Anesthesiologists, Chicago, 1975, pp. 327–328.
38. Berkowitz, B.A., Ngai, S.H., Yang, J.C., Hempstead, B.S., and Spector, S.: The disposition of morphine in surgical patients. Clin. Pharmacol. Ther., *17*:629, 1975.
39. Harper, M.H., Hickey, R.F., Cromwell, T.H., and Linwood, S.: The magnitude and duration of respiratory depression produced by fentanyl and fentanyl plus droperidol in man. J. Pharmacol. Exp. Ther., *199*:464, 1976.
40. Murphy, M.R., and Hug, C.C., Jr.: Dose independent pharmacokinetics of fentanyl. Anesthesiology, *57*:A347, 1982.
41. Bailey, P.L., Wilbrink, J., Zwanikken, P., Pace, N.L., and Stanley, T.H.: Anesthetic induction with fentanyl. Anesth. Analg., *64*:48, 1985.
42. Neal, E.A., Meffin, P.J., Gregory, P.B., and Blaschke, T.F.: Enhanced bioavailability and decreased clearance of analgesics in patients with cirrhosis. Gastroenterology, *77*:96, 1979.
43. Pond, S.M., Tong, T., Benowitz, N.L., Jacaob, P., Rigod, J.: Presystemic metabolism of meperidine to normeperidine in normal and cirrhotic subjects. Clin. Pharmacol. Ther., *30*:183, 1981.
44. McHorse, T.S., Wilkinson, G.R., Johnson, R.F., and Schenker, S.: Effect of acute viral hepatitis in man on the disposition and elimination of meperidine. Gastroenterology, *68*:775, 1975.
45. Coral, I.M., Moore, A.R., and Strunin, L.: Plasma concentrations of fentanyl in normal surgical patients and those with severe renal and hepatic disease. Br. J. Anaesth., *52*:101P, 1980.
46. Don, H.F., Dieppa, R.A., and Taylor, P.: Narcotic analgesics in anuric patients. Anesthesiology, *42*:745, 1975.
47. Hug, C.C., Jr., DeLange, S., and Burm, A.G.L.: Alfentanil pharmacokinetics in cardiac surgical patients before and after cardiopulmonary bypass (CPB). Anesth. Analg., *62*:266, 1983.
48. Hug, C.C., Jr., and Moldenhauer, C.C.: Pharmacokinetics and dynamics of fentanyl infusions in cardiac surgical patients. Anesthesiology, *54*:A45, 1982.
49. Koska, A.J., Romagnoli, A., and Kramer, W.G.: Effect of cardiopulmonary bypass on fentanyl distribution and elimination. Clin. Pharmacol. Ther., *29*:100, 1981.
50. Koren, G., Crean, P., Goresky, G., Klein, J., Villamater, J., MacLeod, S.M.: Irreversible binding of fentanyl to the cardiopulmonary bypass. Anesth. Analg., *63*:175, 1984.
51. Bovill, J.G., Sebel, P.S., Blackburn, C.L., and Heykants, J.: Kinetics of alfentanil and sufentanil: a comparison. Anesthesiology, *55*:A174, 1981 (Abstr.)
52. Meuldermans, W.E.G., Hurkmans, R.M.A., and Heykants, J.J.P.: Plasma protein binding and

distribution of fentanyl, sufentanil, alfentanil and lofentanil in blood. Arch. Int. Pharmacodyn. Ther., 257:4, 1982.

53. Smith, N.T., Dec-Silber, H., Harrison, W.K., Sanford, T.J., and Gillig, J.: A comparison among morphine, fentanyl and sufentanil anesthesia for open-heart surgery: induction, emergence and extubation. Anesthesiology, 57(3S):A-291, 1982 (Abstr.)

54. Kay, B., and Rolly, G.: Duration of action of analgesic supplements to anesthesia. A double-blind comparison between morphine, fentanyl and sufentanil. Acta Anaesthesiol. Belg., 28:25, 1977.

55. Bovill, J.G., Sebel, P.S., Blackburn, C.L., and Heykants, J.: The pharmacokinetics of alfentanil (R 39209): a new opioid analgesic. Anesthesiology, 57:439, 1982.

56. Camu, F., Gepts, E., Rucquio, M., and Heykants, J.: Pharmacokinetics of alfentanil in man. Anesth. Analg., 61:657, 1982.

57. de Lange, S., and de Bruijn, N.: Alfentanil-oxygen anaesthesia: plasma concentration and clinical effects during variable rate continuous infusion for coronary artery surgery. Br. J. Anaesth., 55:S183, 1983.

58. Wagner, J.G.: A safe method for rapidly achieving plasma concentration plateaus. Clin. Pharmacol. Ther., 16:691, 1974.

59. Hug, C.C., Jr., and Stanski, D.R.: Editorial: Alfentanil—A kinetically predictable narcotic analgesic. Anesthesiology, 57:435, 1982.

60. Hug, C.C., Jr., and Stanski, D.R.: In reply. Anesthesiology, 59:257, 1983.

61. Bentley, J.B., Finely, J.H., Humphrey, L.R., Gandolfi, A.J., and Brown, B.R.: Obesity and alfentanil pharmacokinetics. Anesth. Analg., 62:251, 1983.

Chapter 5

PHARMACOLOGY OF NARCOTIC ANALGESICS

CENTRAL NERVOUS SYSTEM (CNS)

Narcotic analgesics activate opioid receptors in all body organ systems that possess these organelles.[1-4] Structures and pathways that involve pain contain the highest concentrations of opioid receptors.[1-7] Narcotic or electrical stimulation of opioid receptors in these structures results in analgesia that can be antagonized with the use of naloxone or other narcotic antagonists. Stimulation of peri-aqueductal gray receptors (with morphine, electricity, or endogenous opiate-like peptides) results in a barrage of impulses that move caudally from the brain. This activity ultimately results in the inhibition of the transmission of nociceptive information from peripheral nerves into the spinal cord.[8,9] The integrity of certain neurotransmitter systems connecting the pain-inhibiting system in the brain to the spinal cord seems to be necessary for opioids to exert their full analgesic action. Satoh and Takagi found that blockade with morphine of the transmission of spinal cord potentials evoked by painful stimulation is inhibited by high spinal cord transection.[9]

Unfortunately, this theory of *"descending inhibition"* does not entirely explain the analgesic action of morphine or other opioids. The substantia gelatinosa of the spinal cord also possesses a dense collection of opiate receptors.[10,11] Direct application of narcotics to these receptors creates intense analgesia. Opiate receptors have been found in the substantia gelatinosa of the caudal spinal trigeminal nucleus, the nucleus that receives pain fibers from the face and hands via branches of the 5th, 7th, 9th, and 10th cranial nerves.[12] Undoubtedly, narcotics produce analgesia by acting at receptors both in the spinal cord and in higher centers. Within the brain stem, opiate receptors are highly concentrated in the solitary nuclei that receive visceral sensory fibers from the 9th and 10th cranial nerves and the area postrema. Stimulation of the solitary nuclei depresses gastric secretion and the cough reflex and causes orthostatic hypotension. Stimulation of the area postrema with its chemoreceptor trigger zone results in nausea and vomiting.

The clinical implications of opiate receptor physiology are just beginning to be understood. Morphine and most opioids are effective in relieving dull, boring, poorly localized, visceral-type pain, but are not nearly as effective in influencing highly localized somatic pain.[12] Lateral thalamic nuclei are involved with highly localized pain, whereas medial thalamic nuclei mediate poorly localized and emotionally influenced pain. As might be expected, higher concentrations of opiate receptors are found in medial than in lateral thalamic nuclei.

Opioid receptor occupancy is closely correlated with the production and regulation of analgesia and anesthesia in rats.[13] Increasing doses of the highly potent synthetic mu receptor-stimulating opioid, lofentanil, produce increasing levels of analgesia and opioid receptor occupation in this species; finally, at 25 to 30% receptor occupancy, anesthesia is achieved.[13] Results from this and numerous other studies in man and other animals confirm that increasing doses of opioids, particularly mu receptor-stimulating opioids, produce increasing levels of analgesia, unconsciousness, and absence of all somatic responses to any painful or surgical stimulus if the dose of the opioid is sufficiently high, e.g., 2 to 3 g of fentanyl in the dog.[13–23]

Incomplete amnesia, however, remains an occasional problem with low and high doses of opioid-based anesthesia. In virtually all patients, recall of pain is rare. A most likely reason for either or both awareness and inadequate anesthesia during narcotic-analgesic based anesthesia is the difficulty in reliably predicting the appropriate dose of opioid for each patient. Generally, healthier patients (i.e., ASA classes I and II) with normal or high cardiac output require larger doses of narcotics for anesthesia than do patients who have serious metabolic disease, cardiovascular limitations, or reduced cardiac output.[15,16,21,22,24,25] In addition, age influences the ability of a given dose of fentanyl or of any opioid to produce unconsciousness. Younger patients, particularly those individuals less than 40 years of age, require the administration of more narcotics than do older patients to produce unconsciousness.[25] Opioid receptor kinetics may be different in older patients. Smoking and alcohol consumption may also influence anesthetic requirements.[26] Undoubtedly, differences in body fat, plasma protein binding, fat solubility, hepatic metabolism, renal excretion, and regional perfusion also influence requirements for opioids.

How and why all these factors influence opioid analgesic and anesthetic requirements in man is unknown. If data obtained in rat receptor-binding studies are applicable, however, the answer may lie in determining and ensuring that the percent of CNS opioid receptor occupation necessary for anesthesia is achieved in every patient.[13] This goal will undoubtedly be difficult to attain for many reasons, not the least of which relates to variability of opioid requirements in the same individual. Indeed, acute tolerance, as seen with barbiturates, may occur with opioids.[23,27] Awakening or absence of analgesia can take place at plasma opioid levels higher than those associated with initial loss of consciousness or onset of analgesia.[27]

When an opioid is used in large doses as a complete anesthetic, or when it is used with supplements, such as nitrous oxide or other intravenous compounds, there are few reliable, measurable clinical indications of amnesia. This fact, too, contributes to the problem of inadequate anesthesia. Profound analgesia and apnea can easily be achieved with opioids without producing anesthesia.[14–16,20–22] Although the administration of supplements (nitrous oxide, diazepam, or droperidol) or of larger doses of narcotic anesthetics increases the likelihood of amnesia, its occurrence is not guaranteed.[25,28] Furthermore, undesirable side-effects, such as prolonged postoperative respiratory depression and cardiovascular depression, are frequently experienced after the administration of some supplements.[15,29–31]

In any event, the reported frequency of awareness with fentanyl anesthesia in man is comparable to that with inhalation agent-based techniques.[31–38] Nonetheless, concern about the occurrence of awareness remains legitimate. Hypertension and traumatic neurosis (consisting of repetitive nightmares, anxiety, preoccupation with death, and patient resistance to talking about recall) can occur.[31,35] Awareness associated with anesthesia is best dealt with by informing patients of its possibility preoperatively and by discussing frankly and openly such an episode postoperatively. Direct explanation may be most helpful to a reluctant and fearful patient.[31]

Reports of awareness and inadequate anesthesia after morphine are mainly anecdotal; thus, their true incidence is unknown. Awareness seems more common, however, in patients undergoing coronary artery surgery, especially in individuals without previous congestive heart failure.[39,40] In the relatively fit patient, much larger doses (up to 11 mg/kg) of morphine may be required to abolish awareness and to produce adequate surgical anethesia.[41] Morphine (2 mg/kg) given to healthy, unpremedicated volunteers does not reliably produce amnesia or unconsciousness; the addition of 70% nitrous oxide is required.[42]

A factor contributing to immediate awareness during anesthesia with morphine used alone is the prolonged induction time required because of its poor lipid solubility.[39,43] Although the time can be shortened by concomitant use of a barbiturate, cardiovascular depression commonly results.[44]

Awareness is less frequent with high doses of fentanyl. Even without prior use of drugs with amnesic properties (e.g., diazepam and scopolamine), 50% of patients become amnesic to visual stimuli after the administration of fentanyl (6 to 7 μg/kg).[45] In one report, awareness occurred only during the second of 2 fentanyl administrations that occurred 6 days apart; doses of fentanyl were comparable (75.8 and 72 μg/kg), although diazepam was given during the first, but not the second, administration of anesthetic. In another report, a 41-year-old woman receiving fentanyl (90 μg/kg) for elective mitral valve replacement was aware of sounds and conversation during the sternotomy. Apart from a few such anecdotal reports, data are as yet insufficient either to quantify the incidence of awareness during fentanyl anesthesia or to compare it with similar doses of morphine.

The neurophysiologic state produced by large doses of narcotic-analgesics differs from the state of general anesthesia obtained with volatile anesthetics, which produce a dose-related generalized depression of the CNS.[46–48] High-dose fentanyl anesthesia produces an EEG response that is characterized by high voltage, slow delta waves and is consistent with deep surgical anesthesia; high-dose administration of meperidine (e.g., 400 mg) yields a similar result.[47] The EEG pattern consistent with fentanyl administration is not altered by nitrous oxide or surgical stimulation. In contrast to the continuum of EEG changes ending in burst suppression and an isoelectric ("flat") EEG tracing seen with increasing dosage of conventional anesthetic agents, a "ceiling effect" is reached with fentanyl.[48] Increasing the dosage from 50 to 150 μg/kg does not further alter the EEG.[49] Although the EEG effects of still higher doses of fentanyl in man have not been studied, recent findings suggest that opioids produce "anesthesia" by blocking afferent input rather than by causing generalized depression of the CNS.[46] Opioids also differ from potent anesthetics in that they do not produce muscular relaxation and may occasionally cause muscle rigidity.[50]

CARDIOVASCULAR SYSTEM

The cardiovascular effects of opioid administration reflect a complex interplay of actions that affect the heart, blood vessels, CNS, and other regions. Thus, cardiovascular dynamics in most normal adults breathing oxygen are not significantly altered by the administration of morphine in doses as high as 1 to 3 mg/kg.[14] It is important to note that different opioids may affect the heart and peripheral vasculature in different ways in both normal and disease-affected individuals.

Heart Rate

Therapeutic doses of most opioids slow the heart.[14,15,17–22,51–56] Morphine decreases heart rate, through a combination of central vagal nucleus stimulation[39,52] and direct depression of cardiac action at the sinus and atrioventricular nodes.[52–55] Fentanyl also stimulates the central vagal nucleus and depresses the sinoatrial and atrioventricular nodes, but may decrease central sympathetic tone to the heart as well.[56–58]

Morphine- or fentanyl-induced bradycardia can be almost, but not totally, prevented by pretreatment with atropine or other belladonna or belladonna-like drugs.[19] Curiously, second and subsequent intravenous doses of most narcotics seem to cause less bradycardia than does the initial dose;[59] this may represent a form of "acute tolerance." Bradycardia after opioid delivery is related to the dose of the drug, the speed of injection, and the presence or absence of premedication with a belladonna drug.[21,56,59] Indeed, without prior administration of atropine, decreases in heart rate are commonly of sufficient magnitude to reduce cardiac output in the dog after injection of fentanyl and in man after the administration of any of the pure agonist opioids (e.g., morphine and fentanyl), especially when higher doses are used.[19] The incidence of bradycardia may be minimized by slow administration of opioids, especially during induction of anesthesia and when preceded by administration of a belladonna-like compound.[19,21,39] Alternatively, injection of a small (2 mg) dose of pancuronium before induction of anesthesia with opioids may not only attenuate the expected bradycardia but may also actually result in a small increase in heart rate.[39,60] Once induced, bradycardia can be treated with atropine, but even large doses of atropine (1 to 2 mg) can prove ineffective.[39]

Tachycardia sometimes follows the injection of a narcotic-analgesic, and has been attributed to opioid-induced increases in circulating catecholamines, histamine, or other hormones.[59,61–66] Such hormonal changes occur more commonly with morphine than with fentanyl, which may explain why tachycardia more frequently accompanies morphine administration.[66,67] Tachycardia most frequently occurs with meperidine use.[68,69] The reason for this frequency is not totally clear, but it may be related to the structural similarity of meperidine to atropine; to histamine release or as a toxic manifestation of CNS excitation; or to preconvulsant CNS stimulation.[18] Indeed, continued administration of any opioid to mammals (even those mechanically ventilated) may ultimately prove fatal. Such demise is caused by a marked increase in central autonomic activity with concomitant large increases in concentrations of circulating catecholamines and in cerebral and total body oxygen demand, a demand that ultimately outstrips supply.[18] Usual clinical doses of meperidine, the therapeutic index of which is only 4.7 (in contrast to 70 for morphine and 277 for fentanyl), may result in blood and brain levels that are toxic to some patients, in whom an increase in heart rate may be the first warning of trouble.[18,49]

Cardiac Output

Cardiac output in man or animals is minimally affected by morphine[14,15,44,47,62,70–73] or fentanyl[17–22] when given slowly. This fact is true irrespective of dose, provided hydration is adequate, intravenous atropine or other belladonna premedication is used, other intravenous or inhalation anesthetic supplements are avoided, and ventilation is assisted or controlled to maintain normal values of Pa_{CO_2}. Under these conditions, both drugs cause minimal or no depression of myocardial mechanics.[17,62,74,75] In contrast, meperidine, alphaprodine, and piritramide do not preserve cardiac output, regardless of experimental conditions, because they are all myocardial depressants.[17,18,22,51,74–77] Among the older opioids, methadone appears to have little effect on cardiac output and most other cardiovascular variables.[78] The newer pure agonist opioids, sufentanil and alfentanil, resemble fentanyl in their effects on cardiac output, heart rate, and other parameters at comparable doses.[18,51,79–84]

Among the less extensively studied agonist-antagonist compounds, pentazocine decreases contractility and cardiac output in patients with ischemic heart disease.[85] Butorphanol, in doses of 0.03 or 0.06 mg/kg, does not significantly alter any cardiovascular variable in healthy volunteers,[86] and increases cardiac index and pulmonary artery pressure in patients with cardiac disease.[87] The desirability of these latter changes is not clear.

Blood Pressure

Hypotension

Morphine-nitrous oxide anesthesia is occasionally associated with hypotension, which can be severe.[18,44,66,70,88] Hypotension (systolic blood pressure below 70 mm Hg) was reported in 10% of a group of patients undergoing cardiac valvular surgery.[88] Although 1 patient in the series sustained a myocardial infarction presumably the result of morphine-induced hypotension, the incidence of severe hypotension with morphine-nitrous oxide was similar to that with halothane-nitrous oxide in the same study.[50] The rate of administration and the underlying disease of the patient may each be important causes of hypotension associated with morphine use. In the aforementioned series of patients with valvular heart disease, the minimum rate of administration of morphine was 5 mg/minute. In patients with coronary artery disease, hypotension occurs when morphine is infused at 10 mg/minute,[2] but not when the infusion rate is limited to 5 mg/minute.[89]

Morphine use can cause hypotension. This hypotensive state is not ordinarily associated with significant myocardial depression, although in healthy volunteers, morphine (2 mg/kg given intravenously) does prolong the pre-ejection period, an indicator of isovolemic cardiac contractility.[47] Hypotension has been attributed to changes in the distribution of regional blood flow, but is more probably caused by a decrease in systemic vascular resistance secondary to histamine release.[66,71] Morphine administered intravenously in doses of 10 mg can cause hypotension with significant increases in plasma histamine concentrations.[66,72,73,90–99] The recent development of a sensitive and specific assay for histamine and of specific histamine receptor antagonists has enabled further appraisal of the role of histamine in these effects.[65,96] Morphine alone in doses of 1 mg/kg given intravenously is associated with marked increases in plasma histamine levels (Fig. 5–1) and cardiac index, and with decreases in blood pressure and vascular resistance.

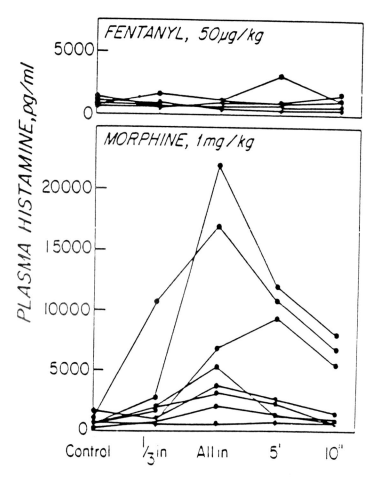

Fig. 5–1. Individual data for plasma histamine from arterial blood samples in patients exposed to morphine (1mg/kg) or fentanyl (50 μg/kg). (Reprinted from Rosow, C.E., Moss, J., Philbin, D.M., and Savarese, J.J.: Histamine release during morphine and fentanyl anesthesia. Anesthesiology, 56:93, 1982, with permission.)

Similar cardiovascular changes occur in patients pretreated with either diphenhydramine (a histamine H_1 antagonist) or cimetidine (a histamine H_2 antagonist). In patients pretreated with both H_1 and H_2 antagonists, however, these responses are significantly attenuated despite comparable increases in plasma histamine concentrations.[96] These data strongly suggest that many of the hemodynamic effects of morphine are attributable to histamine release and indicate potential means for their prevention. In contrast, hypotension rarely occurs with high-dose fentanyl anesthesia, perhaps because, unlike morphine, fentanyl does not cause histamine release (Fig. 5–1).[66] Although the effects of large (anesthetic) doses of meperidine on plasma histamine concentrations have not been studied, limited clinical data suggest that the effect of the drug is probably much like that of morphine.[67,68]

Morphine reduces venous and arterial tone and decreases venous return to the heart in both animals and man, thus contributing to hypotension.[14,72,73,91–93,97,98] The dose-related degree of venous pooling significantly increases the amount of blood or crystalloid fluid required to maintain adequate ventricular filling pressure

(Table 5–1).[46,93] The reduced venous return to the heart after large doses of morphine has been attributed to hepatic sequestration of plasma[97,98] and to venous dilatation related to the preservatives in commercial preparations of the drug.[46] The vasodilatation may also be the result of the action of morphine directly on vascular smooth muscle or indirectly through histamine release.[66,92] Clinical experience suggests that fentanyl produces none or fewer of these changes.[67]

HYPERTENSION

Hypertension may occur during cardiac surgery in patients anesthetized with morphine. For example, hypertension (defined as a rise in systolic blood pressure to over 200 mm Hg or to 60 mm Hg above the preoperative level) was observed in 36% of patients undergoing coronary artery surgery with morphine anesthesia (2 mg/kg).[16,68,88,99] The precise mechanism remains to be defined, although suggestions include light or inadequate anesthesia, reflex responses, and stimulation of the renin-angiotensin mechanism.[44,45,70,100] Hypertension during or after sternotomy is probably the most common cardiovascular disturbance that occurs during high-dose fentanyl anesthesia for cardiac surgery.[39,101,102] For reasons that are not clear, the reported incidence of hypertension varies. Stanley, et al., reported no change in cadiovascular variables after surgical stimulation.[21,103] Other investigators report post-sternotomy hypertension values that range from 10 to 100% in patients given fentanyl (50 to 121 μg/kg).[45,101,102,104] Possible reasons for these differences include the rate of administration of the drug; the degree of beta-adrenergic and calcium channel blockade present; the timing, dosage, and type of muscle relaxant used; and differences in opioid requirements between populations.[79,104] In an investigation comparing patients undergoing coronary artery surgery in Salt Lake City, Utah, with those undergoing the same procedure in Leiden, The Netherlands, post-sternotomy hypertension was observed in only 10% of patients from Salt Lake City receiving fentanyl (75 μg/kg), but was noted in 80% of Dutch patients, despite higher dosage (121 μg/kg).[104] Still higher doses (130 to 140 μg/kg) reduced the incidence of hypertension in the Dutch patients. Unfortunately, prolonged postoperative respiratory depression is likely to follow such doses of fentanyl.[104] Satisfactory control of blood pressure can be achieved with the use of lower doses of fentanyl (50 μg/kg), together with vasodilatory therapy.[101] Note, however, that the risk of intraoperative awareness is increased with such doses of fentanyl, but not with doses of 120 μg/kg or higher.[105,106] A maximal dose of fentanyl (100 μg/kg) has been recommended by some clini-

Table 5–1. Blood Requirements During Surgery and for the First Postoperative Day.*

Pathology	Anesthetic	Mean Blood Requirements (ml)	
		Intraoperative	Postoperative
Aortic valve disease	Morphine	2822†	1091†
	Halothane	988	767
Coronary artery disease	Morphine	2763†	1481
	Halothane	1726	708

*Sixty-one patients anesthetized with morphine (1 to 4 mg/kg) plus oxygen or halothane (0.1 to 1.5%) plus 30% nitrous oxide and oxygen during aortic valve replacement or coronary artery bypass surgery.
†p<0.05, Student's paired *t*-test when compared to halothane values. (From Stanley, T.H., Gray, N.H., Isern-Amaral, J.H., et al.: Comparison of blood requirements during morphine and halothane anesthesia for open-heart surgery. Anesthesiology, *41*:34, 1974.)

cians.[45] Hypertension, if encountered, is then controlled by vasodilator therapy with sodium nitroprusside or by the addition of a potent inhalation agent; the latter often decreases myocardial contractility, which may not be desirable.[45,49] Other investigators reject any limitation of the dosage of fentanyl.[39,104] If minimal postoperative respiratory depression is desired, however, fentanyl dosage should be limited to 80 to 100 μg/mg, with supplementary low (0.1 to 0.5%) concentrations of isoflurane or another inhalation agent to control arterial blood pressure.

Cardiovascular Effects of Supplemental Agents

Various supplemental agents have been used in conjunction with narcotics to reduce the incidence of awareness; to control hypertension; and, by decreasing the opioid dosage, to minimize postoperative respiratory depression.[15,21,39,40,70,107–116] Unfortunately, some impairment of cardiovascular stability seems an inevitable concomitant. The supplement is commonly nitrous oxide, which when used alone has minimal effects on cardiovascular dynamics; it does, however, depress myocardial contractile force in dogs.[107,108] Used in combination with opioids, e.g., morphine, meperidine, and fentanyl, nitrous oxide can significantly impair cardiac function—decreasing cardiac output (Fig. 5–2) and blood pressure and increasing systemic vascular resistance.[15,19,22,39,109,111,112,114] The mechanism of the cardiovascular depressant action of nitrous oxide in the presence of opioids is unknown. Interestingly, the degree of depression seems unrelated to the plasma concentration of opioid.[111]

Similarly, diazepam, by itself innocuous cardiovascularly, causes marked car-

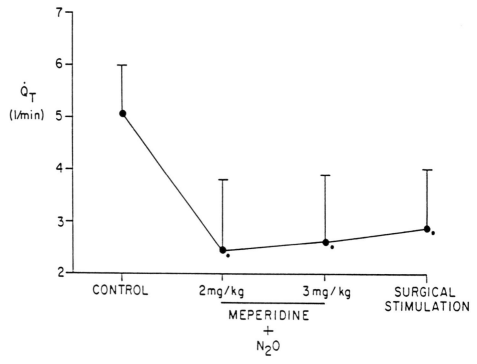

Fig. 5–2. Cardiac output before and after meperidine-N_2O anesthesia before and after surgical stimulation. ($p < 0.01$, one-way analysis of variance.)

diac depression in patients also receiving either morphine or fentanyl (Fig. 5–3).[21,110] Comparable interactions may be anticipated with other benzodiazepines. Among other intravenous supplements studied, only scopolamine and droperidol do not produce significant cardiovascular depression when combined with opioids, although droperidol may decrease systemic vascular resistance and arterial blood pressure.[110,113,114]

Among the potent inhalation anesthetics, even low concentrations of halothane after the delivery of large doses of morphine may produce marked cardiovascular depression in patients with coronary artery disease.[115] Combinations of fentanyl and enflurane, however, may or may not do so, depending on the dosage of each agent.[116] Results generated from analogous studies of fentanyl and isoflurane used together are not yet available.

RESPIRATORY SYSTEM

Respiratory Depression

Opioids act on medullary and pontine respiratory centers to produce dose-related depression of all components of respiratory function: rate, tidal and minute volumes, rhythmicity, responsiveness to carbon dioxide (Fig. 5–4), and respiratory reflexes.[97,117–122] Respiratory rate usually slows before tidal volume. In most instances, the respiratory effects of opioids are maximal between 5 and 30 minutes

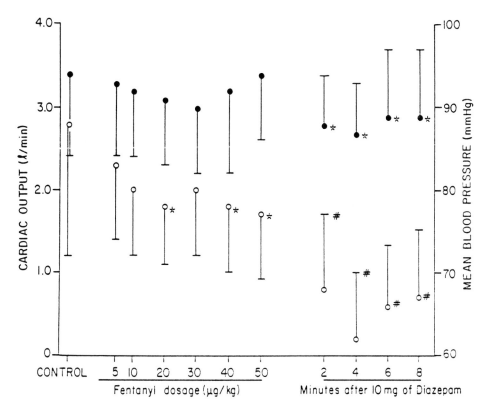

Fig. 5–3. Cardiac output (○) and mean arterial (●) blood pressure before and after large doses of fentanyl and fentanyl plus diazepam (mean ± SD). (*p < 0.05; #p < /-1. one-way analysis of variance.)

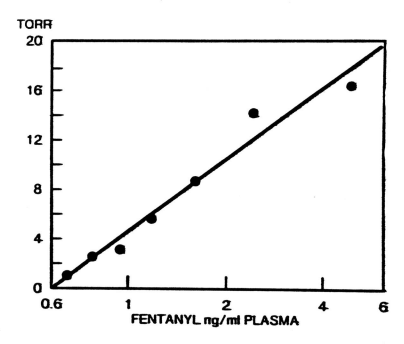

Fig. 5–4. Elevation of end-tidal P_{CO_2} above normal (torr or mm Hg) versus plasma fentanyl concentration (mg/ml) of plasma. (Reprinted from McClain, D.A., and Hug, C.C., Jr.: Intravenous fentanyl kinetics. Clin. Pharmacol. Ther., 28:106, 1980; and Hug, C.C., Jr.: The Pharmacokinetics of Fentanyl. Janssen Pharmaceutica Library, 1982.)

after intravenous injection, although some degree of depression may persist, particularly with morphine use, but also after the administration of fentanyl. Thus, respiratory responses to hypercarbia may be depressed 3 to 4 hours after the administration of fentanyl (5 to 10 μg/kg) (Fig. 5–5) in contrast to the much shorter duration of analgesia with the same dose.[111,118,121,123,124] With the higher doses of fentanyl and morphine used in cardiac surgery, respiratory depression can persist for many hours, necessitating ventilatory support for 12 to 24 hours after surgery.

Respiratory depression may follow even the moderate doses of opioids used for preoperative medication.[122] Concurrent use of other agents (thiopental and nitrous oxide) may or may not (droperidol) be a further depressant to the respiratory system.[122,123,125]

Recurrence of respiratory depression after adequate spontaneous ventilation has been observed following delivery of small doses of fentanyl.[126–128] This recurrence may be due to decreased stimulation in the postoperative period, or (as described by some, but not all, investigators) to secondary increases in plasma fentanyl concentrations related to enterohepatic recirculation.[129,130]

Reversal of Respiratory Depression

Opioid-induced respiratory depression can be reversed by the use of opioid antagonists, e.g., naloxone. Note, however, that respiratory depression may recur if the antagonist is shorter acting than the agonist, and that the analgesic effects may also be reversed.[131]

Extreme caution must be exercised when administering naloxone, especially

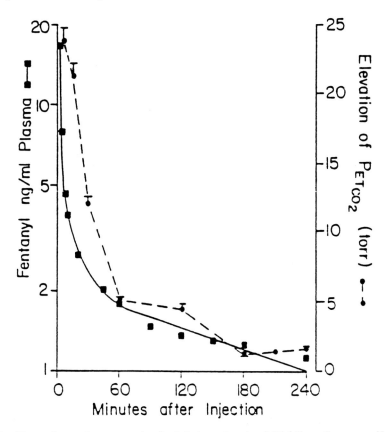

Fig. 5–5. Plasma fentanyl concentration (ng/ml plasma) and end-tidal $PaCO_2$ (torr or mg Hg) versus time after bolus doses of 5 to 10 µg/kg of fentanyl administered intravenously in man. (Reprinted from McClain, D.A., and Hug, C.C., Jr.: Anesthesiology, *51*:S29, 1979.)

to reverse the depressant effects of opioids given in high doses. Intense pressor responses have been reported with this drug, not only for opioid reversal in animals and man, but also after its use during enflurane anesthesia.[17,132–137] Severe pulmonary edema and multiple premature atrial contractions may accompany the hypertension.[138] These cardiovascular responses to naloxone, given to dogs that were anesthetized with halothane, nitrous oxide, and morphine but that did not undergo surgery, caused tachycardia, hypertension, and sharp rises in coronary blood flow and myocardial oxygen consumption, despite the absence of pain. The enflurane-anesthetized patients mentioned previously were also pain-free after naloxone administration.[137] Naloxone may cause the release of catecholamines when it is administered after opioids. However induced, the effects can be extremely dangerous, especially in patients with coronary artery disease. Therefore, this author believes that opioid antagonists must not be used to reverse the respiratory effects of high doses of opioids in patients with cardiovascular disease. This prescription does not necessarily apply to other patients. Indeed, there may be a place for naloxone administration to enable neurologic assessment, e.g., to guide therapy when brain damage is suspected after the use of large doses of opioids for neurosurgical operations. In any case, the risk of severe hypertension must be balanced against the advantages of rapid recovery whenever naloxone is used as an opioid antagonist.

Effects of Agonist-Antagonist Narcotic Compounds

Opioid antagonists have been studied for 70 years, but few such drugs have had significant clinical impact.[139–149] The first opioid agonist-antagonist to be used widely in man was pentazocine, the N-dimethylallyl derivative of phenazocine, the analgesic potency of which is one third to one fifth that of morphine.[147,148] Unfortunately, equipotent doses of each drug produce similar degrees of respiratory depression. Although the potential for abuse is less than that with morphine,[148] prolonged use of pentazocine can lead to physical dependence.[147] In addition, dysphoric side-effects are common, especially in elderly patients.

More recently, two totally different synthetic agonist-antagonist analgesics, butorphanol (levo-N-cyclobutylmethyl-3,14 β-dihydroxymorphinan) and nalbuphine ((-)-3-hydroxy-N-propargylmorphinan tartrate), have become available. The respiratory depression produced by butorphanol (2 mg intravenously) is similar to that with morphine (10 mg intravenously), although increasing doses of butorphanol do not cause the dose-related increases in depression that are seen with morphine use.[86] During cardiac catheterization, equianalgesic doses of butorphanol and morphine produce comparable respiratory depression.[87]

Nalbuphine is an agonist-antagonist analgesic structurally related to the opioid, oxymorphine, and the opioid antagonist, naloxone. As with butorphanol, single doses of nalbuphine cause the same respiratory depression as caused by equianalgesic doses of morphine.[149] Curiously, however, with cumulative doses the degree of depression is dose-related only to a "ceiling" of 30 mg/70 kg; at higher doses, further depression of respiration does not occur. A similar effect has been reported for nalorphine.[150] This phenomenon, which may occur with the use of all agonist-antagonist analgesics, is presumably due to the antagonist properties of these drugs, and may become therapeutically significant with higher doses or after accidental overdosage.

Muscle Rigidity

Opioid-induced muscle rigidity during anesthesia, first reported 30 years ago, was generally ignored until the introduction of neuroleptanalgesia.[43,151,152] Some rigidity was observed in 80% of patients receiving droperidol and fentanyl.[50] Other subjects consistently noted chest wall rigidity 60 to 90 seconds after receiving single doses of fentanyl (0.5 to 0.8 mg intravenously).[153]

When it occurs, opioid-induced rigidity is characterized by increased thoracic and abdominal muscle tone, which progresses to severe stiffness. This "wooden chest" can greatly hamper ventilation of the nonparalyzed anesthetized patient. Rigidity usually begins just as the patient is losing consciousness, but may be experienced by conscious patients.[154] Rapid opioid injection seems to increase the severity, thus suggesting the advisability of slow administration.[95,97,155] The phenomenon seems accentuated by concomitant use of nitrous oxide.[156–158]

The mechanism of this muscle rigidity remains obscure, but may be related to opioid-induced catatonia. This rigidity is not caused by a direct action on muscle fibers, because rigidity can be decreased or prevented by pretreatment with or concomitant use of muscle relaxants.[159] Creatinine phosphokinase levels do not rise, thus indicating that minimal or no muscle damage occurs.[157] Opioids do not significantly affect nerve conduction, and monosynaptic spinal reflexes associated with muscle stretch receptors are only minimally depressed.[156–158] Rigidity has been attributed to stimulation at a single site in the CNS, perhaps the caudate nucleus.[160,161] In the rat, this stimulation results in activation of extensor α-motoneurons.[162–164]

Bronchial Effects

Opioids have different effects on the peripheral respiratory tract. When $Paco_2$ is kept normal after administration of morphine, pulmonary dead space decreases. When $Paco_2$ is allowed to rise, pulmonary dead space remains unchanged by morphine.[165] High doses of morphine (and probably of many other opioids) decrease bronchial ciliary motion.[166] Fentanyl has antimuscarinic, antihistaminergic, and antiserotonergic actions, and may be preferable to morphine for use in patients with asthmatic or bronchospastic disease processes.[167]

RENAL SYSTEM

Morphine, delivered in doses of 10 to 30 mg, exerts a significant antidiuretic effect.[168,169] Although release of antidiuretic hormone (ADH) has been implicated, large doses of morphine and fentanyl do not stimulate ADH release in man.[103,168,169] Morphine may induce ADH release in unusual circumstances (e.g., nausea and vomiting) or during surgical stimulation in lightly anesthetized patients.[170] Morphine does, however, increase blood levels of ADH in the dog; it also reduces urine output and increases urine osmolarity, despite minimal effects on cardiovascular dynamics.[171]

The antidiuretic effect of morphine in man seems hemodynamically determined; its primary cause is a reduction in glomerular filtration rate.[168,169] Thus, in a comparison of anesthetics, intraoperative and postoperative urine output determinations did not differ in 61 patients undergoing similar open heart operations with high-dose morphine or halothane anesthesia.[93] When given slowly and intravenously, morphine (2 mg/kg) also did not affect glomerular filtration rate, urine osmolarity, or urine output in volunteers when $Paco_2$ was held to a normal level by controlled ventilation and cardiovascular dynamics were maintained with adequate amounts of intravenous fluids.[172] If arterial blood pressure and cardiac output were reduced, however, either by the addition of nitrous oxide (60%) or by more rapid administration of morphine, these renal variables were also markedly diminished.[172]

Finally, narcotics may increase detrusor and urethral sphincter tone, which can result in urinary retention in urinary bladders that have not been catheterized.[164,169,171,172,173]

GASTROINTESTINAL SYSTEM

Opioids may cause nausea and vomiting through several mechanisms.[174] They may directly stimulate the emetic chemoreceptor trigger zone located in the area postrema of the medulla.[174] Changes in posture—from side to side, supine to sitting, or sitting to standing—may also contribute to nausea and vomiting. Inhibition of gastrointestinal tract motility with delayed passage of its contents may also be a factor.[175–180] Finally, opioids can induce vomiting by causing an increased volume of secretions in the gastrointestinal tract.[181] Because neither vomiting nor nausea ordinarily occurs during induction of anesthesia with larger doses of narcotics, such doses may depress CNS emetic zones. In addition, although opioids decrease bowel motility, and hence are often used to treat diarrhea and dysentery, they also delay gastric emptying by contracting the proximal portion of the duodenum.[175,182] Indeed, similar contractions throughout the gastrointestinal tract, with increases in resting smooth muscle tone and even spasm, may occur with use of all opioids.[176,177] The causative mechanisms probably involve both CNS and direct gastrointestinal actions, undoubtedly the result of stimulation of opiate receptors.[178,179,183]

Opioids increase stomach, pancreatic, biliary, and salivary gland secretions through both central and peripheral actions.[184,185] They simultaneously increase biliary duct pressure, thereby causing right upper quadrant pain both pre- and postoperatively.[186,187] This action would seem to contraindicate the use of opioids in biliary surgery, although the occurrence of tachyphylaxis to biliary pressure changes with repeated doses seems to render them safe for such operations.[186,188,189]

THE SURGICAL STRESS RESPONSE

The stress of anesthesia and especially of trauma commonly triggers sudden release of the so-called stress hormones, catecholamines, cortisol, growth hormones, glucagon, and antidiuretic hormone (ADH), while simultaneously inhibiting release of insulin.[47,190–199] The resultant hyperglycemia, together with increases in the levels of circulating free fatty acids, lactate, pyruvate, glycerol, and 3-hydroxybutyrate, are all indicators of increased catabolism. The magnitude of these changes is directly proportional to the severity of the operative trauma; these changes are much greater during intra-abdominal than superficial surgical procedures, and are greatest with heart surgery involving cardiopulmonary bypass.[190–192,199] The stress response is considered undesirable because it promotes hemodynamic instability and intra- and postoperative catabolism. Its modification by opioids seems desirable.

Morphine appears to modify the surgical stress response in a dose-related fashion.[194–199] Small doses inhibit the release of ACTH, which is at least part of the pituitary-adrenal response to surgical stress.[194,195] Larger doses (0.33 mg/kg) cause a significant decrease in the quantity of blood lactate but not of pyruvate.[196] Still larger doses (1 mg/kg) suppress surgically induced increases in plasma cortisol, but not of human growth hormone during major abdominal operations.[197] Morphine may, however, actually increase some stress-responding hormones, e.g., catecholamines, ADH, and renin.[61,200] Thus, in cardiac surgery with high-dose morphine anesthesia (4 mg/kg), plasma concentrations of cortisol and growth hormone are increased during cardiopulmonary bypass (but not in the pre-bypass period).[197–199] Increases in plasma catecholamine concentration continue after bypass and into the postoperative period.[198]

Plasma catecholamine concentrations are increased in dogs by an action of morphine that affects release mechanisms in the adrenal medulla and to a lesser extent in sympathetic nerve endings.[61,200,201] This occurrence may explain the positive inotropic action of morphine in dogs; the effect is blocked by beta-adrenergic blocking drugs or previous adrenalectomy.[62] Morphine-induced catecholamine release also occurs in man.[63–65] The extent of release is not only dose-related (e.g., urinary excretion of norepinephrine [NE] is greater with low than with high blood levels of morphine), but also appears dependent on the functional state of the sympathetic nervous system (e.g., urinary NE excretion is greater in patients with hypertension than in otherwise similar normotensive patients),[63,64] and on the pre-induction plasma levels of NE (e.g., if low, they may show a small rise after morphine; if higher, they tend to sustain decreases).[63,64,202] Similar changes occur with inhalational agents.

Although morphine alone stimulates ADH secretion in animals, humans require the addition of surgical stimulation.[203–205] Thus, in patients undergoing cardiac surgery with nitrous oxide-morphine (1 mg/kg) anesthesia, the amount of plasma ADH rises significantly before cardiopulmonary bypass and increases further during bypass.[205] Plasma renin activity also increases markedly in such patients and is closely correlated with simultaneous increases in mean arterial pressure.[69,100]

Fentanyl and some of its newer congeners seem even more effective than morphine in modifying hormonal responses to surgery. The use of fentanyl (50 μg/kg) with nitrous oxide abolishes the hyperglycemic response to prolonged gynecologic surgery and reduces concomitant plasma cortisol and growth hormone responses more effectively than does halothane-nitrous oxide.[206] Similar results occur with large doses of fentanyl for gastric surgery.[207]

In patients about to undergo coronary artery surgery, plasma NE levels are significantly elevated after infusion of fentanyl (15 to 30 μg/kg), but return to control values after 50 μg/kg have been delivered.[208] Plasma epinephrine or dopamine levels remain unchanged. In contrast, fentanyl in doses of 50 μg/kg or more prevents increases in plasma catecholamine concentrations during cardiac surgery, although marked increases may occur during cardiopulmonary bypass.[39,190,209,210] The increases are probably in response to the significant physiologic abnormalities of hemodilution, hypothermia, and nonpulsatile flow during this period. There is also some evidence that vasopressin and catecholamine responses to cardiopulmonary bypass can be significantly attenuated by the use of pulsatile flow.[211]

Anesthesia with fentanyl (60 to 100 μg/kg) prevents the increase in levels of plasma ADH, renin, and aldosterone before cardiopulmonary bypass.[103,210] These changes contrast markedly with the significant *increases* of these hormones that occur in similar patients anesthetized with morphine.[205] During bypass, however, the level of plasma ADH rises significantly despite the use of high doses (more than 100 μg/kg) of fentanyl.[103] High-dose fentanyl anesthesia usually (but not always) prevents increases in blood glucose, plasma cortisol, and growth hormone concentrations throughout open heart operations.[190,209,210,212]

Thus, fentanyl appears somewhat more effective than morphine in reducing the surgical stress response. Whether this discrepancy is the result of differences in pharmacologic actions or in potency has not been determined. Other opioids have been less well studied. Papaveretum (extract of opium) is significantly less effective than fentanyl,[212] whereas the new narcotics, alfentanil and sufentanil, seem more effective.[213]

The *mechanism* by which large doses of opioids inhibit the stress response to surgical trauma is unknown. Whatever the cause, the pituitary release of ACTH (and perhaps other stress hormonal precursors) is probably involved, because ACTH secretion is reduced by high doses of opioids.[199] Interestingly, decreases in plasma human growth hormone concentrations produced by morphine (4 mg/kg) are totally reversible after ACTH administration.[199] Because endogenous opioid-like peptides play an important regulatory role in the secretion of several pituitary hormones, possibly through release of neurotransmitters (e.g., dopamine) that either regulate the secretion directly or release inhibiting factors, these exogenous opiates may have similar actions of inhibition or stimulation.[214–216]

Techniques of opioid analgesia, particularly those that involve the use of high doses of fentanyl, can help to diminish the surgical stress response. This response, admirable for "fight or flight" reactions, may be totally inappropriate in patients undergoing certain forms of cardiovascular surgery, e.g., coronary artery bypass grafting for ischemic heart disease. Increases in plasma catecholamine concentrations in these patients increase myocardial work and further compromise an already damaged myocardium. Increased protein catabolism caused by elevated plasma levels of the stress hormones may also delay postoperative recovery. Modification of these metabolic responses should reduce morbidity and mortality; however "stress-free anesthesia," although an attractive biochemical concept, is still of unproven clinical benefit. Reductions in the metabolic responses to anesthesia and surgery are short-lived, and with morphine, at least, postoperative nitrogen balance is not improved.[198,203,208] Whether the same is true after delivery of high doses of fentanyl or of the newer synthetic opioids remains to be documented.

NEW AGONIST OPIOIDS

Two new synthetic fentanyl derivatives are now undergoing clinical investigation as anesthetics and analgesic supplements. They may prove to have certain advantages over the currently available compounds in some situations.

Sufentanil

Sufentanil is an N-4 substituted derivative of fentanyl (Fig. 5–6). Its chemistry was first described in 1976.[217] Animal experiments have shown that sufentanil is extremely potent; in the tail-withdrawal reflex of rats, it is 4521 times as potent as morphine.[218]

Sufentanil is also very safe; the LD_{50} ratio in rats is 25,111 (morphine is 69

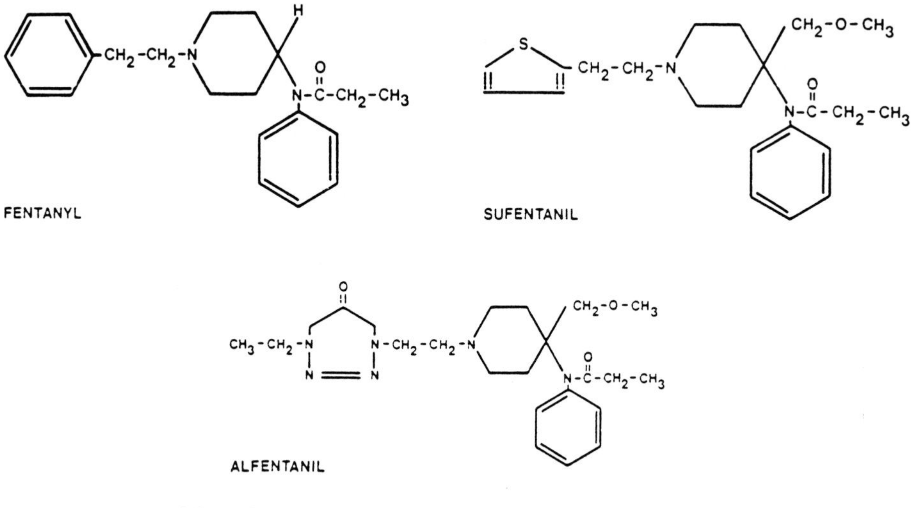

Fig. 5–6. Structural formulas of fentanyl, alfentanil, and sufentanil.

and fentanyl is 277).[218] Dogs have survived intravenous doses of 5 mg/kg without respiratory assistance and with complete recovery after 24 hours. Infusions of very high doses of sufentanil (40 μg/kg/minute) in atropine-medicated, mechanically ventilated dogs produce scant change in cardiovascular dynamics.[51] In Sprague-Dawley rats, sufentanil is capable of decreasing the minimal alveolar concentration (MAC) of halothane by more than 90% at an infusion rate of 1 μg/kg/minute.[219] These data may indicate an important difference between sufentanil and fentanyl, as the latter is only capable of reducing the MAC of enflurane in dogs by a maximum of 65% after a loading dose of 270 μg/kg followed by an infusion of 3.2 μg/kg/minute.[220] The validity of comparing the results of these studies, however, which involve different species with different inhalation agents, may be debatable. Furthermore, the significance of MAC reduction of inhalation agents by opioids in animals other than subhuman primates and humans is open to question because of the marked differences (decrease) in sensitivity of dogs, rats, and virtually all other mammals to most, if not all, narcotic analgesics when compared with humans.[23]

On the basis of clinical experience in humans with the use of sufentanil alone and in supplemented balanced anesthesia, sufentanil has been found to be 5 to 10 times as potent as fentanyl, and doses as high as 10 μg/kg have produced little change in cardiovascular dynamics.[221–223] In a study in which the effects of sufentanil (0.7 μg/kg) and fentanyl (7 μg/kg) on general and coronary hemodynamics were compared, no differences could be detected between the two drugs.[224] No differences in cardiovascular or hormonal effects could be detected between sufentanil (2 μg/kg) or fentanyl (20 μg/kg) as an anesthetic supplement during hysterectomy.[223] Van de Walle and colleagues, however, compared sufentanil (0.8 μg/kg/hour) with fentanyl (7.15 μg/kg/hour) as anesthetic supplements and found that sufentanil provided greater cardiovascular stability.[222]

Because sufentanil given in very large doses produces minimal hemodynamic changes in dogs, the drug has been suggested as an alternative opioid anesthetic to fentanyl.[51] Some investigators have now evaluated this agent to determine its value as a complete anesthetic.[225,226] Sufentanil (15 μg/kg) with air/O$_2$, when used as an anesthetic for cardiac surgery, produced no significant changes in cardiovascular dynamics.[225] There was also a lesser incidence of hypertension related to sternotomy with sufentanil (15 μg/kg) (10% of patients required vasodilator therapy) than with fentanyl (70 μg/kg) (50% of patients required vasodilator therapy).[225] In a study in which fentanyl (mean total dose of 122 μg/kg) was compared with sufentanil (mean total dose of 12.9 μg/kg), a similar reduction in intraoperative hypertension was found with the newer opioid.[226] In addition, speed of induction was faster with sufentanil. In a double-blind comparison with fentanyl, however, Rosow, et al., found that sufentanil did not provide better "hemodynamic stability" in patients undergoing coronary artery surgery.[227] Despite the use of as much as 30 μg/kg of sufentanil (equivalent to 150 to 300 μg/kg of fentanyl), most patients receiving both opioids had hypertensive responses to sternotomy or aortic manipulation that necessitated the use of supplemental inhalation anesthesia or vasodilator therapy.

The electroencephalographic responses to sufentanil anesthesia consist of high voltage, slow delta waves, and are indistinguishable from those described for fentanyl.[228] This similarity is in keeping with the like pharmacologic profiles of the two compounds. As yet, little information is available regarding the hormonal and substrate responses to sufentanil anesthesia, but sufentanil apparently blocks some hormonal "stress" responses (e.g., antidiuretic hormone) during cardiac surgery, including cardiopulmonary bypass. During cardiopulmonary bypass with sufentanil anesthesia, however, large increases in plasma catecholamine concentrations, similar to those described during fentanyl anesthesia, occurred.[229]

Results of investigations of the peripheral circulation and central hemodynamics after sufentanil and morphine anesthesia in dogs have shown that peripheral infusion was better maintained with sufentanil and was unaltered by beta blockade.[230,231] In addition, central hemodynamics were more stable after sufentanil than morphine anesthesia. Thus, sufentanil has certain advantages over morphine; comparisons were not made with fentanyl in these studies.

Alfentanil

Alfentanil is a less potent, shorter-acting drug than fentanyl;[232] its chemical structure is shown in Figure 5–6. In the tail-withdrawal test in rats, it is approximately one-quarter to one-third as potent as fentanyl and has one-third the duration of action, with a safety ratio LD_{50}/ED_{50} of 1080.[232] Results of hemodynamic studies in ventilated dogs show that the acute toxicity of alfentanil is between that of morphine and that of fentanyl and that myocardial function and cardiovascular dynamics remain essentially unchanged at low doses (160 µg/kg).[18] When delivered in doses of 5 mg/kg, alfentanil results in transient cardiac stimulation (increases in left ventricular contractility, aortic blood flow velocity, and acceleration).[18] Peripheral and pulmonary vascular resistance values also were increased, as were heart rate and cardiac output. De Bruijn and colleagues also found evidence of transient increases in myocardial contractility in dogs, but not with the use of lower doses of alfentanil (200 µg/kg).[233]

The respiratory effects of alfentanil have been compared with those of fentanyl in rabbits.[234] Alfentanil has an earlier peak effect and shorter duration of action than does fentanyl, but otherwise the respiratory effects of the two drugs are similar. In human volunteers, small doses of alfentanil (1.6 to 6.4 µg/kg) produced transient depression of ventilation, with no change in mean ventilatory response to carbon dioxide 30 minutes after injection.[235]

Small doses of alfentanil (0.8 to 1.0 mg) have been used for anesthetic supplementation for minor surgery in spontaneously breathing patients and during balanced anesthesia for laparoscopic surgery (0.05 mg/kg).[236,237] Anesthesia was described as adequate (no movement or evidence of awareness); heart rate and arterial blood pressure remained unchanged; and recovery was fast. There was, however, a high incidence of side-effects: movement, apnea, difficulty in assisting ventilation, and nausea and vomiting in the patients having minor surgery.

Alfentanil has been compared with fentanyl for use with nitrous oxide in patients undergoing short, outpatient procedures.[238] The authors found that alfentanil was superior to fentanyl (with respect to speed of postoperative recovery), whether administered in a bolus or with a continuous infusion technique; continuous infusion of alfentanil resulted in the fastest postoperative recovery. In patients undergoing longer operations (1.5 to 2.5 hours) with nitrous oxide-alfentanil or nitrous oxide-fentanyl anesthesia in which both opioids were given in small equianalgesic bolus injections throughout surgery, recovery was significantly slower in patients receiving alfentanil.[239] These data suggest that frequent bolus administration of alfentanil for longer operations may result in accumulation of the drug. Furthermore, the question of whether the compound has advantages over fentanyl for other than short operations is raised. A study designed to compare fentanyl and alfentanil administered as a continuous infusion for longer operations might be valuable in settling this question.

Alfentanil (35 to 150 μg/kg) also has been investigated as an anesthetic induction agent in patients with and without significant cardiac disease.[240] Induction time was fast (45 to 140 seconds), and cardiovascular variables, including heart rate, systemic and pulmonary arterial blood pressures, and cardiac output, changed minimally throughout the induction sequence, even after endotracheal intubation. In addition, when anesthetic induction was followed by halothane (0.2 to 1.0%) and nitrous oxide (60%) administration, all patients were extubated on the operating room table and responded to verbal command upon entrance to the recovery room. No patient demonstrated evidence of respiratory depression at any time in the postoperative recovery period. The only problem noted in the findings of this study was a high incidence of chest wall rigidity. Similar findings, minimal change in heart rate and blood pressure and a rapid recovery after anesthetic induction and endotracheal intubation, have been reported by Black, et al.[241] Moldenhauer, et al., however, found that use of alfentanil may result in significant hypotension when used as an induction agent with succinylcholine in patients identified as ASA class II to IV.[242] Apparently, more experience is necessary before the value, if any, of alfentanil as an induction agent can be established.

Alfentanil has also been compared with fentanyl for the treatment of postoperative pain by using an on-demand analgesia computer.[243] Both drugs produced good pain relief. The mean rate of infusion of fentanyl was 0.88 μg/minute and that of alfentanil was 8.1 μg/minute (a ratio of 1:9.2); these rates correlate well with the estimated ratios of potency (3:1) and duration of action (3:1).

Alfentanil-oxygen anesthesia has been evaluated for use in patients undergoing coronary surgery.[244] Frequent bolus doses were used to keep the patients adequately anesthetized during surgery; the mean total dose requirement was 1.22 mg/kg. This technique resulted in shorter induction and recovery times than with fentanyl; however, a high incidence of hypertension during surgery was observed. The administration of alfentanil by continuous infusion as a complete anesthetic seems more appropriate. Initial experience with doses on the order of 50 μg/kg for induction, with subsequent infusion of approximately 8 μg/kg/hour during cardiac surgery, has produced encouraging results.[245] In this study, de Lange and de Bruijn showed that alfentanil, infused at continuous but variable rate, was far superior to alfentanil given in bolus amounts on multiple occasions in terms of prevention of hemodynamic stimulation (hypertension and tachycardia) or depression (hypotension) and in hastening recovery in patients after coronary artery surgery.[245] Indeed, these authors, having experience with multiple high-dose fentanyl and sufentanil techniques, as well as extensive clinical experience with alfentanil for all types of cardiac surgery, believe that alfentanil given by continuous but variable infusion is the ideal opioid anesthetic for patients undergoing coronary artery surgery.[245]

Alfentanil is a short-acting opioid analgesic that will probably occupy a unique place as an analgesic supplement for short operative procedures. It is potentially useful for anesthetic induction as well as for longer operations, either as a supplement or as a complete anesthetic if given by continuous intravenous infusion.

REFERENCES

1. Stoelting, R.K.: Opiate receptors and endorphins their role in anesthesiology. Anesth. Analg., *59*:874, 1980.
2. Cousins, M.J., and Mather, L.E.: Intrathecal and epidural administration of opioids. Anesthesiology, *61*:276, 1984.
3. Pert, C.B., and Snyder, S.H.: Opiate receptor: demonstration in nervous tissue. Science, *179*:1011, 1973.
4. Terenius, L.: Characteristics of the "receptor" for narcotic analgesics in synaptic plasma membrane fractions from rat brain. Acta Pharmacol. Toxicol., (Copenh.), *13*:377, 1973.
5. Paternak, G.W., and Childers, S.R.: Opiates, opioid peptides and their receptors. *In* Critical Care: State of the Art. Vol. V. Edited by W.M. Shoemaker, Society of Critical Care Medicine, 1984.
6. Yaksh, T.L., and Howe, J.R.: Opiate receptors and their definition by antagonists. Anesthesiology, *56*:246, 1982.
7. Yaksh, T.L.: Spinal opiate analgesia: characteristics and principles of action. Pain, *11*:293, 1981.
8. Mayer, D.J., Wolfle, T.L., Akil, H., Carden, B., and Liebeskind, J.C.: Analgesia from electrical stimulation in the brainstem of the rat. Science, *174*:1351, 1971.
9. Satoh, M., and Takagi, H.: Enhancement by morphine of the central descending inhibitory influence on spinal sensory transmission. Eur. J. Pharmacol., *14*:60, 1971.
10. Yaksh, T.L., and Rudy, T.A.: Studies on the direct spinal action of narcotics in the production of analgesia in the rat. J. Pharmacol. Exp. Ther., *202*:411, 1977.
11. Yaksh, T.L., Frederickson, R.C.A., Huang, S.P., and Rudy, T.A.: In vivo comparison of the receptor populations acted upon in the spinal cord by morphine and pentapeptides in the production of analgesia. Brain Res., *148*:516, 1978.
12. Goldstein, A.: Opiate receptors. Life Sci., *14*:615, 1974.
13. Stanley, T.H., Leysen, J., Niemegeers, J.E., and Pace, N.L.: Narcotic dosage and central nervous system opiate receptor binding. Anesth. Analg., *62*:705, 1983.
14. Lowenstein, E., Hallowell, P., Levine, F.H., Daggett, W.M., Austin, G., and Laver, M.B.: Cardiovascular response to large doses of intravenous morphine in man. N. Engl. J. Med., *281*:1389, 1969.
15. Stoelting, R.K., and Gibbs, P.S.: Hemodynamic effects of morphine and morphine-nitrous oxide in valvular heart disease and coronary artery disease. Anesthesiology, *38*:42, 1973.
16. Hasbrouk, J.D.: Morphine anesthesia for open heart surgery. Ann. Thorac. Surg., *10*:364, 1970.
17. Freye, E.: Cardiovascular effects of high dosages of fentanyl, meperidine and naloxone in dogs. Anesth. Analg., *53*:40, 1974.
18. De Castro, J., Van de Water, A., Wouters, L., Xhonneux, R., Reneman, R., and Kay, B.: Comparative study of cardiovascular, neurological and metabolic side effects of eight narcotics in dogs. (Parts I, II and III). Acta Anesthesiol. Belg., *30*:5, 1979.
19. Liu, W.S., Bidwai, A.V., Stanley, T.H., and Loeser, E.A.: Cardiovascular dynamics after large doses of fentanyl and fentanyl plus N₂O in the dog. Anesth. Analg., *55*:168, 1976.
20. De Castro, J.: Analgesic anesthesia based on the use of fentanyl in high doses. Anesthesia, *1*:87, 1977.
21. Stanley, T.H., and Webster, L.R.: Anesthetic requirements and cardiovascular effects of fentanyl-oxygen and fentanyl-diazepam-oxygen anesthesia in man. Anesth. Analg., *57*:411, 1978.
22. Stanley, T.H., Bidwai, A.V., Lunn, J.K., and Hodges, M.R.: Cardiovascular effects of nitrous oxide during meperidine infusion in the dog. Anesth. Analg., *56*:836, 1977
23. Bailey, P., Stanley, T.H., and Port, J.D.: Fentanyl anesthesia in dogs. Anesth. Analg., In press.
24. Stanley, T.H., and Lathrop, G.D.: Urinary excretion of morphine during and after valvular and coronary-artery surgery. Anesthesiology, *46*:166, 1977.
25. Bailey, P.L., Wilbrink, J., Zwanikken, P., Pace, N.L., and Stanley, T.H.: Anesthetic induction with fentanyl. Anesth. Analg., *64*:48, 1985.
26. Stanley, T.H., and de Lange, S.: The influence of patient habits on dosage requirements during high dose fentanyl anesthesia. Can. Anaesth. Soc. J., *3*:368, 1984.
27. Shafter, A., White, P.G., Schuttler, J., and Rosenthal, H.H.: Use of a fentanyl infusion in the intensive care unit: tolerance to its anesthetic effect. Anesthesiology, *59*:245, 1983.
28. Stanley, T.H., Liu, W.S., and Lathrop, G.D.: The effects of morphine and halothane anaesthesia on urine norepinephrine during surgery for congenital heart disease. Can. Anaesth. Soc. J., *23*:58, 1976.
29. Bedford, R.F., and Wollman, H.: Postoperative respiratory effects of morphine and halothane anesthesia: a study in patients undergoing cardiac surgery. Anesthesiology, *43*:1, 1975.
30. Stoelting, R.K., Gibbs, P.S., Creasser, C.W., and Peterson, C.: Hemodynamic and ventilatory responses to fentanyl, fentanyl-droperidol, and nitrous oxide in patients with acquired valvular heart disease. Anesthesiology, *42*:319, 1975.

31. Mark, J.B., and Greenberg, L.M.: Intraoperative awareness and hypertensive crisis during high-dose fentanyl-diazepam-oxygen anesthesia. Anesth. Analg., 62:698, 1983.
32. Tomichek, R.C., Rosow, C.E., Philbin, D.M., Moss, J., Teplick, R.S., and Schneider, R.C.: Diazepam-fentanyl interaction–hemodynamic hormonal effects in coronary artery surgery. Anesth. Analg., 62:881, 1983.
33. Sebel, P.S., and Bovill, J.G.: Editorial—Opioid anaesthesia—Fact or fallacy? Br. J. Anaesth., 54:1149, 1982.
34. Wilson, S.L, Vaughan, R.W., and Stephen, C.R.: Awareness, dreams and hallucinations associated with general anesthesia. Anesth. Analg., 54:609, 1975.
35. Saucier, N., Walts, L.F., and Moreland, J.R.: Patient awareness during nitrous oxide, oxygen and halothane anesthesia. Anesth. Analg., 62:239, 1983.
36. Hilgengerg, J.C.: Intraoperative awareness during high-dose fentanyl-oxygen anesthesia. Anesthesiology, 54:341, 1981.
37. Mummanemi, N., Rao, T.L.K., and Montoya, A.: Awareness and recall with high-dose fentanyl oxygen anesthesia. Anesth. Analg., 59:948, 1980.
38. Blacher, R.S: On awakening paralyzed during surgery. A syndrome of traumatic neurosis. JAMA, 234:67, 1975.
39. Stanley, T.H.: The pharmacology of intravenous narcotic anesthetics. *In* Anesthesia. Edited by R.D. Miller. New York, Churchill Livingstone, 1981, pp. 425–449.
40. Sebel, P.S., Bovill, J.G., Boekhorst, R.A.A., and Rog, N.: Cardiovascular effects of high-dose fentanyl anaesthesia. Acta Anaesthesiol. Scand., 26:308, 1982.
41. Stanley, T.H., Gray, N.H., Stanford, W., and Armstrong, R.: The effects of high-dose morphine on fluid and blood requirements in open-heart operations. Anesthesiology, 38:536, 1973.
42. Wong, K.C., Martin, W.E., Hornbein, T.F., Freund, F.G., and Everett, J.: The cardiovascular effects of morphine sulfate with oxygen and with nitrous oxide in man. Anesthesiology, 38:542, 1973.
43. Kitahata, L.M., and Collins, J.G.: Narcotic Analgesics in Anesthesiology. Baltimore, Williams and Wilkins, 1982.
44. Stoelting, R.K.: Influence of barbiturate anesthetic induction on circulatory responses to morphine. Anesth. Analg., 56:615, 1977.
45. Knight, P.R., Pandit, S.K., Bolles, R., Kothary, S.P., Hill, A.B., Nahrwold, M.N., and Cohen, P.J.: Amnesia to visual stimulation after large doses of fentanyl. Anesthesiology, 53:S2, 1982.
46. Sebel, P.S., Bovill, J.G., Wauquier, A., and Rog, P.: Effects of high-dose fentanyl anesthesia on the electroencephalogram. Anesthesiology, 55:203, 1981.
47. Pearcy, W.C., Knott, J.R., and Bjurstrow, R.O.: Studies on nitrous oxide, meperidine and levalorphan with unipolar electroencephalography. Anesthesiology, 18:310, 1957.
48. Winters, W.D., Mori, K., Spooner, C.E., and Bauer, R.O.: The neurophysiology of anesthesia. Anesthesiology, 28:65, 1967.
49. Bovill, J.G., Sebel, P.S., and Stanley, T.H.: Opioid analgesics in anesthesia: with special reference to their use in cardiovascular anesthesia. Anesthesiology, 61:731, 1984.
50. Corssen, G., Domino, E.F., and Sweet, R.B.: Neuroleptanalgesia and anesthesia. Anesth. Analg., 43:748, 1964.
51. Reddy, P., Liu, W.S., Port, D., Gillmor, S., and Stanley, T.H.: Comparison of haemodynamic effects of anaesthetic doses of alphaprodine and sufentanil in the dog. Can. Anaesth. Soc. J., 27:345, 1980.
52. Urthaler, F., Isobe, J.G., and James, T.N.: Direct and vagally medicated chronotropic effects of morphine studied by selective perfusion of the sinus node of awake dogs. Chest, 68:222, 1975.
53. De Silva, R.A., Verrier, R.L., and Lown, B.: Protective effect of vagotonic action of morphine sulfate on ventricular vulnerability. Cardiovasc. Res., 12:167, 1978.
54. Kennedy, B.L., and West, T.C.: Effects of morphine on electrically-induced release of autonomic mediators in the rabbit sinoatrial node. J. Pharmacol. Exp. Ther., 157:149, 1967.
55. Urthaler, F., Isobe, J.H., Gilmour, K.E., and James, T.N.: Morphine and autonomic control of the sinus node. Chest, 64:203, 1973.
56. Reitan, J.A., Stangert, K.B., Wymore, M.L., and Martucci, R.W.: Central vagal control of fentanyl-induced bradycardia during halothane anesthesia. Anesth. Analg., 57:31, 1978.
57. Laubie, M., Schmitt, H., and Drouillat, M.: Central sites and mechanisms of the hypotensive and bradycardic effects of the narcotic analgesic agent fentanyl. Naunyn Schmiedebergs Arch. Pharmacol., 296:255, 1977.
58. Laubie, M., and Schmitt, S.: Action of the morphinometic agent, fentanyl, on the nucleus tractus solitarii and the nucleus ambiguus cardiovascular neurons. Eur. J. Pharmacol., 67:403, 1980.
59. Liu, W.S., Bidwai, A.V., Lunn, J.K., and Stanley, T.H.: Urine catecholamine excretion after large doses of fentanyl, fentanyl and diazepam, and fentanyl, diazepam and pancuronium. Can. Anaesth. Soc. J., 24:371, 1977.

60. Kelman, G.R., and Kennedy, B.R.: Cardiovascular effects of pancuronium in man. Br. J. Anaesth., *43*:335, 1971.
61. Kayaalp, S.O., and Kaymakcalaw, S.: Studies on the morphine-induced release of catecholamines from the adrenal glands in the dog. Arch. Int. Pharmacodyn. Ther., *172*:139, 1968.
62. Vasko, J.S., Henney, R.P., and Brawley, R.K.: Effects of morphine on ventricular function and myocardial contractile force. Am. J. Physiol., *210*:329, 1966.
63. Stanley, T.H., Isern-Amaral, J., and Lathrop, G.D.: The effects of morphine anesthesia on urine norepinephrine during and after coronary artery surgery. Can. Anaesth. Soc. J., 22:478, 1975.
64. Stanley, T.H., Isern-Amaral, J., and Lathrop, G.D.: Urine epinephrine excretion in patients undergoing mitral or aortic valve replacement with morphine anesthesia. Anesth. Analg., *54*:509, 1975.
65. Balasaroswathi, K., Glisson, S.N., El-Etr, A., and Piffari, R.: Serum epinephrine and norepinephrine during valve replacement and aorto-coronary bypass. Can. Anaesth. Soc. J., 25:198, 1978.
66. Rosow, C.E., Moss, J., Philbin, D.M., and Savarese, J.J.: Histamine release during morphine and fentanyl anesthesia. Anesthesiology, 56:93, 1982.
67. Bovill, J.G., Sebel, P.S., and Stanley, T.H.: Opioid analgesics in anesthesia: with special reference to their use in cardiovascular anesthesia. Anesthesiology, *61*:731, 1984.
68. Stanley, T.H., and Liu, W.S.: Cardiovascular effects of nitrous oxide-meperidine anesthesia before and after pancuronium. Anesth. Analg., 56:669, 1977.
69. Foldes, F.F., Shiffman, H.P., and Kronfeld, P.P.: The use of fentanyl, meperidine or alphaprodine for neuroleptanesthesia. Anesthesiology, 35:35, 1970.
70. Lowenstein, E.: Morphine "anesthesia"—perspective. Anesthesiology, 35:363, 1971.
71. Priano, L.L., and Vatner, S.F.: Morphine effects on cardiac output and regional blood flow distribution in conscious dogs. Anesthesiology, 55:236, 1981.
72. Henney, R.P., Vasko, J.S., Brawley, R.K., Oldham, N.H., and Morrow, A.G.: The effects of morphine on the resistance and capacitance vessels of the peripheral circulation. Am. Heart J., 72:242, 1966.
73. Ward, J.M., McGrath, R.C., and Weil, J.V.: Effect of morphine on the peripheral vascular response to sympathetic circulation. Am. J. Cardiol., 29:659, 1972.
74. Strauer, B.: Contractile responses to morphine, piritramide, meperidine and fentanyl: a comparative study of effects on the isolated ventricular myocardium. Anesthesiology, 37:304, 1972.
75. Patschke, D., Gethmann, J.W., Hess, W., Tarrow, J., and Waibel, H.: Hamodynamic Koronardurchblutung und myocardialer Sauerstoffverbrauch unter hohen Fentanyl und Piritramidosen. Anaesthesist, 25:309, 1976.
76. King, B.D., Elder, J.D., and Dripps, R.D.: The effect of intravenous administration of meperidine upon the circulation of man and the circulatory response to tilt. Surg. Gynecol. Obstet., *94*:591, 1952.
77. Sugioka, D., Boniface, K.J., and Davis, D.A.: The influence of meperidine on myocardial contractility in the intact dog. Anesthesiology, *18*:623, 1957.
78. Stanley, T.H., Liu, W.S., Webster, L.R., and Johansen, R.: Haemodynamic effects of intravenous methadone anaesthesia in dogs. Can. Anaesth. Soc. J., 27:52, 1980.
79. de Lange, S., Stanley, T.H., Boscoe, M., and Pace, N.: Comparison of sufentanil-O_2 and fentanyl-O_2 anesthesia in man. Anesthesiology, 56:112, 1982.
80. Sebel, P.S., and Bovill, J.G.: Cardiovascular effects of sufentanil anesthesia: a study in patients undergoing cardiac surgery. Anesth. Analg., *61*:115, 1982.
81. Kay, B., and Pleuvry, B.: Human volunteer studies of alfentanil (R39209), a new short-acting narcotic analgesic. Anaesthesia, 35:952, 1980.
82. de Lange, S., Stanley, T.H., and Boscoe, M.J.: Alfentanil-oxygen anaesthesia for coronary artery surgery. Br. J. Anaesth., 53:1291, 1981.
83. de Lange, S., de Bruijn, H., and Stanley, T.H.: Alfentanil-oxygen anesthesia: comparison of continuous infusion and frequent bolus techniques for coronary artery surgery. Anesthesiology, 55:A43, 1981.
84. Nauta, J., Koopman, D., Spierdijk, J., van Kleef, J., de Lange, S., and Stanley, T.H.: Alfentanil, a new narcotic anesthetic induction agent. Anesth. Analg., *61*:267, 1982.
85. Jewitt, D.E., Maurer, B.J., Sonnenblick, E.J., and Shillingford, J.P.: Pentazocine: effect on ventricular muscle and hemodynamic changes in ischemic heart disease. Circulation, 44(Suppl. II):118, 1971.
86. Nagashima, H., Karamanian, A., Malovany, R., Radnay, P., Ang, M., Koener, S., and Foldes, F.F.: Effects of intravenous butorphanol and morphine. Clin. Pharmacol. Ther., *19*:738, 1976.
87. Popio, K.A., Jackson, D.H., Ross, A.M., Schreiner, B.F., and Yu, P.N.: Hemodynamic and respiratory effects of morphine and butorphanol. Clin. Pharmacol. Ther., 23:281, 1978.
88. Conahan, T.J., Ominsky, A.J., Wollman, H., and Stroth, R.: A prospective random comparison of halothane and morphine for open-heart anesthesia: one year's experience. Anesthesiology, 38:528, 1973.

89. Lappas, D.G., Geha, D., Fischer, J.E., Laver, M.B., and Lowenstein, E.: Filling pressures of the heart and pulmonary circulation of the patient with coronary-artery disease after large intravenous doses of morphine. Anesthesiology, 42:153, 1975.

90. Bennett, G.M., and Stanley, T.H.: Cardiovascular effects of fentanyl during enflurane anesthesia in man. Anesth. Analg., 58:179, 1979.

91. Jaffe, J.H., and Martin, W.R.: Opioid analgesics and antagonists. *In* The Pharmacological Basis of Therapeutics. 6th Ed. Edited by A.G. Gilman, L.S. Goodman, and A. Gilman. New York, MacMillan, 1980, pp. 494–534.

92. Lowenstein, E., Whiting, R.B., and Bittar, D.A.: Local and neurally mediated effects of morphine on skeletal muscle vascular resistance. J. Pharmacol. Exp. Ther., 180:359, 1972.

93. Stanley, T.H., Isern-Amaral, J., Gray, N.H., and Patton, C.P.: Comparison of blood requirements during morphine and halothane anesthesia for open-heart surgery. Anesthesiology, 41:34, 1974.

94. Feldberg, W., and Paton, W.D.M.: Release of histamine from skin and muscle in the cat by opium alkaloids and other histamine liberators. J. Physiol. (Lond.), 114:490, 1951.

95. Eckenhoff, H.E., and Oech, S.R.: The effects of narcotics and antagonists upon respiration and circulation in man. Clin. Pharmacol. Ther., 1:483, 1960.

96. Philbin, D.M., Moss, J., Akins, C.W., Rosow, C.E., Kono K., Scheider, R.C., Verlee, T.R., and Savarese, J.J.: The use of H_1 and H_2 histamine agonists with morphine anesthesia: a double-blind study. Anesthesiology, 55:212, 1981.

97. Greene, J.F., Jackman, A.P., and Krohn, K.A.: Mechanism of morphine-induced shifts in blood volume between extracorporeal reservoir and the systemic circulation under conditions of constant blood flow and vena caval pressures. Circ. Res., 42:479, 1978.

98. Greene, J.F., Jackman, A.P., and Parsons, G.: The effects of morphine on the mechanical properties of the systemic circulation in the dog. Circ. Res., 42:474, 1978.

99. Arens, J.F., Benbow, B.P., Ochsner, J.L., and Gheard, R.: Morphine anesthesia for aorto-coronary bypass procedures. Anesth. Analg., 51:901, 1972.

100. Bailey, D.R., Miller, E.D., Kaplan, J.A., and Rogers, P.W.: The renin-angiotension-aldosterone system during cardiac surgery with morphine-nitrous oxide anesthesia. Anesthesiology, 42:538, 1975.

101. Waller, J.L., Hug, C.C., Nagle, D.N., and Craver, J.M.: Hemodynamic changes during fentanyl-oxygen anesthesia for aortocoronary bypass operations. Anesthesiology, 55:212, 1981.

102. Edde, R.R.: Hemodynamic changes prior to and after sternotomy in patients anesthetized with high-dose fentanyl. Anesthesiology, 55:444, 1981.

103. Stanley, T.H., Philbin, D.M., and Coggins, C.H.: Fentanyl-oxygen anaesthesia for coronary artery surgery: cardiovascular and antidiuretic hormone responses. Can. Anaesth. Soc. J., 26:168, 1979.

104. de Lange, S., Stanley, T.H., and Boscoe, M.: Fentanyl-oxygen anesthesia: comparison of anesthetic requirements and cardiovascular responses in Salt Lake City and Leiden, Holland. Proceedings of the Seventh World Congress of Anaesthesiology. Edited by M. Zindler, and E. Rugheimer. Amsterdam, Excerpta Medica, 1980, p.313.

105. Hilgenberg, J.C.: Intraoperative awareness during high-dose fentanyl oxygen anesthesia. Anesthesiology, 54:341, 1981.

106. Mummaneni, N., Rao, T.L.K., and Montoya, A.: Awareness and recall with high-dose fentanyl-oxygen anesthesia. Anesth. Analg., 59:948, 1980.

107. Goldberg, A.H., Sohn, Y.Z., and Phear, W.P.Z.: Direct myocardial effects of nitrous oxide. Anesthesiology, 43:61, 1975.

108. Craythorne, N.W.B., and Darby, T.D.: The cardiovascular effects of nitrous oxide in the dog. Br. J. Anaesth., 37:560, 1965.

109. McDermott, R.W., and Stanley, T.H.: The cardiovascular effects of low concentrations of nitrous oxide during morphine anesthesia. Anesthesiology, 41:89, 1974.

110. Stanley, T.H., Berman, L., Loeser, E.A., Kawamura, R., and Sentker, C.R.: Cardiovascular effects of diazepam and droperidol during morphine anesthesia. Anesthesiology, 44:255, 1975.

111. Lunn, J.K., Webster, L.R., Stanley, T.H., and Woodward, A.: High dose fentanyl anesthesia for coronary artery surgery: plasma fentanyl concentration and influence of nitrous oxide on cardiovascular responses. Anesth. Analg., 58:390, 1979.

112. Bennett, G.M., and Stanley, T.H.: Comparison of the cardiovascular effects of morphine N_2O and fentanyl N_2O balanced anesthesia before and after pancuronium in man. Anesthesiology, 51:S138, 1979.

113. Bennett, G.M., Loeser, E.A., and Stanley, T.H.: Cardiovascular effects of scopolamine during morphine-oxygen and morphine-nitrous oxide anesthesia in man. Anesthesiology, 46:255, 1977.

114. Stoelting, R.K., Gibbs, P.S., Creasser, C.W., and Peterson, C.: Hemodynamic and ventilatory responses to fentanyl, fentanyl-droperidol, and nitrous oxide in patients with acquired valvular heart disease. Anesthesiology, 42:319, 1975.

115. Stoelting, R.K., Creasser, C.E., and Gibbs, P.S.: Circulatory effects of halothane added to morphine anesthesia in patients with coronary artery disease. Anesth. Analg., 53:449, 1974.

116. Bennett, G.M., and Stanley, T.H.: Cardiovascular effects of fentanyl during enflurane anesthesia in man. Anesth. Analg., *58*:179, 1979.

117. Harper, M.H., Hickey, R.F., Cromwell, T.H., and Linwood, S.: The magnitude of respiratory depression produced by fentanyl and fentanyl plus droperidol in man. J. Pharmacol. Exp. Ther., *199*:464, 1976.

118. Kaufmann, R.D., Agleh, K.A., and Belville, J.W.: Relative potencies and duration of action with respect to respiratory depression of intravenous meperidine, fentanyl and alphaprodine in man. J. Pharmacol. Exp. Ther., *208*:73, 1979.

119. Belville, J.W., and Seed, J.L.: The effects of drugs on the respiratory response to carbon dioxide. Anesthesiology, *21*:727, 1960.

120. Hug, C.C., Jr., and Murphy, M.R.: Fentanyl disposition in cerebrospinal fluid and plasma and its relationship to ventilatory depression in the dog. Anesthesiology, *50*:342, 1979.

121. Weil, J., McCullough, R., Kline, J., and Sodal, I.: Diminished ventilatory response to hypoxia and hypercapnea after morphine in normal man. N.Engl. J. Med., *292*:1103, 1975.

122. Eckenhoff, J., and Helrich, M.: The effects of narcotics, thiopental and nitrous oxide upon respiration and the respiratory response to hypercapnea. Anesthesiology, *19*:240, 1958.

123. Goroszeniuk, J.C., Whitman, J.C., and Morgan, M.: Uses of methohexitone, fentanyl and nitrous oxide for short operative procedures. Anaesthesia, *32*:209, 1977.

124. Helrich, M., Eckenlroff, J., Jones, R., and Rolph, W.D.: Influence of opiates on respiratory response of man to thiopental. Anesthesiology, *17*:459, 1956.

125. Kallos, T., and Smith, T.: The respiratory effects of Innovar given for premedication. Br. J. Anaesth., *41*:303, 1969.

126. Becker, L.D., Paulson, B.A., Miller, R.D., Severinghaus, J.W., and Eger, E.J.: Biphasic respiratory depression after fentanyl-droperidol or fentanyl alone used to supplement nitrous oxide anesthesia. Anesthesiology, *44*:291, 1976.

127. McQuay, H.J., Moore, R.A., Paterson, G.M.C., and Adam, A.P.: Plasma fentanyl concentrations and clinical observations during and after operation. Br. J. Anaesth., *51*:543, 1979.

128. Stoekel, H., Hengstman, J.G., and Schuttler, J.: Pharmacokinetics of fentanyl as a possible explanation for recurrence of respiratory depression. Br. J. Anaesth., *51*:741, 1979.

129. Schleimer, R., Benjamini, E., and Eisele, J.: Pharmacokinetics of fentanyl as determined by radioimmunoassay. Clin. Pharmacol. Ther., *23*:188, 1978.

130. Murphy, M.R., Olson, W.A., and Hug, C.C.: Pharmacokinetics of ^{3}H-fentanyl in dogs anesthetized with enflurane. Anesthesiology, *50*:13, 1979.

131. Foldes, F.F., and Torda, T.A.G.: Comparative studies of narcotics and narcotic antagonists in man. Acta Anaesthesiol. Scand., *9*:121, 1965.

132. Patschke, D., Eberlein, H.J., Hess, W., Tarnow, J., and Zimmerman, G.: Antagonism of morphine with naloxone in dogs. Cardiovascular effects with special references to the coronary circulation. Br. J. Anaesth., *49*:525, 1977.

133. Freye, E.: Die Anwendung hohen Dosen von fentanyl und naloxone in der anaesthesie. Anaesthesist, *24*:145, 1975.

134. Tanaka, G.Y.: Hypertensive reaction to naloxone. JAMA, *228*:25, 1974.

135. Azar, I., and Turndorf, H.: Severe hypertension and multiple atrial premature contraction following naloxone administration. Anesth. Analg., *58*:524, 1979.

136. Michaelis, L.L., Hickey, P.R., Clark, T.A., and Dixon, W.M.: Ventricular irritability associated with the use of naloxone. Ann. Thorac. Surg., *18*:608, 1974.

137. Azar, I., Patel, A.K., and Phau, C.O.: Cardiovascular responses following naloxone administration during enflurane anesthesia. Anesth. Analg., *60*:237, 1981.

138. Flacke, J.W., Flacke, W.E., and Williams, G.D.: Active pulmonary edema following naloxone reversal of high-dose morphine anesthesia. Anesthesiology, *47*:376, 1977.

139. Pohl, J.: Uber das N-allylnorecodeine, einen Antagonisten des Morphins. J. Exp. Pathol. Ther., *17*:370, 1915.

140. McCawley, W.L., Hart, E.R., and Marsh, D.F.: The preparation of N-allylnormorphine. J. Am. Chem. Soc., *63*:314, 1941.

141. Weijlard, J., and Erickson, A.E.: N-allylnormorphine. J. Am. Chem. Soc., *64*:869, 1942.

142. Unna, K.: Antagonist effect of *N*-allylnormorphine upon morphine. J. Pharmacol. Exp. Ther., *70*:27, 1943.

143. Hart, E.R., and McCawley, W.L.: The pharmacology of *N*-allylnormorphine as compared with morphine. J. Pharmacol. Exp. Ther., *82*:339, 1944.

144. Schnider, O., and Hellerback, J.: Synthese von Morphinan. Helv. Chem. Acta, *33*:1437, 1950.

145. Pearl, J., Stander, H., and McKean, D.B.: Effects of analgesics and other drugs on mice in phenylquinone and rotarod test. J. Pharmacol. Exp. Ther., *167*:9, 1969.

146. Perrine, T.D., Atwell, L., Tice, I.B., Jacobson, A.E., and May, E.L.: Analgesic activity as determined by the Nilsen method. J. Pharm. Sci., *61*:86, 1972.

147. Jasinski, D.R., Martin, W.R., and Hoeldtke, R.D.: Effects of short- and long-term administration of pentazocine in man. Clin. Pharmacol. Ther., *11*:385, 1970.

148. Fraser, H.F., and Rosenberg, D.E.: Studies on the human addiction liability of 2-hydroxy-5,9-dimethyl-2-(3,3-dimethylallyl)-6,7-benzomorphan (Win 20,228): a weak narcotic antagonist. J. Pharmacol. Exp. Ther., *143*:149, 1964.

149. Romagnoli, A., and Keats, A.S.: Ceiling effect for respiratory depression by nalbuphine. Clin. Pharmacol. Ther., 27:478, 1980.

150. Keats, A.S., and Telford, J.: Studies of analgesic drugs. X. Respiratory effects of narcotic antagonists. J. Pharmacol. Exp. Ther., *151*:126, 1966.

151. Hamilton, W.K., and Cullen, S.C.: Effect of levallorphan tartrate upon opiate induced respiratory depression. Anesthesiology, *14*:550, 1953.

152. Janis, K.M.: Acute rigidity with small intravenous doses of Innovar: a case report. Anesth. Analg., *51*:375, 1972.

153. Grell, F.L., Koons, D.A., and Danson, J.S.: Fentanyl in anesthesia: a report of 500 cases. Anesth. Analg., *59*:523, 1970.

154. Nauta, J., de Lange, S., Koopman, D., Spierdijk, J., van Kleef, J., and Stanley T.H.: Anesthetic induction with alfentanil: a new short-acting narcotic analgesic. Anesth. Analg., *61*:267, 1982.

155. Holderness, M.C., Chase, P.E., and Drips, R.D.: A narcotic analgesic and butyrophenone with nitrous oxide for general anesthesia. Anesthesiology, 24:336, 1963.

156. Freund, F.G., Martin, W.E., Wong, K.C., and Hornbein, T.F.: Abdominal muscle rigidity induced by morphine and nitrous oxide. Anesthesiology, 38:358, 1973.

157. Georgis, S.D., Hoyt, J.L., and Sokoll, M.D.: Effects of Innovar and Innovar plus nitrous oxide on muscle tone and H-reflex. Anesth. Analg., 50:743, 1971.

158. Sokoll, M.D., Hoyt, J.L., and Georgis, S.D.: Studies in muscle rigidity, nitrous oxide, and narcotic analgesic agents. Anesth. Analg., *51*:16, 1972.

159. Hill, A.B., Nahrwald, M.D., de Rosayro, A.M., Knight, J.P., Jones, R.M., and Bolles, R.E.: Prevention of rigidity during fentanyl-oxygen induction of anesthesia. Anesthesiology, 55:452, 1981.

160. Koffer, K.B., Berney, S., and Horrykiewicz, O.: The role of the corpus striatum in neuroleptic and narcotic-induced catalepsy. Eur. J. Clin. Pharmacol., 47:81, 1978.

161. Freye, E., and Kuchinsky, K.: Effects of fentanyl and droperidol on the dopamine metabolism of the rat striatum. Pharmacology, *14*:1, 1976.

162. Jurna, I., Ruzdic, N., Nell, T., and Grossmann, W.: The effect of 2-methyl-*p*-tyrosine and substantia nigra lesion on spinal motor activity in the rat. Eur. J. Pharmacol., *20*:341, 1972.

163. Kuchingsky, K.: Opiate dependence. *In* Progress in Pharmacology. Edited by H. Grobecker, G.F. Kahl, W. Klaus, and K. Wein. Stuttgart, Gustav Fischer, 1977, pp. 1–39.

164. Steg, G.: Efferent muscle innervation and rigidity. Acta Physiol. Scand. (Supp.), *61*:5, 1964.

165. Cooper, D.Y., and Lambertson, C.J.: Effect of changes in tidal volume and alveolar carbon dioxide on physiological dead space. Anesthesiology, *18*:160, 1957.

166. Van Dongen, K., and Leusink, H.: The action of opium-alkaloids and expectorants on the ciliary movements in the air passages. Arch. Int. Pharmacodyn. Ther., *93*:261, 1953.

167. Toda, N., and Hatano, Y.: Contractile responses of canine tracheal muscle during exposure to fentanyl and morphine. Anesthesiology, *53*:93, 1980.

168. Papper, S., and Papper, E.M.: The effects of pre-anesthetic, anesthetic and post-operative drugs on renal function. Clin. Pharmacol. Ther., 5:205, 1964.

169. Deutch, S., Bastron, R.D., Pierce, E.C., and Vandam, L.D.: The effects of anesthesia with thiopentone, nitrous oxide, narcotic and neuromuscular blocking drugs on renal function in normal man. Br. J. Anaesth., *41*:807, 1969.

170. Philbin, D.M., Wilson, N.E., Sokolshi, I., and Coggins, C.: Radioimmunoassay of antidiuretic hormone during morphine anaesthesia. Can. Anaesth. Soc. J., 23:290, 1976.

171. Bidwai, A.V., Stanley, T.H., and Bloomer, H.A.: Effects of anesthetic doses of morphine on renal function in the dog. Anesth. Analg., 54:357, 1975.

172. Stanley, T.H., Gray, N.H., Bidwai, A.V., and Lordem, R.: The effects of high dose morphine and morphine plus nitrous oxide on urinary output in man. Can. Anaesth. Soc. J., *21*:379, 1974.

173. Porter, J.M., McGregor, F., Jr., and Aconopura, A.J.: Renal function following abdominal aortic aneurysmectomy. Surg. Gynecol. Obstet., *123*:819, 1966.

174. Wang, S.C., and Glaviano, V.V.: Locus of emetic action of morphine and hydergine in dogs. J. Pharmacol. Exp. Ther., *111*:329, 1954.

175. Abbott, W.O., and Pendergrass, E.P.: Intubation studies of the human small intestine. V. The motor effects of single clinical doses of morphine sulfate in normal subjects. AJR, 35:289, 1936.

176. Daniel, E.E., Sutherland, W.H., and Bogoch, P.: Effects of morphine and other drugs on motility of the terminal ileum. Gastroenterology, *36*:510, 1959.

177. Garrett, J.M., Suer, W.G., and Moertel, C.G.: Colonic motility in ulcerative colitis after opiate administration. Gastroenterology, 53:93, 1967.

178. Parolaro, D., Sala, M., and Gori, E.: Effect of intra-cerebroventricular administration of morphine upon intestinal motility in rat and its antagonism with naloxone. Eur. J. Pharmacol., *46*:329, 1977.

179. Steward, J.J., Weisbrodt, N.W., and Burks, T.F.: Center and peripheral actions of morphine on intestinal transit. J. Pharmacol. Exp. Ther., 205:547, 1978.
180. Chapman, W.P., Rowlands, E.N., and Jones, C.M.: Multiple-balloon kymographic recording of the comparative action of Demerol, morphine and placebo on the motility of the upper small intestine in man. N. Engl. J. Med., 243:171, 1950.
181. Reynolds, A.K., and Randall, L.O.: Morphine and allied drugs. Toronto, University of Toronto Press, 1957.
182. Jaffee, J.H., and Martin, R.: Opioid analgesics and antagonists. In The Pharmacological Basis of Therapeutics. Edited by A.G. Gilman, L.S. Goodman, A. Gilman. New York, MacMillan, 1980, pp. 503–534.
183. Polak, J.M., Sullivan, S.N., Bloom, S.R., Facer, P., and Pearce, A.: Enkephalin-like immunoreactivity in the human gastrointestinal tract. Lancet, I:972, 1977.
184. Weinstock, M.: Peripheral tissue. In Narcotic Drugs. Edited by D.H. Clouet. New York, Plenum Press, 1971, pp. 394–407.
185. Roze, C., Chariot, J., De La Tour, J., Souchard, M., Vaille, C., and Debray, C.: Methadone blockade of 1-deoxy-glucose-induced pancreatic secretion in the rat. Gastroenterology, 74:215, 1978.
186. Rodnay, P.A., Bodman, E., Mankikar, D., and Roberts, T.M.: The effect of equianalgesic doses of fentanyl, morphine, meperidine and pentazocine on common bile duct pressure. Anaesthesist, 29:26, 1980.
187. Salik, J.O., Siegel, C.I., and Mendeloff, A.I.: Biliary duodenal dynamics in man. Radiology, 106:1, 1977.
188. Canellas, J., Roquebert, J., DuMartin, A., and Limoge, A.: Action sur le sphincter d'oddi du cobaye d'un analgesique, dun neuroleptique et de leur association. C. R. Soc. Biol. (Paris), 159:1538, 1965.
189. Murphy, P., Salomon, J., and Roseman, D.L.: Narcotic anesthetic drugs: their effect on biliary dynamics. Arch. Surg., 115:710, 1980.
190. Stanley, T.H., Bermar, L., Green, O., and Robertson, D.: Plasma catecholamine and cortisol responses to fentanyl-oxygen anesthesia for coronary artery operations. Anesthesiology, 53:250, 1980.
191. Madsen, S.N., Engquist, A., Badwai, I., and Kehlet, H.: Cyclic AMP, glucose and cortisol in plasma during surgery. Horm. Metab. Res., 8:483, 1976.
192. Clarke, R.S.J.: The hyperglycaemic response to different types of surgery and anaesthesia. Br. J. Anesth., 42:45, 1970.
193. Clarke, R.S.J., Hohnston, H., and Sheridan, B.: The influence of anaesthesia and surgery on plasma cortisol, insulin and free fatty acids. Br. J. Anaesth., 42:295, 1979.
194. McDonald, R., Evans, F., Weise, V., and Patrick, R.W.: Effects of morphine and nalorphine on plasma hydrocortisone levels in man. J. Pharmacol. Exp. Ther., 125:241, 1959.
195. Briggs, F., and Munson, P.: Studies on the mechanism of stimulation of ACTH secretion with the aid of morphine as a blocking agent. Endocrinology, 57:205, 1955.
196. Di Fazio, C.A., and Chen, P.: The influence of morphine on excess lactate production. Anesth. Analg., 50:211, 1971.
197. George, J.M., Reier, C.E., Larense, R.R., and Rower, M.M.: Morphine anesthesia blocks cortisol and growth hormone response to surgical stress in humans. J. Clin. Endocrinol. Metab., 38:736, 1974.
198. Brandt, M.R., Korshin, J., Prange Hansen, A., Hummer, L., Madsen, S.N., Ryog, I., and Kehlet, H.: Influence of morphine anesthesia on the endocrine-metabolic response to open-heart surgery. Acta Anaesthesiol. Scand., 22:400, 1978.
199. Reier, C.E., George, J.M., and Kilman, J.W.: Cortisol and growth hormone response to surgical stress during morphine anesthesia. Anesth. Analg., 52:1003, 1973.
200. Fennessey, M.R., and Ortiz, A.: The behavioral and cardiovascular actions of intravenously administered morphine in the conscious dog. Eur. J. Pharmacol. 3:177, 1968.
201. Klingman, G.E., and Maynert, E.W.: Tolerance to morphine. III. Effects on catecholamines in the heart, intestine and spleen. J. Pharmacol. Exp. Ther., 136:300, 1962.
202. Roizen, M.F., Horrigan, R.W., and Frazer, B.M.: Anesthetic doses blocking adrenergic (stress) and cardiovascular responses to incision—MAC BAR. Anesthesiology, 54:390, 1981.
203. Glariman, N.H., Mattie, L.R., and Stephenson, W.F.: Studies on the antidiuretic action of morphine. Science, 117:225, 1953.
204. De Bodo, R.C.: The antidiuretic action of morphine and its mechanisms. J. Pharmacol. Exp. Ther., 82:74, 1944.
205. Philbin, D.M., Wilson, N.E., Sokoloski, J., and Coggins, C.: Radioimmunoassay of antidiuretic hormone during morphine anaesthesia. Can. Anaesth. Soc. J., 23:290, 1976.
206. Hall, G.M., Young, C., Holdcroft, A., and Alaghband-Zadeh, J.: Substrate mobilisation during surgery: a comparison between halothane and fentanyl anaesthesia. Anaesthesia, 33:924, 1978.

207. Cooper, G.M., Patterson, J.L., Ward, I.D., and Hall, G.M.: Fentanyl and the metabolic response to gastric surgery. Anaesthesia, *36*:667, 1981.
208. Hicks, H.C., Mowbray, A.G., and Yhab, E.O.: Cardiovascular effects of and catecholamine responses to high dose fentanyl-O$_2$ for induction of anesthesia in patients with ischemic coronary disease. Anesth. Analg., *60*:563, 1981.
209. Sebel, P.S., Bovill, J.G., Schellekens, A.P.M., and Hawker, C.D.: Hormonal effects of high-dose fentanyl anaesthesia: a study in patients undergoing cardiac surgery. Br. J. Anaesth. *53*:941, 1981.
210. Kono, K., Philbin, D.M., Coggins, C.H., Moss, J., Rosow, C.E., Schneider, R.C., and Slater, F.E.: Renal function and stress response during halothane or fentanyl anesthesia. Anesth. Analg., *60*:552, 1981.
211. Philbin, D.M., Levine, F.H., Kono, K., Coggins, C.H., Moss, J., Slater, E.E., and Buckley, M.J.: Attenuation of the stress response to cardiopulmonary bypass by the addition of pulsatile flow. Circulation, *64*:808, 1981.
212. Walsh, E.S., Paterson, J.L., O'Riordan, J.B.A., and Hall, G.M.: Effects of high-dose fentanyl anaesthesia on the metabolic and endocrine response to cardiac surgery. Br. J. Anaesth., *53*:1155, 1981.
213. de Lange, S., Boscoe, M.J., Stanley, T.H., de Bruijn, N., Philbin, D.M., and Coggins, C.H.: Antidiuretic and growth hormone responses during coronary artery surgery with sufentanil-oxygen and alfentanil-oxygen anesthesia in man. Anesth. Analg., *61*:434, 1982.
214. Bruni, J.F., van Vugt, D., Marshall, S., and Meites, J.: Effects of naloxone, morphine and methionine enkephalins on serum prolactin, luteinizing hormone, follicle stimulating hormone, thyroid stimulating hormone and growth hormone. Life Sci., *21*:461, 1977.
215. Fishman, J.: The opiate and the endocrine system. *In* The Basis of Addiction. Edited by J. Fishman. Berlin, Dhalern Konferenzen, Abkon Verlagsgesellschaft, 1978, pp. 257–279.
216. Beaumont, A., and Hughes, J.: Biology of opioid peptides. Annu. Rev. Pharmacol. Toxicol., *19*:245, 1979.
217. Van Bever, W.F.M., Niemegeers, C.J.E., and Schellekens, K.H.L.: N-4 substituted 1(2-arylethyl) 4-piperdinyl-N-phenylpropanamides, a novel series of extremely potent analgesics with unusually high safety margin. Arzneimittel forschung, *26*:1548, 1973.
218. Van Bever, W.F.M., Niemegeers, C.J.E., Schellekens, K.H.L., and Janssen, P.A.G.: Sufentanil potent and extremely safe intravenous morphine-like compound in mice, rats and dogs. Arzneimittel forschung, *26*:1551, 1976.
219. Hecker, B.A., Lake, C.L., Di Fazio, C.A., Mosciki, M.S., and Engle, B.S.: The decrease of the minimal alveolar anesthetic concentration produced by sufentanil in rats. Anesth. Analg., *62*:987, 1983.
220. Murphy, M.R., and Hug, C.C.: The anesthetic potency of fentanyl in terms of its reduction of enflurane MAC. Anesthesiology, *57*:485, 1982.
221. De Castro, J.: Practical applications and limitations of anesthesia. A review. Acta Anaesthesiol. Belg. *3*:107, 1976.
222. Van de Walle, J., Lauwers, P., and Adriaensen, H.: Double blind comparison of fentanyl and sufentanil in anesthesia. Acta Anaesthesiol. Belg., *27*:129, 1976.
223. Rolly, G., Kay, B., and Cockx, F.: A double blind comparison of high doses of fentanyl and sufentanil in man. Influence on cardiovascular, respiratory and metabolic parameters. Acta Anaesthesiol. Belg., *30*:247, 1979.
224. Larsen, R., Sonntag, H., Schenk, H.D., Radke J., and Hilfiker, O.: Die Wirkung von Sufentanil und Fentanyl auf Hamodynamik, Koronardurchbluting und myocardialen Metabolismus des Menschen. Anaesthesist, *29*:277, 1980.
225. Sebel, P.S., and Bovill, J.G.: Cardiovascular effects of sufentanil anesthesia: a study in patients undergoing cardiac surgery. Anesth. Analg., *61*:115, 1982.
226. Howie, M.B., McSweeney, T.D., Lingam, R.P., and Moschke, S.P.: A comparison of fentanyl-O$_2$ and sufentanil-O$_2$ for cardiac anesthesia. Anesth. Analg., *64*:877, 1985.
227. Rosow, C.E., Philbin, D.M., Moss, J., Keegan, C.R., and Scheider, R.C.: Sufentanil vs fentanyl: I. Suppression of hemodynamic responses. Anesthesiology, *59*:A323, 1983.
228. Bovill, J.G., Sebel, P.S., Wauquier, A., and Rog, P.: Electroencephalographic effects of sufentanil anaesthesia in man. Br. J. Anaesth. *54*:45, 1982.
229. Sebel, P.S., Bovill, J.G., Fiolet, J., Touber, J., and Philbin, D.: Hormonal responses to sufentanil anesthesia. Anesth. Analg., *61*:214, 1982.
230. Berthelsen, P., Eriksen, J., Ahn, N.C., and Rasmussen, J.P.: Peripheral circulation during sufentanil and morphine anesthesia. Acta Anaesthesiol. Scand., *24*:241, 1980.
231. Eriksen, J., Berthelsen, P., Ahn, N.C., and Rasmussen, J.P.: Early response of central hemodynamics to high doses of sufentanil or morphine in dogs. Acta Anaesthesiol. Scand., *25*:33, 1981.
232. Niemegeers, C.J.E., and Janssen, P.A.J.: Alfentanil, a particularly short-acting intravenous narcotic analgesic. Drug Dev. Res. *1*:83, 1981.

233. de Bruijn, N., Christian, C., Fagraeus, L., Freedman, B., Davis, G., Hamm, D., Everson, C., Pellom, G., and Wechsler, A.: The effects of alfentanil on global ventricular mechanics. Anesthesiology, 59:A33, 1983.

234. Brown, J.H., Pleuvry, B., and Kay, B.: Respiratory effects of a new opiate analgesic (R 39209) in the rabbit: comparison with fentanyl. Br. J. Anaesth. 52:1101, 1980.

235. Kay, B., and Pleuvry, B.: Human volunteer studies of alfentanil (R 39209), a new short-acting narcotic analgesic. Anaesthesia, 35:952, 1980.

236. Kay, B., and Stephenson, D.K.: Alfentanil (R 39209): initial clinical experience with a new narcotic analgesic. Anaesthesia, 35:1197, 1980.

237. Van Leeuwen, L., and Deen, L.: Alfentanil, a new potent and very short-acting morphinomimetic for minor operative procedures: a pilot study. Anaesthesist, 30:115, 1981.

238. Coe, V., Shafer, A., and White, P.F.: Techniques for administering alfentanil during outpatient anesthesia—a comparison with fentanyl. Anesthesiology, 59:A347, 1983.

239. Stanley, T.H., Pace, N.L., Liu, W.S., Gillmor, S.T., and Willard, K.F.: Alfentanil-N_2O vs fentanyl-N_2O balanced anesthesia: comparison of plasma hormonal changes, early postoperative respiratory function, and speed of postoperative recovery. Anesth. Analg., 62:285, 1983.

240. Nauta, J., de Lange, S., Koopman, D., Spierdijk, J., van Kleef, J., and Stanley, T.H.: Anesthetic induction with alfentanil: a new short-acting narcotic analgesic. Anesth. Analg., 61:267, 1982.

241. Black, T.E., Kay, B., and Healy, T.E.J.: Alfentanil prevents the stress response to intubation. Anesthesiology, 59:A87, 1983.

242. Moldenhauer, C.C., Griesemer, R.W., Hug, C.C., and Holbrook, G.W.: Hemodynamic changes during rapid induction of anesthesia with alfentanil. Anesth. Analg., 62:276, 1983.

243. Kay, B.: Postoperative pain relief. Use of an on-demand analgesia computer (ODAC) and comparison of the rate of use of fentanyl and alfentanil. Anaesthesia, 36:949, 1981.

244. de Lange, S., Stanley, T.H., and Boscoe, M.J.: Alfentanil-oxygen anaesthesia for coronary artery surgery. Br. J. Anaesth., 53:1291, 1981.

245. de Lange, S., and de Bruijn, N.: Alfentanil-oxygen anaesthesia: plasma concentration and clinical effects during variable rate continuous infusion for coronary artery surgery. Br. J. Anaesth., 55:S183, 1983.

Chapter 6

THE BARBITURATES

HISTORY

Barbituric acid was first prepared in 1864 by the Nobel prize-winning German organic chemist, J.F.W. Adolph von Baeyer (1835–1971). There are several anecdotes regarding the derivation of the term barbituric acid, the consensus being that the word is a conjugation of *Barbara* and *urea*.[1] Although the origination of urea is understandable in that urea is required for the formation of barbituric acid, the only mystery remains in identifying the relationship of von Baeyer to the name Barbara.

The first sedative barbiturate, diethylbarbituric acid or barbital, was reported by Fischer and von Mering in 1903. This hypnotic enjoyed clinical success, but it was not until water-soluble salts were synthesized that intravenous barbiturates became widely available. The first intravenously administered barbiturate was somnifene, a mixture of the diethylamines of diethyl and diallyl barbituric acids. Redonnet described the pharmacologic characteristics of somnifene in 1920, and the French co-workers Bardet and Bardet were the first to use this intravenous barbiturate in clinical practice in 1921.[2–4]

Hexobarbital (Evipan-Na), the first ultra-short-acting barbiturate, was synthesized by Kropp and Taub and was introduced clinically in 1932 by Weese and Scharpf in Germany.[5,6] Hexobarbital was the intravenous anesthetic of choice for 3 years until Tabern and Volwiler synthesized a series of sulfur-containing barbiturates, of which thiopental (Pentothal-Na) was part. A sulfur analogue of pentobarbital (Nembutal), thiopental was clinically introduced in 1934 by John Lundy at the Mayo Clinic and Ralph Waters at the University of Wisconsin (see Chapter 1).[7,8] Hexobarbital continues to be used extensively in most European countries; recently, however, for reasons that are not clearly understood, hexobarbital has gradually failed to maintain its position in the pharmaceutical market. Many other barbiturate derivatives have been synthesized and used clinically, but none enjoy the general popularity of thiopental. The history and a description of the barbiturates are detailed in the book by R. Charles Adams and the volume co-authored by John W. Dundee and Gordon M. Wyant.[9,10]

CHEMISTRY AND PHYSICAL PROPERTIES

Chemical Structure and Solubility

The hypnotic barbiturates used in clinical practice are barbituric acid compounds with substitutions of the hydrogen on the carbon at position 5 with alkyl or aryl groups. Barbituric acid and water are formed by the condensation of malonic acid and urea (Fig. 6–1A). The resulting pharmacologically inactive

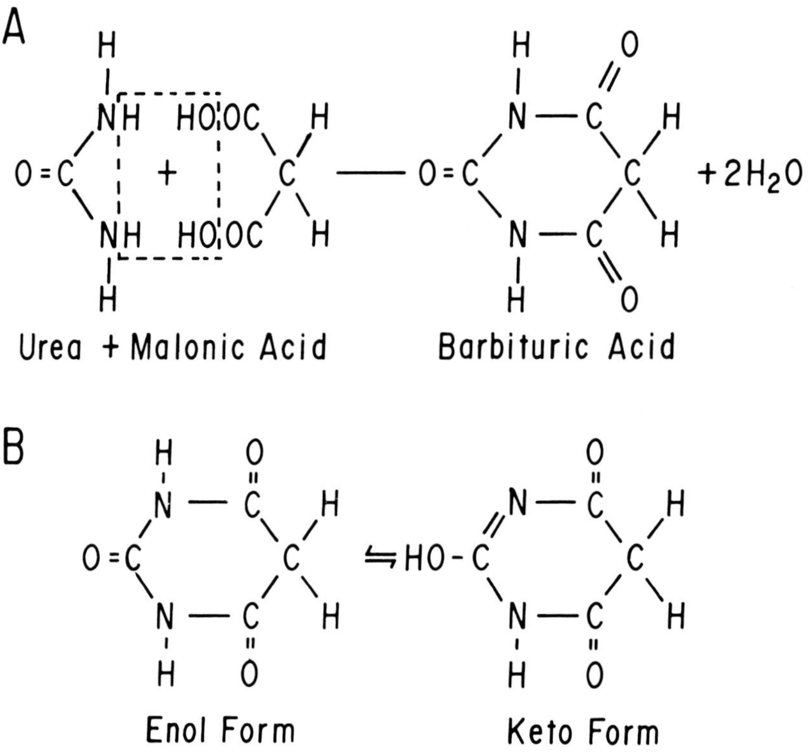

Fig. 6–1. *A,* formation of barbituric acid by the combination of urea and malonic acid. *B,* the two forms of barbituric acid, enol and keto.

barbituric acid exists in the keto and enol forms (Fig. 6–1B). Most barbiturates are in the enol form and are weak acids. The barbiturates in common use and their chemical constitution are listed in Table 6–1.[11] Most barbiturates are essentially insoluble in water; in the enol form, however, when the weak acids are substituted with sodium, water-soluble salts are created. Most of these water-soluble salts are not stable over extensive periods of time.[11]

Structure-Activity Relationship

Multiple substitutions to the basic inactive barbituric acid structure (Table 6–1) confer pharmacologic activity. The central nervous system (CNS) effects are related to the structural alterations. In general, the addition of alkyl or aryl groups at position 5 produces hypnotic and sedative effects.[11] A phenyl group at C5 or one of the nitrogens of the barbituric acid produces anticonvulsant activity. Increases in length (to as many as five carbons) of one or both alkyl side-chains at C5 increases hypnotic potency. Dundee and Wyant tabulated the relationship of chemical structure to pharmacodynamic response (Table 6–2).[10] A sulfur atom in position C2 usually produces a drug of rapid action. The addition of a methyl or ethyl group in position 1 may produce a more rapid effect, but excitatory phenomena may also occur during drug administration. These reactions are tremor, hypertonus, and involuntary movement. Perhaps the best illustration of these structure-activity relationships is the comparison of pentobarbital and thiopental (Fig. 6–2): the substitution of a sulfur for the oxygen at position C2

Table 6–1.   Chemical Structure of Some Important Barbiturates

Barbiturate	Trade Name	R_1	R_2	R_3	X
Amobarbital	Amytal	Ethyl	Isopentyl	H	O
Barbital	Neuronidia	Ethyl	Ethyl	H	O
Butabarbital	Butisol	Ethyl	Sec-butyl	H	O
Hexobarbital	Sombulex	Methyl	1-cyclohexen-1-yl	CH_3	O
Methohexital *	Brevital	Allyl	1-methyl-2-pentynyl	CH_3	O
Pentobarbital	Nembutal	Ethyl	1-methylbutyl	H	O
Phenobarbital	Luminal	Ethyl	Phenyl	H	O
Secobarbital	Seconal	Allyl	1-methylbutyl	H	O
Thiamylal	Surital	Allyl	1-methylbutyl	H	S
Thiopental *	Pentothal	Ethyl	1-methylbutyl	H	S

*Drugs commonly used as intravenous anesthetics.

Table 6–2.   Relationship of Chemical Grouping to Clinical Action of Barbiturates

Group	Substituents		Group Characteristics when Given Intravenously
	Position 1	Position 2	
Oxybarbiturates	H	O	Delay in onset of action, degree depending on 5 and 5′ side-chains. Useful as basal hypnotics. Prolonged action.
Methylated oxybarbiturates	CH_3	O	Usually rapid acting with fairly rapid recovery. High incidence of excitatory phenomena.
Thiobarbiturates	H	S	Rapid acting, usually smooth onset of sleep, fairly prompt recovery.
Methylated thiobarbiturates	CH_3	S	Rapid onset of action and very rapid recovery but with so high an incidence of excitatory phenomena as to preclude use in clinical practice.

(From Dundee, J.W.: Intravenous Anaesthesia. Edinburgh, Churchill Livingstone, 1974, with permission.)

transforms the rather slow onset and prolonged hypnotic effect of pentobarbital to the rapid-acting, shorter-lasting hypnotic thiopental.[10]

Chemical Classification

The chemical classification of barbiturates includes four groups, according to substitutions at positions C1 and C2 (Table 6–2). These classifications also have implications for the CNS effects (vide supra). The *oxybarbiturates* have oxygen at C2. The *thiobarbiturates* replace the oxygen with sulfur. *Methylated oxybarbiturates* have a methyl group at C3 and retain the oxygen at C2. *Methylated thiobarbiturates* have a methyl group at C1 and sulfur at C2. These alterations in chemical structure produce important differences in the actions of these compounds, as well as changes in metabolism. For example, methylation of an oxybarbiturate alters the resulting compound so that it biotransforms more rapidly in the liver. Thus, methohexital (a methylated thiobarbiturate) more rapidly clears from the blood than does thiopental (a thiobarbiturate).

Site and Mechanisms of Action

The precise mechanism of action of barbiturates on the CNS is not yet known; in fact, it appears there are multiple sites and more than one mechanism of action. Way and Trevor summarized the selectivity of actions of barbiturates on CNS neurophysiologic systems as two general types of effects at specific synapses: (1) facilitation of enhancement of the synaptic actions of *inhibitory* neurotransmitters, and (2) *blockade* of the synaptic actions of *excitatory* neurotransmitters.[12,13] There appear to be "target" sites of barbiturates at specific synapses of neural tracts in the CNS. The major inhibitory neurotransmitter in the CNS is γ-aminobutyric acid (GABA). It appears that barbiturates enhance GABA.[14] The barbiturates modulate GABA at a receptor site that is different from that of the benzodiazepines, which also produce a sedative-hypnotic effect by increasing GABA. The site of the effect on GABA has been labeled a "sedative-convulsant" receptor.[14] It appears that the barbiturate-GABA responses alter ionic conductance and not chloride channels, although this is neither the sole site nor the sole mechanism of the CNS effect of barbiturates.[15] These drugs also inhibit synaptic transmission of excitatory neurotransmitters such as L-glutamate and acetylcholine.[12] The actions of barbiturates to block excitatory CNS transmission are specific for synaptic ion channels, unlike the nonspecific action of local and volatile anesthetics.[12,16–18] Thus, rather than a single site or mechanism of CNS action,

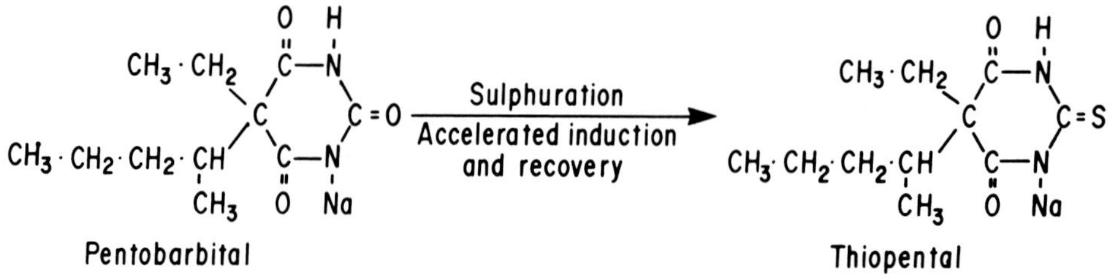

Pentobarbital → Sulphuration / Accelerated induction and recovery → Thiopental

Fig. 6–2. Sulphuration changes pentobarbital to thiopental, and enhances onset and reduces duration of hypnotic effect. (From Dundee, J.W.: Intravenous Anaesthesia. Edinburgh, Churchill Livingstone, 1974, p. 26, with permission.)

barbiturates produce their sedative-hypnotic effects at various sites and by different mechanisms, some of which are still unknown.

Stereospecific Actions

Barbiturates, like many drugs, are optically active compounds (Fig. 6–3).[19] They exhibit enantiomorphism, the phenomena by which optical isomers exist; each isomer rotates polarized light in different directions (commonly referred to as d and l, or + and -). The molecules of the compounds are otherwise identical, with the same chemical and physical properties. The fundamental importance of this fact is that the stereo isomers of barbiturates have different CNS potency,

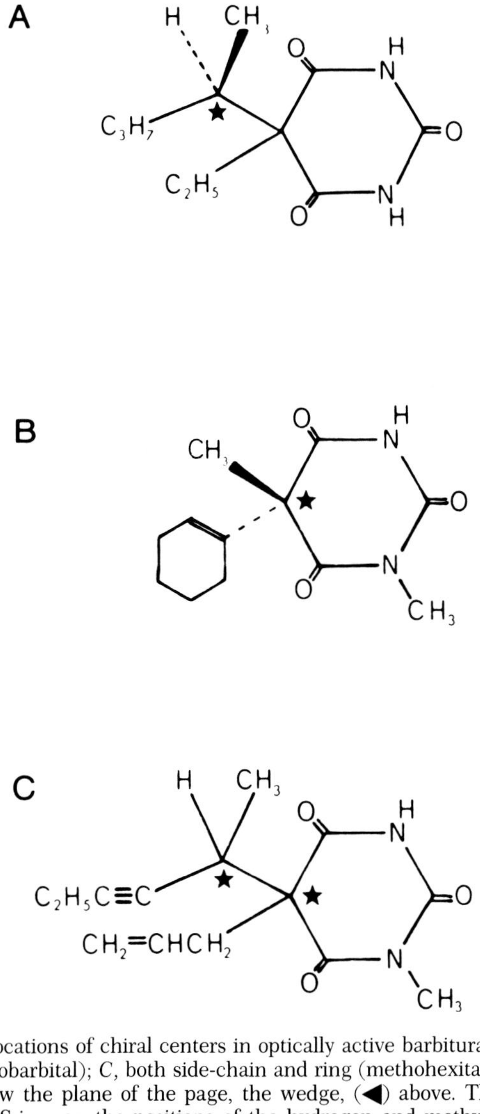

Fig. 6–3. Alternative locations of chiral centers in optically active barbiturates. *A,* side-chain (pentobarbital); *B,* ring (hexobarbital); *C,* both side-chain and ring (methohexital). Dashed line (---), the atom or group lies below the plane of the page, the wedge, (◄) above. The pentobarbital isomer illustrated is R. In the S-isomer, the positions of the hydrogen and methyl group attached to the chiral center would be reversed. (From Andrews, P.R., and Mark, L.C.: Structural specificity of barbiturates and related drugs. Anesthesiology, 57:314, 1982, with permission.)

which is suggestive of the existence of stereo-specific sites of CNS action of the barbiturates.[12,19] For example, the racemic mixture of pentobarbital has isomers that produce different actions in cultured mammalian neurons.[20] In fact, the (+) isomers are predominantly excitatory and the (-) isomers are inhibitory. The existence of stereo-specific receptor sites of "target" membrane sites is consistent with the hypothesis that barbiturates do have specific sites of CNS action. The overall CNS activity of a particular barbiturate depends on the collective effects of the drug isomers at each particular receptor site. Thus, the action of the barbiturate reflects the combined effect of the isomers at their particular CNS site of action. Similarly, the duration of action depends on the duration of the relative effects of each isomer at its receptor site.

Cerebral Metabolism

Barbiturates, like other CNS depressants, have potent effects on cerebral metabolism (Table 6–3). In general, the effects of barbiturates are summarized as a dose-related depression of cerebral metabolic oxygen consumption rate ($CMRO_2$) and of cerebral blood flow (CBF).[21-23] The barbiturates affect the metabolism of functioning neurons; these drugs depress cerebral activity and metabolism presumably by decreasing membrane excitability and impulse traffic. There is a resultant decrease in ATP production.[24] The relationship of depressed metabolism to drug dosage was shown in dogs in whom circulation at high thiopental doses was preserved by an extracorporeal circulation pump.[25] When the results of the electroencephalogram (EEG) became isoelectric, no further decrements in $CMRO_2$ occurred (Fig. 6–4). These findings support the hypothesis that metabolism and function are coupled. Thus, the effect of barbiturates on cerebral metabolism is a depression of cerebral function; less oxygen is required and $CMRO_2$ is diminished. With the reduced $CMRO_2$, there is a reduction in cerebral perfusion, presumably by preserved cerebral autoregulation.[23] Thus, with reduced $CMRO_2$, cerebral vascular resistance increases and CBF decreases. The ratio of CBF to $CMRO_2$ is unchanged (Table 6–3). With the reduction in CBF, there is a decrease in intracranial pressure (ICP) after the administration of barbiturates. Even though the systemic mean blood pressure (MBP) determination decreases, barbiturates do not compromise the overall cerebral perfusion pressure (CPP). The CPP is not affected because CPP = MBP - ICP and ICP decreases more relative to the decrease in MBP after barbiturate use.[26]

Table 6–3.   Relative Effects of Intravenous Anesthetic Drugs on Cerebral Blood Flow (CBF) and Metabolic Oxygen Consumption Rate ($CMRO_2$)

Drug	CBF	$CMRO_2$	$CBF/CMRO_2$
Barbiturates	↓↓*	↓↓	—
Benzodiazepines	↓	↓	?
Narcotics	↓	↓	—
Droperidol	↓	?—	↓
Ketamine	↑↑↑	?—	↑

*Key: ↑↑↑, greatly increased; ↑↑, moderately increased; ↑, mildly increased; ?↑, possibly increased (data not firm); —, no change; ↓, mildly decreased; ↓↓, moderately decreased. (From Michenfelder, J.D.: The cerebral circulation. *In* The Circulation in Anaesthesia: Applied Physiology and Pharmacology. Edited by C. Prys-Roberts. Oxford, Blackwell Scientific, 1980, pp. 209–225, with permission.)

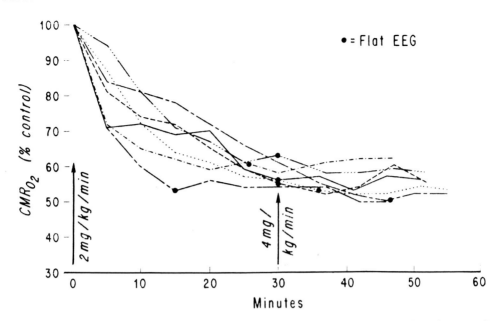

Fig. 6–4. Individual $CMRO_2$ values plotted as percentages of control (initial) values determined before initiating thiopental infusion but after establishing partial bypass. In each dog, $CMRO_2$ decreased progressively until EEG became isoelectric. $CMRO_2$ then stabilized and, despite continued infusion of thiopental, did not decrease further. (From Stuleken, E.H., Milde, J.H., Michenfelder, J.D., and Tinker, J.H.: The nonlinear responses of cerebral metabolism to low concentrations of halothane, enflurane, isoflurane, and thiopental. Anesthesiology, *46*:28, 1977, with permission.)

Metabolism

Barbiturates are metabolized in the liver. Most of the metabolites are inactive, water-soluble, and excreted in the urine. Barbiturates are biotransformed by four processes: (1) oxidation at C5; (2) N-dealkylation; (3) desulfuration of the thiobarbiturates; and (4) destruction of the barbituric acid ring.[27,28] Oxidation is the most important pathway, producing polar alcohols, ketones, phenols, or carboxylic acids. These metabolites are excreted in the urine or as glucuronic acid conjugates. The barbituric acid ring is so stable in vivo that hydrolytic cleavage of the ring is insignificant in the metabolism of barbiturates. Drugs that induce the oxidative microsomes enhance the metabolism of barbiturates; chronic administration of barbiturates will also induce the enzymes.[28] Thus, biotransformation of barbiturates may be enhanced in patients taking drugs that are known to induce hepatic microsomes. The hepatic enzyme induction of barbiturates is responsible for the recommendation that they not be administered to patients with acute intermittent porphyria. Barbiturates may precipitate an attack by stimulating γ-amino levulinic acid (ALA) synthetase, the enzyme responsible for the production of porphyrins.[29]

Hepatic metabolism accounts for the elimination of all barbiturates with the exception of barbital. Renal excretion is important in elimination of barbital; 60 to 90% of that drug is excreted unchanged by the kidneys.[30] Thirty percent of phenobarbital is excreted in the urine, but trivial amounts of other barbiturates are excreted unchanged by the kidney. The alkalinization of urine with bicarbonate enhances the renal excretion of phenobarbital; as pH increases, the concentration of the undissociated form of phenobarbital decreases, enhancing excretion across the lipid tubular epithelium.[30,31]

PHARMACOKINETICS

The plasma disappearance of a drug (Fig. 6–5) reflects its composite distribution to all tissues from the blood, the hepatic elimination, and the renal excretion of the compound. Mathematically, the plasma decay may be described and fit to models that express disappearance as time per concentration constants. The mathematical expression of plasma drug disappearance with the use of these models is the foundation for the pharmacokinetic description of a drug. Simply defined, the *pharmacokinetics* of a drug is what the body does to a drug and the *pharmacodynamics* is what the drug does to the body. Reliance upon pharmacokinetics alone to predict pharmacodynamic responses may prove disappointing, but often pharmacokinetics can explain clinical observations of drug effect. For example, patients given doses of methohexital are alert sooner after administration

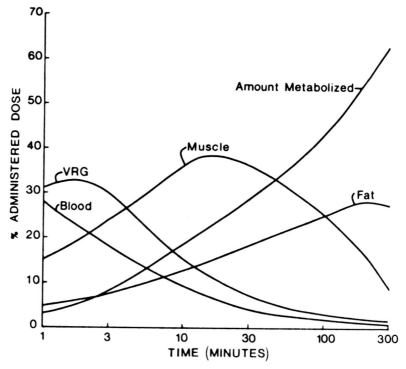

Fig. 6–5.   After delivery of an intravenous bolus, the percent of thiopental remaining in blood rapidly decreases as drug moves from blood to body tissues. Time to attainment of peak tissue levels is a direct function of tissue capacity for barbiturate relative to blood flow. Thus, a larger capacity or smaller blood flow is related to a longer time to a peak tissue level. Initially, most thiopental is taken up by the vessel-rich group (VRG) of tissues because of its high blood flow. Subsequently, drug is redistributed to muscle and to a lesser extent to fat. Throughout this period, small but substantial amounts of thiopental are removed and metabolized by the liver. Unlike removal by the tissues, this removal is cumulative. Note that the rate of metabolism equals the early rate of removal by fat. The sum of this early removal by fat and metabolism is the same as the removal by muscle. (From Saidman, L.J.: Uptake, distribution and elimination of barbiturates. *In* Anesthetic Uptake and Action. Edited by E.I. Eger. Baltimore, Williams and Wilkins, 1974, with permission.)

than those individuals given thiopental because methohexital has a greater rate of total body clearance.

The pharmacokinetic behavior of barbiturates commonly used in anesthesia is detailed in Table 6–4.[32] Of these commonly administered barbiturates, it is apparent that methohexital has the fastest rate of plasma clearance whereas pentobarbital has the slowest rate. Because the volumes of distribution at steady state are not significantly different, the differences in pharmacokinetics among the barbiturates relate to different rates of hepatic metabolism (clearance). Thus, methohexital has a high rate of hepatic biotransformation and pentobarbital has a low rate. On the basis of these pharmacokinetic data, blood levels of pentobarbital and the CNS effects of the drug would be predicted to persist longer after pentobarbital use than after methohexital administration; such is the case.

PHARMACODYNAMICS

Barbiturates produce the clinical effects of sedation and sleep. In sufficient doses, they produce CNS depression that is termed general anesthesia and is attended by loss of consciousness, amnesia, and respiratory and cardiovascular depression. Barbiturates are used to induce general anesthesia because of their prompt, predictable hypnotic effects. Although the response to pain and other noxious stimulation during general anesthesia appears to be obtunded, results of pain studies (tibial pressure in man) reveal that barbiturates may actually decrease the pain threshold.[33] This antanalgesic effect only occurs at low blood levels of barbiturates, such as with small induction doses of thiopental or after emergence from thiopental when the blood levels are low. Antanalgesia is also noted with the use of pentobarbital.[33] The amnesic effects of barbiturates have not been well studied, but any such effect is decidedly less pronounced than that produced by benzodiazepines. Both the respiratory and the cardiovascular depressant effects of barbiturates are negligible in low sedative doses. With higher doses, however, respiratory depression is significant. Respiratory depression results from the central effects of barbiturates, whereas cardiovascular effects are a result of both central and peripheral (direct vascular and cardiac) effects.[34]

Onset of Central Nervous System (CNS) Effects

Barbiturates produce CNS effects when they enter the brain from the blood. This process is often termed crossing the blood-brain barrier. CBF (approximately 20% of the cardiac output) is apparently maintained and there is normal circu-

Table 6–4.   Barbiturate Pharmacokinetics

Drug	Distribution half-lives (min)	Elimination half-life (hr)	Clearance $(ml/kg^{-1}/min^{-1})$	V_D^{ss}* $(1\ kg^{-1})$
Thiopental	2.4–3.3 (rapid)† 47.0 (slow)	5.1–11.5	1.6–4.3	1.5–3.3
Methohexital	4.8–6.2 (rapid) 60.0 (slow)	1.5–4.0	9.9–12.1	1.13–2.1
Pentobarbital	240.0 (slow)	17.2–50.0	0.36–0.48	0.99–1.94

*V_D^{ss} = volume of distribution at steady state.
†Values for each pharmacokinetic parameter represent the range of mean values reported in 13 individual studies. (From Stanski, D.R.: Pharmacokinetics of barbiturates. *In* Pharmacokinetics of Anaesthesia. Edited by C. Prys-Roberts and C.C. Hug, 1984, with permission.)

lation with drug mixing in the right and left circulations. There are several well-known factors that help to determine the rapidity with which a drug enters the cerebral spinal fluid (CSF) and brain tissue.[31]

Lipid Solubility. Drugs with high lipid solubility cross the blood-brain barrier rapidly and produce their pharmacologic effect. Lipid-soluble drugs cross the cell membranes quickly. Most barbiturates exist in an un-ionized form (vide infra). Therefore, the degree of lipid solubility of that un-ionized form of the drug determines the rapidity with which a drug crosses the blood-brain barrier. Thiopental has a partition coefficient (defined as the ratio of concentration in methylene chloride to concentration in water) of 580 in contrast to only 39 for pentobarbital.[35] Thus, thiopental crosses the blood-brain barrier more rapidly than does pentobarbital as illustrated in Figure 6–6.[36,37]

Degree of Ionization. Only the un-ionized form of a drug passes the blood-brain barrier because only the un-ionized form can traverse the cellular membranes. The degree of ionization of a compound depends on the dissociation constant (pKa) of the compound and the physiologic pH.[35] The pKa of a drug is the pH at which 50% of a weak acid (like the barbiturates) is ionized. Weak acids become more ionized as pH increases. At the physiologic pH of 7.4 (most barbiturates have pKa at or around 7), a relatively large proportion of the drugs exist in an un-ionized form. Crossing of the blood-brain barrier is then facilitated. For example, thiopental has a pKa of 7.6.[35] Therefore, approximately 50% of the drug is un-ionized at physiologic pH, which accounts in part for the rapid accumulation of CSF after intravenous administration.[35,38] Methohexital is 75% un-ionized at pH 7.4, a fact that may explain the slightly more rapid effect of this drug when compared to the effect of thiopental.[11] As pH decreases, for example, with poor perfusion, barbiturates have a larger proportion of un-ionized drug available to

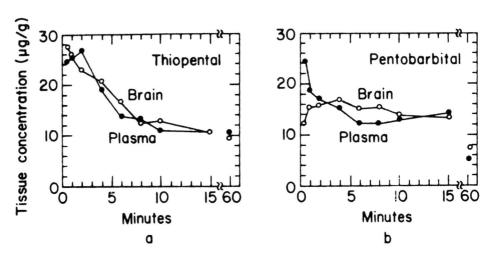

Fig. 6–6. Plasma and brain concentrations of thiopental (*a*) and pentobarbital (*b*) after intravenous injection in rats. The dose for both drugs was 15 mg/kg. Each point represents the mean value for four male rats. Note that early (< 3 minutes) there is a better plasma-brain equilibration with thiopental than pentobarbital, the primary reason being thiopental is 60 times more lipid soluble. (From Granik, S.J.: Induction of the synthesis of δ-amino-levulinic acid synthetase in liver parenchyma cells in culture by chemicals that induce acute porphyria. Biol. Chem., 238:PC2247, 1963; and Goldstein, A., Aronow, L., and Kalman, S.M. (eds.): Principles of Drug Action: The Basis of Pharmacology. New York, Harper & Row, 1968, with permission.)

cross the blood-brain barrier. There are obvious resulting clinical consequences. Patients with acidosis require that less barbiturate be administered because more of a given dose would cross the blood-brain barrier, whereas patients with alkalosis might require an increased dose.

Protein Binding. Barbiturates are highly bound to albumin and other plasma proteins. Because only unbound drug (free drug) can cross the blood-brain barrier, an inverse relationship exists between the degree of plasma protein binding and the rapidity of drug passage across the blood-brain barrier. Drugs have different degrees of protein binding, and in general the thiobarbiturates are more highly bound than are the oxybarbiturates.[39] The degree of protein binding of a drug is influenced by the physiologic pH and disease states, which alter the absolute amount of protein. Most barbiturates tend to experience peak protein binding at or around pH 7.5, and slightly fewer drugs have most bound at a more acidic or basic pH.[40] Disease states such as hepatic cirrhosis or chronic renal disease may reduce the total availability of plasma albumin which could reduce the absolute amount of protein available for binding. This situation may be more theoretical than real in terms of actual pharmacologic importance because there are many more protein molecules than drug molecules in most patients. Another possible consideration is whether other drugs that are highly protein bound can displace barbiturates from albumin. In theory, this sequence could also occur, although an important clinical effect is unlikely to occur again because of the enormous amount of protein available for drug binding.

Plasma Drug Concentration. The final factor governing the rapidity of drug penetration of the blood-brain barrier is the plasma drug concentration. The more drug there is in the plasma, the more drug that diffuses into the CSF and brain. The two primary determinants of the plasma concentration are the *dose* administered and the *rate* (speed) of administration. The higher the dose and the more rapidly it is administered, the more rapid is the effect. For example, as the dose of thiopental over the same time is increased, an increased percentage of patients are anesthetized.[41] A dose of 2 mg/kg produced anesthesia in 20% of patients, whereas a dose of 2.4 mg/kg produced anesthesia in 80% of patients. Similarly, the speed of injection influences the effect of thiopental.[42] When an initial dose of thiopental of approximately 2.75 mg/kg was used, a significantly (p < 0.001) smaller amount of drug was required to produce anesthesia when the dose was given over 5 seconds as opposed to over 15 seconds. Thus, the dose and rate of intravenous administration can profoundly affect the onset of barbiturate CNS effect.

Placental Transfer

The factors governing CNS uptake or passage across the blood-brain barrier (vide supra) also dictate the passage of barbiturates across the placenta. These factors are lipid solubility, protein binding, degree of ionization, and drug plasma concentration (dose and speed of administration). The factors responsible for placental transfer of barbiturates have been reviewed in detail.[43–45] All barbiturates cross the placenta. The transfer of drugs used for intravenous anesthesia are of greatest concern, however, because they are administered in doses that are sufficient to anesthetize the mother and depress the infant.[41] Thiopental rapidly crosses the placenta. In fact fetal blood levels of this drug are detectable within 15 seconds of maternal administration.[46] Fifty-eight percent of maternal blood levels (after 120 to 180 mg of thiopental) can be found in fetal blood at delivery.[47] The longer the time interval from administration, the lower the fetal blood level, presumably because of redistribution of the drug in both maternal and fetal circulations. In fact, maternal redistribution may be the most significant determinant of fetal blood level.[48] Equilibrium of maternal and fetal blood levels is achieved within 3 minutes (Fig. 6–7), which means fetal and maternal blood levels parallel each other after that time.[46]

Neonatal depression after barbiturate use is related to the dose; higher doses of the drug are associated with higher maternal and fetal blood levels and lower newborn Apgar scores.[49] In 1956, Crawford showed the good association of maternal and fetal blood levels of thiopental, as well as that, with greater operation time, thiopental levels in the maternal and fetal circulations were reduced.[50] Thus, if sufficient time passes after a *single* administration, the fetal blood level is low and sedative-hypnotic effects should be reduced in the newborn. When properly administered, as for anesthesia induction for cesarean section, thiopental has little or no clinically apparent depressant effects on the newborn.[49,51] With *repeated* administrations, there are higher maternal and fetal blood levels of barbiturates.[49] This increased level can lead to newborn depression and is the basis for recommendations against repeated administrations to the mother before delivery.

Termination of Effect

Factors that determine the rate of onset of drug effects also affect their termination, because there is an equilibrium between brain concentration and

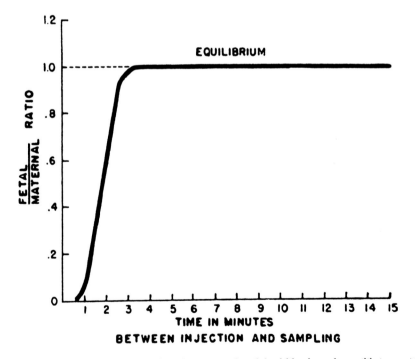

Fig. 6–7. Concentrations of thiopental in the maternal and fetal blood reach equilibrium within 3 minutes. Diagram based on data of McKechnie and Converse. (From Moya, F., and Thorndike, V.: Passage of drugs across the placenta. Am. J. Obstet. Gynecol., *84*:1778, 1962, with permission.)

plasma concentration. Thus, lipid solubility, degree of ionization, and CSF drug concentration affect the movement of drugs from the CSF to plasma. Protein binding is less important because there is usually no protein in the CSF, although there certainly is protein in the brain to which drugs may be bound. As plasma levels decrease, drug levels in the brain and CSF decrease. Thus, the most important factors in the termination of drug effect are those that govern plasma disappearance of the drug.

In a classic pharmacologic study, Brodie and co-workers conclusively demonstrated that awakening from thiopental occurred because the plasma level rapidly declined.[52] They further demonstrated that the cause of the rapid plasma decay of thiopental was *not metabolism* of the drug, but rather was a *redistribution* of the drug to other tissues throughout the body. Their commentary follows:

> The concentration of pentothal in plasma fell rapidly for the first 30 minutes and then more slowly (Fig. 6–8, typical example). The early sharp decline has been erroneously interpreted as signifying rapid destruction of the drug, thus explaining the quick recovery from anesthesia following the administration of small doses of pentothal. Actually, the early sharp decline might better be interpreted as representing a shift of pentothal from plasma to tissues as the drug is distributed throughout the body. As equilibrium between plasma and tissues is established, further decline in plasma levels becomes dependent only on the rate of metabolism of the drug which, as the second phase of the decline shows, is slow.[52]

Thus, in approximately 100 words and one picture (Fig. 6–8), the explanation was given for the termination of effects not only of thiopental but also of all drugs given intravenously. Many subsequent studies have yielded results that prove the hypothesis correct. The role of metabolism influencing the "second phase" of plasma decline was further elucidated by Saidman and Eger in 1966.[53]

The relationship of plasma drug level to onset and termination of effect as it relates to drug redistribution is illustrated in Figure 6–5. Because the brain receives a large percentage of the cardiac output (it belongs to the vessel-rich group [VRG] of tissues), it is exposed to a concentration of drug

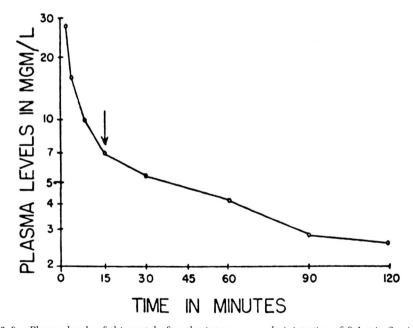

Fig. 6–8. Plasma levels of thiopental after the intravenous administration of 0.4 g in 2 minutes. *Arrow,* point at which subject awakened. (From Brodie, B.B., Mark, L.C., Papper, E.M., Lief, P.A., Bernstein, E., and Rovenstine, E.A.: The fate of thiopental in man and method for its estimation in biological material. J. Pharmacol. Exp. Ther., *98*:85, 1950, with permission.)

that approximates the blood concentration. This large volume also explains the rapid transfer rate of thiopental across the blood-brain barrier to produce sleep within 10 to 15 seconds of thiopental administration. As time passes, the blood level decreases and the drug is taken up by less well-perfused tissues, such as muscle and fat.[54] There is also a constant rate of metabolic clearance; the liver biotransforms a constant proportion or fraction (first-order kinetics) of the drug from the blood. Patients awake from a single dose of thiopental at a point from 5 to 10 minutes after administration because the drug level in the brain has decreased (along with the decline in blood level); drug is redistributed from VRG tissues to less well-perfused tissues. Price predicted that perturbations of the normal circulatory system should alter the normal redistribution of barbiturates.[54] Thus, apprehension, with hyperdynamic circulation, should produce more rapid clearance of barbiturates, and shock would reduce it. This theory is probably true.

If barbiturates are given repeatedly, the termination of effect becomes dependent more on the metabolic clearance and less on redistribution. In fact, if barbiturates are given repeatedly over time and attain a steady-state level, the termination of effect is mostly due to hepatic clearance. This situation occurs because other tissues are saturated with the drug and equilibrium exists. The drugs can no longer redistribute to less well-perfused tissues because they have become saturated and have equilibrated with the same concentration as the plasma. If barbiturates are given repeatedly over a relatively short time, such as during surgery, repeated delivery of fixed identical doses will cause accumulation of the drug in the blood, possibly prolonging the effect (Fig. 6–9).[55] In the first report of thiopental use by Lundy, he found that if the same dose was repeated, respiratory depression persisted. If, however, repeat doses were reduced and were given only after respiration returned, there was minimal postoperative hypoventilation.[56] This finding is a classic description of the cumulative effect of repeated delivery of barbiturate relative to the CNS. In summary, the termination of effect after multiple drug administrations or constant infusion is dependent on the elimination of the drug from the blood more by metabolism than by redistribution.

CLINICAL APPLICATIONS

Barbiturates are used clinically in the practice of anesthesia for premedication as well as for induction and maintenance of anesthesia. Less frequently, barbi-

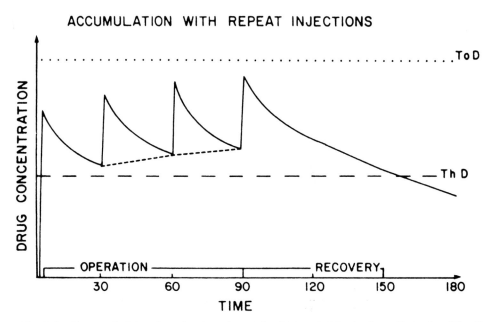

Fig. 6–9. Repeat administration of a given dose at fixed intervals (shorter than elimination t½) will cause drug accumulation. Effect would then be prolonged because the plasma level at the termination of surgery (90 min) is high. ToD = toxic dose level; ThD = therapeutic drug level. (From Reves, J.G., Greene, E.R., Jr., and Mackrell, T.N.: Continuous infusion of intravenous anesthetics: automated IV anesthesia, a rational method of drug administration. *In* New Anesthetic Agents, Devices and Monitoring Techniques. Edited by T.H. Stanley and W.C. Petty. Dordrecht, The Netherlands, Martinus Nijhoff, 1983.)

turates are used to provide cerebral protection to patients at risk of developing incomplete ischemia.[57] Barbiturates are also rarely used to terminate seizure activity in emergency situations.

In the beginning of this chapter (*History*), it was mentioned that the barbiturate hexobarbital no longer enjoys extensive popularity. Because its use today is somewhat limited, details of barbiturate use will focus on those that are now widely accepted. The three barbiturates used most commonly in the United States for intravenous anesthesia and maintenance of anesthesia, thiopental, thiamylal, and methohexital, are listed in Table 6–5 together with important characteristics of each drug. Because thiopental is the most universally accepted standard intravenous barbiturate anesthetic, it is considered the reference compound against which the other two are compared.[51] Thiamylal is closer characteristically to thiopental than is methohexital. Methohexital is 2.5 times more potent than the other two drugs, which accounts for the customary difference in formulation: methohexital is distributed as a 1% salt solution whereas thiopental and thiamylal are formulated as 2.5% salt solutions. Similarly, the usual dose of thiopental (3 to 4 mg/kg) and thiamylal (3 to 4 mg/kg) is about twice that of methohexital (1.0 to 2.0 mg/kg). In dose-effect studies, the ED_{50} (50% effective dose) for thiopental ranged from 2.2 mg/kg to 2.7 mg/kg, and that for methohexital is 1.1 mg/kg.[58,59] Because the ED_{50} induces anesthesia in only 50% of a given group of patients, higher doses are recommended to induce anesthesia reliably in most patients. Barbiturate dosage should be reduced in elderly patients.[60] Despite its greater potency, methohexital has a duration of action that is less than that of thiopental and thiamylal.

There are no important differences between these intravenous anesthetics with regard to their effects on the various organ systems (respiratory, cardiovascular, gastrointestinal, hepatic, and renal), but there are differences in complications with these drugs. Thiopental and thiamylal produce fewer excitatory symptoms with induction. The incidence of cough, hiccough, tremors, and twitching is approximately five times greater after methohexital than after the other two induction agents. Tissue irritation and local complications may occur more frequently with the use of thiopental and thiamylal, however, than with methohexital. In comparative studies, the pain on injection was shown to be greater with methohexital (12%) than with thiopental (9%). Results also show phlebitis occurs more frequently with methohexital use (8%) than with thiopental use (1%).[61] In summary, the primary differences between these compounds are a smoother period of induction with thiopental and thiamylal and a quicker emergence time with methohexital.

THIOPENTAL

Thiopental (Fig. 6–10) has survived the test of time as an intravenous anesthetic drug. Since Lundy introduced it in 1934, thiopental has become the most widely used induction agent, principally because of its rapid hypnotic effect (one arm-brain circulation time), highly predictable effect, lack of vascular irritation, and general overall safety.[62]

Metabolism, Pharmacokinetics, and Duration of Action

Thiopental is oxidized in the liver to form a carboxylic acid metabolite and to a lesser degree hydroxythiopental.[63] These metabolites are inactive. The desul-

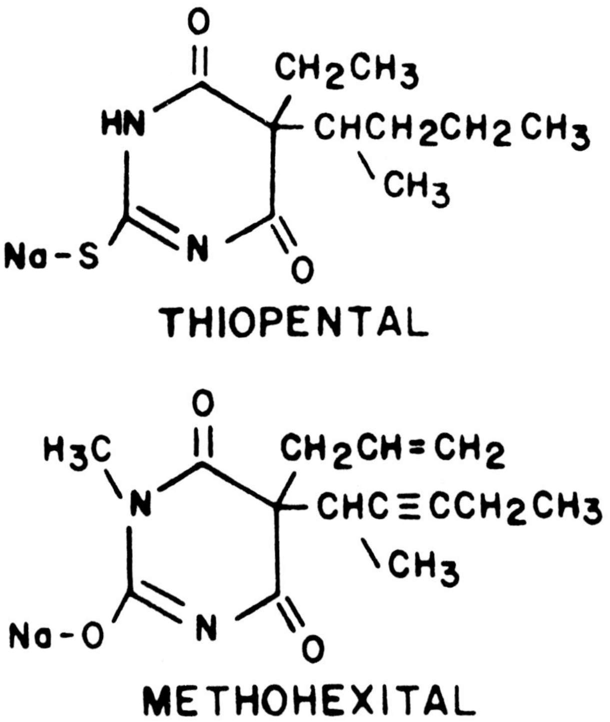

Fig. 6–10.   Structural formula of thiopental and of methohexital.

furation reaction can produce pentobarbital, which is active but is a relatively minor metabolic product.[64] Thiopental has relatively low hepatic extraction (25% of hepatic blood flow).[63]

In usual doses (4 to 5 mg/kg), thiopental exhibits first-order kinetics (i.e., a constant *fraction* of drug is cleared from the body per unit time); however, at very high doses of thiopental (300 to 600 mg/kg), zero-order kinetics occur (i.e., a constant *amount* of drug is cleared per unit time).[11,32,65,66] Table 6–4 is a summary of the pharmacokinetic variables of thiopental and other barbiturates. Thiopental has a distribution half-life ($t\frac{1}{2}$ α) of 2.4 to 3.3 minutes. The rate of total body clearance varies according to sampling times and techniques, from 1.6 to 2.4 ml/kg/minute.[67–71] The elimination half-life varies from 5 to 12 hours.[67–71] The volume of distribution is slightly larger in female patients, causing longer elimination half-lives in this group of patients.[70] Pregnancy also increases the volume of distribution of thiopental, thereby prolonging the elimination half-life.[48] The clearance rate of thiopental is not altered in patients with cirrhosis.[72] Enflurane, nitrous oxide, and surgery do not change the pharmacokinetics of thiopental.[67]

Findings of recent pharmacokinetic analyses confirm those of early classic studies by Brodie, et al., relating awakening from thiopental to rapid redistribution.[52,67,69,70] Awakening is dependent on the dose administered, higher doses prolonging recovery.[73] Awakening may be delayed in older patients, either because of increased CNS sensitivity or alterations in metabolism.[71,74] Young (younger than 13 years) patients seem to have a greater rate of total clearance and a shorter rate of plasma thiopental clearance than do adults, which theoretically might result in earlier awakening, especially after multiple doses of the drug.[75] Conversely, the initial volume of distribution is less in elderly patients when compared to that in young patients, which explains a lower dose requirement for the onset of EEG and hypnotic effects.[76]

Because of its affinity for fat, relatively large volume of distribution, and low rate of hepatic clearance, thiopental can accumulate in tissues, especially if given in large doses over a prolonged period. The accumulation of thiopental was shown to occur in studies conducted by Dundee, et al., in which the plasma drug level increased when repeat doses of drug were given.[77–79] Obese patients are likely to have prolonged clearance half-lives of thiopental.[80] Administration by infusion assures relatively constant blood levels (Fig. 6–11), thus maintaining the hypnotic effect. If large doses (24 mg/kg/hour) are given over a prolonged time, however, drug accumulation will result.[54,66]

Although it was reported that protein binding is apparently related to the dose of thiopental (the higher the dose, the less the drug binding), this concept is not universally accepted.[69,81] If this relationship does exist, it could partially explain the observation that rapid administration of thiopental is more effective than slower administration; however, mass concentration effects and even development of acute tolerance are probably also involved.[42] Protein binding is important because only unbound drug can cross the blood-brain barrier. Approximately 70 to 90% of thiopental is bound to protein, which means that relatively small changes in the degree of protein binding could produce important effects (e.g., if a drug is 90% protein bound, then 10% is active, and if the drug becomes 85% protein bound then 15% is active, rendering 50% more active drug avail-

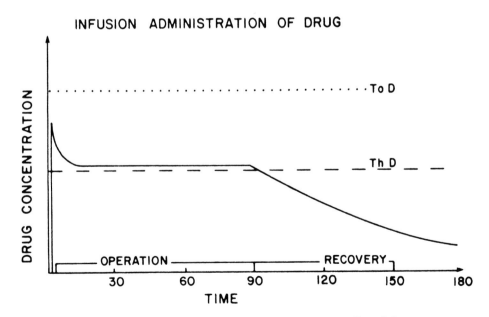

Fig. 6–11. Ideal drug infusion scheme. Drug loading dose is give initially and then a continuous infusion is maintained so that the drug plasma level stays just above the therapeutic level. Emergence from anesthesia should begin with beginning of the recovery period (90 minutes). (From Reves, J.G., Greene, E.R., Jr., and Mackrell, T.N.: Continuous infusion of intravenous anesthetics: automated IV anesthesia a rational method of drug administration. *In* New Anesthetic Agents, Devices and Monitoring Techniques. Edited by T.H. Stanley and W.C. Petty. Dordrecht, The Netherlands, Martinus Nijhoff, 1983.)

able).[4,32,82,83] A possible clinical example is the interaction of thiopental with sulfonamides; sulfonamides may displace thiopental from protein, lowering the dose required for anesthesia.[84] Pathologic states can alter protein binding. For example, renal and hepatic diseases may increase the free fraction of thiopental, making these patients potentially more susceptible to the CNS effects of thiopental.[72,82,85] Protein binding is not altered with advanced age, and therefore differences in the effects of thiopental in the elderly are not due to differences in protein binding.[86]

Pharmacodynamics

RESPIRATORY SYSTEM

Thiopental produces dose-related central respiratory depression. There is also a significant incidence of transient apnea after the administration of thiopental when it is used for induction of anesthesia. In 1952, Patrick and Faulconer produced key evidence that thiopental produced central respiratory depression in a study of seven patients.[87] There was an increase in $PaCO_2$ and a decreased response to inhaled CO_2 and hypoxic gas mixtures. The evidence for central depression was a correlation between EEG depth and minute ventilation; with increased anesthetic depth, there was diminished minute ventilation. Other investigators described the respiratory depressant effects of thiopental on hypoxic and CO_2 response in the dog and in man.[88–90] The time course of respiratory depression has not been fully studied, but it appears that peak respiratory depression, as measured by the slope of CO_2 response and minute ventilation after delivery of thiopental (3.5 mg/kg), occurs 1 to 1.5 minutes after administration. These parameters return to pre-drug levels rapidly, and within 15 minutes the drug effects are barely detectable.[89] Patients with chronic lung disease are slightly more susceptible to the respiratory depression of thiopental.[89] Apnea occurs during anesthesia induction with thiopental in at least 20% of cases, but the duration of apnea is short, approximately 25 seconds.[91] The usual ventilatory pattern with thiopental induction has been described as "double apnea." Initial apnea during drug administration that lasts a few seconds is succeeded by a few breaths of reasonably adequate tidal volume, which is followed by a more lengthy apneic period.[92] During the induction of anesthesia with thiopental, ventilation must be assisted or controlled to provide adequate respiratory exchange.

CARDIOVASCULAR SYSTEM

The hemodynamic changes produced by thiopental have been studied in healthy subjects and in patients with heart disease (Table 6–6).[63,93–106] The principal effect is a decrease in contractility which is related to reduced availability of calcium to the myofibrils.[79,93,94,107] There is also an increase in heart rate.[60,79,93–99,101–106] The cardiac index is unchanged or is reduced, and the mean blood pressure is maintained or is slightly reduced.[42,94–101,103,105,106] Although careful dose-response studies have been carried out, thiopental infusions and lower doses tend to be accompanied by smaller hemodynamic changes than those noted with rapid bolus injections. In the dose range studied, no relationship between plasma thiopental and hemodynamic effect has been found.[60] Early investigations of hemodynamics demonstrated that thiopental (100 to 400 mg) significantly decreased cardiac output (24%) and systemic blood pressure (10%). This decrease

Table 6–5. Characteristics of Barbiturates Used for Intravenous Anesthesia

Characteristics	Thiopental	Thiamylal	Methohexital
Generic name	Thiopental	Thiamylal	Methohexital
Trade name	Pentothal Thionembutal Thiopentone	Surital Thioseconal Thioquinal-barbital	Brevital
Anesthetic properties			
Relative potency	1	1	2.5
Relative duration	1	1	0.5
Usual concentration	2½%	2½%	1%
Induction dose	3–4 mg/kg	1.2–2 mg/kg	75–100 mg
Effects on respiration	Minimum depression with hypnotic dose; moderate with light anesthesia; marked with deep anesthesia; decrease in alveolar ventilation; respiratory acidosis if ventilation unassisted; laryngeal reflex not depressed	Similar to thiopental	Similar to thiopental, but of shorter duration
Effects on circulation	No myocardial depression with hypnotic dose; mild depression with light anesthesia; marked depression with excessive dose; decreased cardiac output and hypotension	Similar to thiopental	Similar to thiopental, except arrhythmia less frequent
Hepatic and renal effects	Minimum, if hypocarbia avoided and with light anesthesia; decreased function with deep anesthesia	Similar to thiopental	Similar to thiopental, but of shorter duration
Effects on gastrointestinal tract	Delay in gastric emptying; mild decrease in intestinal tone and movement	Similar to thiopental	Similar to thiopental
Complications			
Cough/hiccough	5%		25%
Laryngospasm	1%		1%
Tremors; involuntary muscle movement	7%	Similar to thiopental	35%
Hypotension (20 mm Hg or more)	15%		15%
Tissue irritation	May cause sloughing and neuropathy if injected outside the vein; severe arterial spasm if injected into the artery	Similar to thiopental	Less than thiopental (?)

(From Bonica J.J.: Principles and Practice of Obstetric Analgesia and Anesthesia. Chap. 26. Philadelphia, F.A. Davis, 1967, with permission.)

Table 6–6. Hemodynamic Changes (Percent) After Barbiturate Induction

Parameters*	Thiopental	Methohexital
HR	0 to +36%	+40 to +50%
MBP	−18 to +8%	0 to −10%
SVR	0 to 19%	NR
PAP	Unchanged	NR
PVR	Unchanged	NR
LA/PAO	Unchanged	NR
RAP	0 to +33%	0 to +5%
CI	0 to −24%	0 to −12%
SV	−12 to −35%	NR
LVSWI	0 to −26%	NR
RVSWI	NR	NR
dP/dt	−14%	NR
1/PEP^2	−18 to −28%	NR
References	60, 79, 93–101, 103–105	143, 148, 149

*HR = heart rate; MBP = mean blood pressure; SVR = systemic vascular resistance; PAP = mean pulmonary artery pressure; PVR = pulmonary vascular resistance; LA/PAO = left atrial or pulmonary artery occluded pressure; RAP = right atrial pressure; CI = cardiac index; SV = stroke volume; LVSWI = left ventricular stroke work index; RVSWI = right ventricular stroke work index; PEP = pre-ejection period; NR = data not reported. All data from normal patients or patients with compensated ischemic heart disease.

was achieved presumably by reducing venous return because of increased venous capacitance.[107,108] Tracheal intubation after thiopental administration in normal subjects as well as in ischemic heart disease patients is accompanied by marked hypertension and tachycardia.[104–106] Changes in heart rate in response to intubation can be attenuated by the administration of fentanyl (0.01 μg/kg).[105]

Mechanisms for the decrease in cardiac output include (1) direct negative inotropic action, (2) decreased ventricular filling due to increased capacitance, and (3) transiently decreased sympathetic outflow from the CNS.[62,109] The increase in heart rate (10 to 36%) that accompanies thiopental administration probably results from the baroreceptor-mediated sympathetic reflex stimulation of the heart.[110] Thiopental produces dose-related negative inotropic effects, which appear to result from a decrease in calcium influx into the cells with a resultant diminished amount of calcium at sarcolemma sites.[111,112] The difference in the cardiovascular effects associated with thiopental use in healthy subjects relative to those who have compensated heart disease is slight. There was one group of patients, however, who had valvular or congenital heart disease, received 4 mg/kg of thiopental and had a greater (18%) drop in mean blood pressure than other patients.[102] The reasons for this response were not obvious. There is little difference in the responses after thiopental and methohexital administration in heart disease patients (Fig. 6–12).[102] The increase in heart rate (11 to 36%) encountered in patients with coronary artery disease anesthetized with thiopental (1 to 4 mg/kg) is potentially deleterious because of the obligatory increase in myocardial oxygen consumption (MVo$_2$) that accompanies the increased heart rate.[94,101] Patients who have normal coronary arteries have no difficulty in maintaining adequate coronary blood flow to meet the increased MVo$_2$. Even patients with

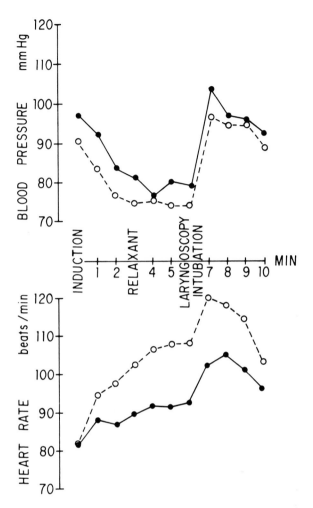

Fig. 6–12. Mean arterial blood pressure and heart rate during the first 10 minutes of anesthesia with thiopental (closed circles) and methohexital (open circles). At minute 3, pancuronium (0.2 mg/ kg) was given. Each line is the mean of 20 patients with heart disease. (From Wyant, G.M., Dobkin, A.B., and Aasheim, G.M.: Comparison of seven intravenous anaesthetic agents in man. Br. J. Anaesth., 29:194, 1957.)

ischemic heart disease can maintain normal lactate metabolism with thiopental induction.[94,101]

Despite the well-known potential for cardiovascular depression when given rapidly in large doses, thiopental has minimal hemodynamic effects in healthy individuals and in those persons with heart disease but in whom the drug is given slowly or by infusion. Very large doses given to produce an isoelectric EEG reduce stroke volume, blood pressure, systemic vascular resistance, and stroke work index.[113] Because the heart rate increases, the cardiac index is maintained during these large infusion doses (75 mg/kg) of thiopental. The use of high doses of thiopental (40 mg/kg) during cardiopulmonary bypass does depress cardiac function so that positive inotropic drugs are required during discontinuation of this procedure.[114] There are no well-documented investigations designed to examine the effects of thiopental in patients with impaired ventricular function, but there likely would be significant reductions in cardiovascular parameters in these patients. When thiopental is given to hypovolemic patients, there is a significant reduction in cardiac output (69%) as well as an important decrease in blood pressure. Patients without adequate compensatory mechanisms, therefore, may have serious hemodynamic depression with thiopental induction.[115] This fact may help to explain the disastrous results of thiopental administration to victims of the attack on Pearl Harbor.[116] Thiopental produces greater reductions in blood pressure and heart rate than diazepam when it is used for induction of anesthesia in ASA class III to IV patients.[117,118]

Clinical Applications

Thiopental is an excellent hypnotic for use as an intravenous anesthesia *induction* drug. The prompt onset (15 to 30 seconds) of action and smooth induction noted with its use make thiopental superior to most other available drugs. The relatively rapid emergence, particularly after short procedures, is also a reason for the widespread use of thiopental in this setting. Thiopental does not possess analgesic properties and therefore it must be supplemented with other analgesic drugs to obtund reflex responses to noxious stimuli during anesthesia and surgical procedures. Thiopental can be used to *maintain* general anesthesia; repeat doses reliably maintain unconsciousness and contribute to amnesia. Thiopental is not a perfect choice, however, to use as the hypnotic component of balanced anesthesia.[119,120] Probably because of the antanalgesic properties noted as drug levels in blood drop, analgesic supplementation is required more often with thiopental than with midazolam when it is used during balanced anesthesia.[120] Benzodiazepine supplementation may provide amnesia more reliably, but awakening after thiopental is more rapid.[119,120] If thiopental is given repeatedly or by continuous infusion for the maintenance of anesthesia, accumulation of the drug in the blood will occur and emergence will then be delayed.

A specialized use of thiopental is *cerebral protection*. Although pentobarbital cerebral protection for global ischemia was once recommended, thiopental is probably the drug of choice.[57] When incomplete cerebral ischemia is encountered or anticipated, however, thiopental may be useful. Thiopental given to produce an isoelectric EEG (40 mg/kg) during open cardiac chamber surgical procedures (operations with a high incidence of regional ischemia presumably from a particulate embolization) proved useful in decreasing the severity of symptoms.[114] Although still considered experimental in man, there is laboratory evidence to support this use of thiopental, the validity of which may yet be proven.[121–127]

Dose Effect and Acute Tolerance

The usual dose of thiopental is 3 to 4 mg/kg given intravenously over 5 to 15 seconds (Table 6–5). The dose should be reduced in elderly individuals, patients in shock, and in any debilitated patients. There is less inter-patient variability in the dose response to barbiturates than to benzodiazepines when used for anesthesia induction, but there still is significant variability in the doses of thiopental required to induce anesthesia.[58] In one large study, the induction dose for healthy patients varied from 2.8 to 9.7 mg/kg.[128] The variability in dose response is related to premedication and age. With increasing premedication and advancing age (Fig. 6–13), less thiopental is required for induction. Also, with more rapid infusion of the drug, less thiopental is required.[42] The surest way to reduce vari-

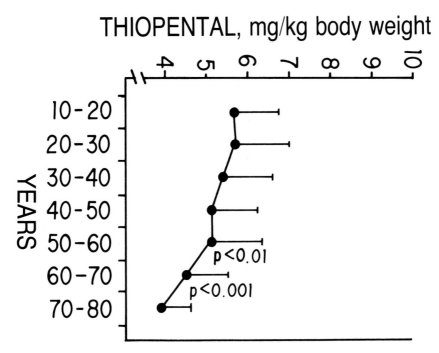

Fig. 6–13. Relationship between age and induction dose of thiopental for 540 patients. Doses are weight related. There is a statistically significant fall in the dose from young to old patients. Standard deviations are shown. (Redrawn from Christensen, J.H., and Andreasen, F.: Individual variation in response to thiopental. Acta Anaesthesiol. Scand., 22:303, 1978.)

ability in dose response is to increase the dose of thiopental; that is, if high doses are given, a higher percentage of patients will be anesthetized. This practice may be unwise, however, for two reasons. First, higher doses of thiopental produce greater respiratory and cardiovascular depression, and secondly, acute tolerance occurs, requiring the administration of even more thiopental.

The development of acute tolerance to thiopental was first described by Brodie and co-workers in 1951.[129] They reported that, after very large doses of thiopental, patients awoke with plasma thiopental levels that were higher than those in subjects given lower doses. Thus, an individual given 33 mg/kg of thiopental was awake and oriented when the plasma thiopental level was 16.8 ng/ml, whereas the same subject given 65 mg/kg (2 times the first dose) awoke when the plasma level was 27 ng/ml. This original demonstration of positive association of induction dose with awakening blood level was shown by other investigators.[77–79] The clinical implication of the development of acute tolerance to thiopental is that lower doses should be used to avoid the possible respiratory and hemodynamic depression that accompany large doses of thiopental. Finally, even though acute tolerance does develop, the duration of sleep after the delivery of thiopental is dose related; if large doses are given, prolonged recovery of normal CNS effects can be expected.[79]

Local Toxicity

Although the incidence of venous and tissue irritation with thiopental use is less than that of many other intravenous anesthetic drugs, it can produce local toxic effects.[61] The sequelae from intravenous thiopental administration vary from local pain and redness to venous thrombosis and tissue necrosis.[130] These effects are more common if a 5% solution rather than a 2% solution is used.[11] It is probably the drug and not the alkalinity of the thiopental solution that causes the irritation. The consequences of accidental arterial injection may be severe.[130] The degree of injury is related to the concentration of the drug. Treatment consists of 1) dilution of the drug by the administration of saline into the artery, 2) heparinization, and 3) brachial plexus block.[51] Overall, the proper administration of thiopental intravenously is remarkably free of local toxicity.

Contraindications

Wood listed the absolute contraindications for thiopental use.[11] First, when there is respiratory obstruction or an inadequate airway, thiopental may worsen respiratory depression. Second, cardiovascular instability or shock precludes its use. Third, status asthmaticus is a condition in which airway control and ventilation may be further decreased by thiopental. Fourth, porphyria may be worsened or acute attacks may be accentuated by the administration of thiopental. Fifth, without proper equipment (intravenous instrumentation) and airway equipment (means of artificial ventilation), thiopental should not be administered.

METHOHEXITAL

Methohexital (Fig. 6–10) is an ultra-short acting methylbarbiturate. It is approximately two to three times more potent than thiopental and has similar actions and uses.[131,132] The greatest distinction between the effects of these drugs with induction are the greater incidence of excitatory movements with induction and pain on injection.[133]

Metabolism, Pharmacokinetics, and Duration of Action

Methohexital is metabolized in the liver by oxidation to an alcohol; there is, incidentally, also *N*-dealkylation. The pharmacokinetics of methohexital were first described completely by Breimer and more recently they were compared to those of thiopental in surgical patients.[134,135] The two barbiturates exhibited similar distribution half-lives, volumes of distribution and protein bindings.[112] A marked difference exists, however, in plasma disappearance (Fig. 6–14) and elimination half-lives (4 hours for methohexital and as many as 12 hours for thiopental). This difference is due to the threefold greater rate of hepatic clearance of methohexital, the mean ranging from 7.8 to 12.5 ml/kg/minute.[43,134] The hepatic extraction ratio of methohexital (clearance/hepatic blood flow) is approximately 0.5, indicating that the liver extracts 50% of the drug presented to it.[135] This ratio contrasts to the lower hepatic extraction ratio of thiopental (0.15). Methohexital may be given rectally and is absorbed rapidly.[136] Mean peak plasma levels occur within 14 minutes after rectal administration and are associated with a rapid hypnotic effect. The therapeutic hypnotic blood level in children is ≥ 2 μg/ml.

The termination of effect after a single administration of methohexital, like thiopental, is from redistribution of the drug to tissue other than the brain. Awakening is dose related—the higher the dose, the longer the emergence time.[73] There is little difference in these two barbiturates with regard to distribution, which may explain the similar wake-up time of methohexital and thiopental (Fig. 6–15).[73,137] There is, however, a difference in the rate of total body clearance,

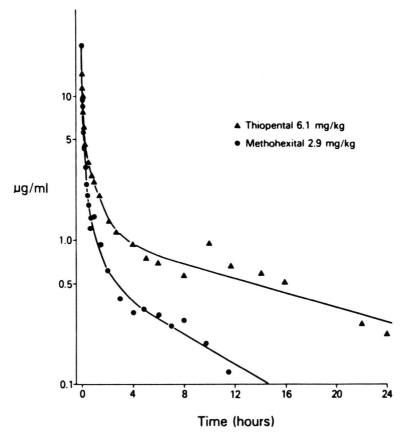

Fig. 6–14. Representative plasma concentration versus time curves for methohexital and thiopental. Symbols indicate the measured concentrations; adjacent lines are the polyexponential functions fit to the data by nonlinear regression. (From Hudson, R.J., Stanski, D.R., and Burch, P.G: Pharmacokinetics of methohexital and thiopental in surgical patients. Anesthesiology, *59*:215, 1983, with permission.)

that of methohexital being higher. This disparity could explain the difference found in the psychomotor skills of patients and the earlier full recovery after methohexital (Fig. 6–15). Sensitive tests of psychomotor skills tend to show better early performance after methohexital than after thiopental use.[138,139] A driving test, however, reveals abnormal skills for as long as 8 hours after anesthesia, suggesting that despite plasma clearance there is residual CNS impairment for about 1 day. Despite these residual effects, methohexital is cleared more rapidly than thiopental, which explains why methohexital is preferred for use by some clinicians when rapid awakening is desirable.

Pharmacodynamics

Respiratory System

Methohexital is a central respiratory system depressant like other barbiturates. Induction doses (1.5 mg/kg) significantly decrease the slope of the ventilatory response to carbon dioxide ($VRCO_2$).[140] This reduction in $VRCO_2$ indicates that methohexital depresses the medullary respiratory center, which modifies venti-

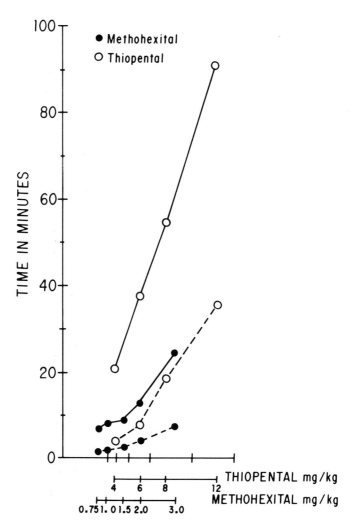

Fig. 6–15. Time (minutes) from induction to opening eyes (---) and time for "full recovery" (_____) after different doses of methohexital and thiopental. (From Carson, I.W., Graham, J., and Dundee, J.W.: Clinical studies of induction agents. XLIII. Recovery from althesin—a comparative study with thiopentone and methohexitone. Br. J. Anaesth., 47:358, 1975, with permission.)

latory response to changing CO_2 tensions. With the induction of anesthesia, there is also a decrease in minute ventilation (V_E), but a minimal effect on respiratory rate; therefore, there is a significant reduction in tidal volume after methohexital use. The time course of these effects was studied in healthy volunteers.[140] The peak reduction in $VRCO_2$ occurred 30 seconds after drug administration and returned to near normal levels within 15 minutes. The peak decrease in V_E occurred 60 seconds after methohexital delivery and also returned to baseline within 15 minutes. Similarly, peak decrements in tidal volume occurred 1 minute after injection and returned to a normal level within 15 minutes. In contrast to the effects on ventilation, patients were awake within about 5 minutes after the administration of methohexital (1.5 mg/kg). There is no difference in the duration of ventilatory depression after methohexital use and after thiopental delivery when the drugs are studied in a similar manner.[89,140]

There is some in vitro evidence that histamine release associated with the use of methohexital may be present to a lesser extent than that triggered by thiopental; whether this laboratory finding has clinical implications is not known.[141] It is possible that methohexital may be preferable to thiopental for use in patients sensitive to histamine (asthmatics) or those with a propensity to release histamine (atopics).

CARDIOVASCULAR SYSTEM

Early claims of less cardiovascular depression with methohexital than with thiopental have not been confirmed.[115] There is little doubt that the cardiovascular depression in patients with cardiac disease is equal when methohexital or thiopental is administered in equipotent doses (Fig. 6–12).[47,102] In patients without cardiac disease, methohexital causes a slight decrease in cardiac output and a compensatory increase in heart rate (Table 6–6). The significant increase in heart rate with methohexital was less than with propanidid, but more than when either althesin or etomidate was used.[142] In hypertensive patients, methohexital caused a fall in arterial pressure that was greater than that noted with thiopental.[143] Used in very large doses (24 mg/kg), methohexital decreases arterial pressure, systemic vascular resistance, and stroke volume, and increases heart rate.[144] Cardiac output is maintained by the compensatory increase in heart rate.

Clinical Applications and Dosage

Methohexital is the only intravenous barbiturate that offers a serious challenge to thiopental.[145] Methohexital is used for the *induction* of anesthesia at a dose of 1 to 2 mg/kg. Induction is swift and so is emergence. Methohexital may also be used as the hypnotic component to *maintain* anesthesia. Methohexital is not an analgesic, and additional opioids or inhalation anesthetic drugs must be combined with methohexital to maintain satisfactory general anesthesia during surgery. Because methohexital is cleared more rapidly than thiopental, it could be superior to thiopental for the maintenance of anesthesia. Certainly awakening times are rapid after the use of methohexital, much faster than with midazolam.[146] Theoretically, because of the greater rate of plasma clearance, methohexital is superior to thiopental for *continuous infusion* during anesthesia.[147] Because methohexital is cleared relatively rapidly after attaining steady state, it is a good drug to use by continuous infusion. There probably are upper limits of safe infusion doses yet to be defined, but seizures have occurred in neurosurgical patients after large doses of methohexital (24 mg/kg).[144] Finally, some clinicians advocate the use of methohexital in pediatric patients as a rectal *premedicant-induction agent*. The dose recommended for this use is 25 mg/kg rectal instillation (10% solution through a 14 French catheter, 7 cm into rectum).[136] With this method of administration, sleep onset is rapid.

Since their first use, barbiturates have been prominent intravenous anesthetic drugs. Thiopental is and has been the most commonly used intravenous anesthetic. Barbiturates are superb hypnotics, although they do depress respiration and can produce hypotension. On the whole, however, the drugs are remarkably free of serious adverse reactions.

REFERENCES

1. Dundee, J.W., and McIlroy, D.A.: The history of the barbiturates. Anaesthesia, 37:726, 1982.
2. Redonnet, T.A.: Recherches comparatives sur l'action pharmacodynamique des derives de l'acide barbiturique. Arch. Int. Pharmacodyn. Ther., 25:27, 1920.

3. Bardet, D.: Sur l'utilisation, comme anesthesique general, d'un produit nouveau, le diethyl-diallylbarbiturate de diethylamine. Bull. Gen. Ther. Med. Chir. Obstet. Pharm., *172*:27, 1921.
4. Bardet, G., and Bardet, D.: Contribution a l'etudes des hypnotiques ureiques; action et utilisation du diethyl-diallyl-barbiturate de diethyl-amine. Bull. Gen. Ther. Med. Chir. Obstet. Pharm., *172*:173, 1921.
5. Weese, H., and Scharpf, W.: Evipan; ein neuartiges Einschlafmittel. Dtsch. Med. Wochenschr., *58*:1205, 1932.
6. Weese, H.: Pharmakologie des intravenoesen Kurznarkotikums Evipan-Na. Dtsch. Med. Wochenschr., *2*:47, 1933.
7. Tabern, T.W., and Volwiler, E.H.: Sulfur-containing barbiturate hypnotics. J. Am. Chem. Soc., *57*:1961, 1935.
8. Wylie, W.D., and Churchill-Davidson, H.C.: A Practice of Anesthesia. Chicago, Year Book, 1972.
9. Adams, R.C.: Intravenous Anesthesia. New York, Paul B. Hoeber, 1944.
10. Dundee, J.W., and Wyant, G.M.: Intravenous Anaesthesia. Edinburgh, Churchill Livingstone 1974.
11. Wood, M.: Intravenous anesthetic agents, *In* Drugs and Anesthesia: Pharmacology for Anesthesiologists. Baltimore, Williams and Wilkins, Baltimore, 1982.
12. Way, W.L., and Trevor, A.J.: Pharmacology of intraveous nonnarcotic anesthetics. *In* Anesthesia, 2nd ed. Vol. II. Edited by Ronald D. Miller. New York, Churchill Livingstone, 1986, pp. 799.
13. Judge, S.E.: Effect of general anaesthetics on synaptic ion channels. Br. J. Anaesth., *55*:191, 1983.
14. Snyder, S.H.: Drug and neurotransmitter receptors in the brain. Science, *224*:22, 1984.
15. Higashi, H., and Nishi, S.: Effect of barbiturates on the gaba receptor of cat primary afferent neurones. J. Physiol., *332*:299, 1982.
16. Richards C.D.: Actions of general anaesthetics on synaptic transmission in the CNS. Br. J. Anaesth., *55*:201, 1983.
17. Richards, C.D., and Smaje, J.C.: Anaesthetics depress the sensitivity of cortical neurones to L-glutamate. Br. J. Pharmacol., *58*:347, 1976.
18. Richards, C.D.: The actions of pentabarbitone, procaine and tetrodotoxin on synaptic transmission in the olfactory cortex of the guinea-pig. Br. J. Pharmacol., *75*:639, 1982.
19. Andrews, P.R., and Mark, L.C.: Structural specificity of barbiturates and related drugs. Anesthesiology, *57*:314, 1982.
20. Huang, L-Y.M., and Barker, J.L.: Pentobarbital: stereospecific actions of (+) and (-) isomers revealed on cultured mammalian neurons. Science, *207*:195, 1980.
21. Messick, J.M., Newberg, L.A., Nugent, M., and Faust, R.J.: Principles of neuroanesthesia for the nonneurosurgical patient with CNS pathophysiology. Anesth. Analg., *64*:143, 1985.
22. Michenfelder, J.G.: The interdependency of cerebral functional and metabolic effects following massive doses of thiopental in the dog. Anesthesiology, *41*:231, 1974.
23. Pierce, E.C., Lambertsen, C.J., Deutsch, S., Chase, P.E., Linde, H.W., Dripps, R.D., and Price, H.L.: Cerebral circulation and metabolism during thiopental anesthesia and hyperventilation in man. J. Clin. Invest., *41*:1664, 1962.
24. Steen, P.A., Newberg, L., Milde, J.H., and Michenfelder, J.D.: Hypothermia and barbiturates: individual and combined effects on canine cerebral oxygen consumption. Anesthesiology, *58*:527, 1983.
25. Stuleken, E.H., Milde, J.H., Michenfelder, J.D., and Tinker, J.H.: The nonlinear responses of cerebral metabolism to low concentrations of halothane, enflurane, isoflurane, and thiopental. Anesthesiology, *46*:28, 1977.
26. Shapiro, H.M., Galindo, A., Wyte, S.R., and Harris, A.B.: Rapid intraoperative reduction of intracranial pressure with thiopentone. Br. J. Anaesth., *45*:1057, 1973.
27. Raventos, J.: The distribution in the body and metabolic fate of barbiturates. J. Pharm. Pharmacol., *6*:217, 1954.
28. Mark, L.C.: Metabolism of barbiturates in man. Clin. Pharmacol. Ther., *4*:504, 1963.
29. Granik, S.: Induction of the synthesis of δ-amino-levulinic acid synthetase in liver parenchyma cells in culture by chemicals that induce acute porphyria. J. Biol. Chem., *238*:PC2247, 1963.
30. Sharpless, S.K.: Hypnotics and sedatives. *In* The Pharmacological Basis of Therapeutics, 4th Ed. Edited by L.S. Goodman and A. Gilman. New York, MacMillan, 1970.
31. Waddell, W.J., and Butler, T.C.: The distribution and excretion of phenobarbital. J. Clin. Invest., *36*:1217, 1957.
32. Stanski, D.R.: Pharmacokinetics of barbiturates. *In* Pharmacokinetics of Anaesthesia. Edited by C. Prys-Roberts and C.C. Hug. Boston, Blackwell Scientific, 1984.
33. Dundee, J.W.: Alterations in response to somatic pain associated with anaesthesia. II. The effect of thiopentone and pentobarbitone. Br. J. Anaesth., *32*:407, 1960.
34. Reves, J.G., and Gelman, S.: Cardiovascular effects of intravenous anesthetic drugs. American Physiological Society, Clinical Physiology Series, *In* Effects of Anesthesia. Edited by B.G. Covino, H.A. Fozzard, K. Rehder, and G.R. Strichartz. 1985, pp. 179.

35. Brodie, B.B., Kurz, H., and Schanker, L.S.: The importance of dissociation constant and lipid-solubility in influencing the passage of drugs into the cerebrospinal fluid. J. Pharmacol. Exp. Ther., *130*:22, 1960.
36. Goldstein, A., and Aronow, L.: The durations of action of thiopental and pentobarbital. J. Pharmacol. Exp. Ther., *128*:1, 1960.
37. Brodie, B.B.: Physiological disposition and chemical fate of thiobarbiturates in the body. Fed. Proc., *11*:632, 1952.
38. Mark, L.C., Burns, J.J., Camponmanes, C.I., Ngai, S.H., Trousof, N., Papper, E.M., and Brodie, B.B.: The passage of thiopental into brain. J. Pharmacol. Exp. Ther., *119*:35, 1957.
39. Saidman, L.J.: Uptake, distribution and elimination of barbiturates. *In* Anesthetic Uptake and Action. Edited by E.I. Eger. Baltimore, Williams & Wilkins, 1974.
40. Goldbaum, L.R., and Smith, P.K.: The interaction of barbiturates with serum albumin and its possible relation to their disposition and pharmacological actions. J. Pharmacol. Exp. Ther., *III*:197, 1954.
41. Stella, L., Torri, G., and Castiglioni, C.L.: The relative potencies of thiopentone, ketamine, propanidid, alphaxalone and diazepam. Br. J. Anaesth., *51*:119, 1979.
42. Aveling, W., Bradshaw, A.D., and Crankshaw, D.P.: The effect of speed of injection on the potency of anaesthetic induction agents. Anaesth. Intensive Care, 6:116, 1978.
43. Moya, F., and Thorndike, V.: Passage of drugs across the placenta. Am. J. Obstet. Gynecol., 84:1778, 1962.
44. Bonica, J.J.: Placental transfer and clinical effects of specific drugs. *In* Principles and Practice of Obstetric Analgesia and Anesthesia. Philadelphia, F.A. Davis, 1967.
45. Flowers, C.E., Jr.: The placental transmission of barbiturates and thiobarbiturates and their pharmacological action on the mother and infant. Am. J. Obstet. Gynecol., 78:730, 1959.
46. McKechnie, F.B., and Converse, J.G.: Placental transmission of thiopental. Am. J. Obstet. Gynecol., 70:639, 1955.
47. Cohen, E.N.: Thiopental, curare and nitrous oxide anesthesia for cesarean section with studies on placental transmission. Surg. Gynecol. Obstet., 97:456, 1953.
48. Morgan, D.J., Blackman, G.L., Paull, J.D., and Wolf, L.J.: Pharmacokinetics and plasma binding of thiopental. II: Studies at cesarean section. Anesthesiology, 54:474, 1981.
49. Kosaka, Y., Takahashi, T., and Mark, L.C.: Intravenous thiobarbiturate anesthesia for cesarean section. Anesthesiology, *31*:489, 1969.
50. Crawford, J.S.: Some aspects of obstetric anaesthesia. Br. J. Anaesth., *28*:146, 1956.
51. Bonica, J.J.: Intravenous anesthetics. *In* Principles and Practice of Obstetric Analgesia and Anesthesia. Philadelphia, F.A. Davis, 1967.
52. Brodie, B.B., Mark, L.C., Papper, E.M., Lief, P.A., Bernstein, E., and Rovenstine, E.A.: The fate of thiopental in man and method for its estimation in biological material. J. Pharmacol. Exp. Ther., 98:85, 1950.
53. Saidman, L.J., and Eger, E.I., II.: The effect of thiopental metabolism on duration of anesthesia. Anesthesiology, 27:118, 1966.
54. Price, H.L.: A dynamic concept of the distribution of thiopental in the human body. Anesthesiology, *21*:40, 1960.
55. Reves, J.G., Greene, E.R. Jr., and Mackrell, T.N.: Continuous infusion of intravenous anesthetics: automated IV anesthesia, a rational method of drug administration. *In* New Anesthetic Agents, Devices, and Monitoring Techniques. Edited by T.H. Stanley, and W.C. Petty. Boston, Martinus Nijhoff, 1983.
56. Lundy, J.S.: Intravenous anesthesia: preliminary report of the use of two new thiobarbiturates. Mayo Clin. Proc., *10*:534, 1935.
57. Michenfelder, J.D.: A valid demonstration of barbiturate-induced brain protection in man—at last. Anesthesiology, *64*:140, 1986.
58. Stella, L., Tori, G., and Castiglioni, C.L.: The relative potencies of thiopentone, ketamine, propanidid, alphazalone and diazepam. Br. J. Anaesth., *51*:119, 1979.
59. Crankshaw, D.P., and Allt-Graham, J.: ED$_{50}$ values for thiopentone, methohexital, propanidid and alfathesin: a clinical experiment. Anaesth. Intensive Care, 6:36, 1978.
60. Christensen, J.H., Andreasen F., and Jansen, J.A.: Pharmacokinetics and pharmacodynamics of thiopentone: a comparison between young and elderly patients. Anaesthesia, 37:398, 1982.
61. Kawar, P., and Dundee, J.W.: Frequency of pain on injection and venous sequelae following the I.V. administration of certain anaesthetics and sedatives. Br. J. Anaesth., 54:935, 1982.
62. Olesen A.S., Huttel, M.S., and Hole, P.: Venous sequelae following the injection of etomidate or thiopentone I.V. Br. J. Anaesth., 56:171 1984.
63. Mark, L.C., Brand, L., Kamvyssi, S., Britton, R.C., Perel, J.M., Landrau, M.A., and Dayton, P.G.: Thiopental metabolism by human liver in vivo and in vitro. Nature, 206:1117, 1965.
64. Furano, E.S., and Greene, N.M.: Metabolic breakdown of thiopental in man determined by gas chromatographic analysis of serum barbiturate levels. Anesthesiology, 24:796, 1963.

65. Stanski, D.R., Mihm, F.G., Rosenthal, M.H., and Kalman, S.M.: Pharmacokinetics of high-dose thiopental used in cerebral resuscitation. Anesthesiology, 53:171, 1980.
66. Turcant, A., Delhumeau, A., Premel-Cabic, A., Granry, J.C., Cottineau, C., Six, P., and Allain, P.: Thiopental pharmacokinetics under conditions of long-term infusion. Anesthesiology, 63:50, 1985.
67. Ghoneim, M.M., and Van Hamme, M.J.: Pharmacokinetics of thiopentone: effects of enflurane and nitrous oxide anaesthesia and surgery. Br. J. Anaesth., 50:1237, 1978.
68. Heikkila, H., Jalonen, J., Arola, M., Kanto, J., and Laaksonen, V.: Midazolam as adjunct to high-dose fentanyl anaesthesia for coronary artery bypass grafting operation. Acta Anaesthesiol. Scand., 28:683, 1984.
69. Morgan, D.J., Blackman, G.L., Paull, J.D., and Wolf, L.J.: Pharmacokinetics and plasma binding of thiopental. I: Studies in surgical patients. Anesthesiology, 54:468, 1981.
70. Christensen, J.H., Andreasen, F., and Jansen, J.A.: Pharmacokinetics of thiopentone in a group of young women and a group of young men. Br. J. Anaesth., 52:913, 1980.
71. Christensen, J.H., Andreasen, F., and Jansen, J.A.: Influence of age and sex on the pharmacokinetics of thiopentone. Br. J. Anaesth., 53:1189, 1981.
72. Pandele, G., Chaux, F., Salvadori, C., Farinotti, M., and Duvaldestin, P.: Thiopental pharmacokinetics in patients with cirrhosis. Anesthesiology, 59:123, 1983.
73. Carson, I.W., Graham, J., and Dundee, J.W.: Clinical studies of induction agents. XLIII. Recovery from althesin—a comparative study with thiopentone and methohexitone. Br. J. Anaesth., 47:358, 1975.
74. Sear, J.W., Cooper, G.M., and Kumar, V.: The effect of age on recovery: a comparison of the kinetics of thiopentone and althesin. Anaesthesia, 38:1158, 1983.
75. Sorbo, S., Hudson, R.J., and Loomis, J.C.: The pharmacokinetics of thiopental in pediatric surgical patients. Anesthesiology, 61:666, 1984.
76. Homer, T.D., and Stanski, D.R.: The effect of increasing age on thiopental disposition and anesthetic requirement. Anesthesiology, 62:714, 1985.
77. Dundee, J.W., Price, H.L., and Dripps, R.D.: Acute tolerance to thiopentone in man. Br. J. Anaesth., 28:344, 1956.
78. Brand, L., Mazzia, V.D.B., Van Poznak, A., Burns, J.J., and Mark, L.C.: Lack of correlation between electroencephalographic effects and plasma concentrations of thiopentone. Br. J. Anaesth., 33:92, 1961.
79. Toner, W., Howard, P.J., McGowan, W.A.W., and Dundee, J.W.: Another look at acute tolerance to thiopentone. Br. J. Anaesth., 52:1005, 1980.
80. Jung, D., Mayersohn, M., Perrier, D., Calkins, J., and Saunders, R.: Thiopental disposition in lean and obese patients undergoing surgery. Anesthesiology, 56:269, 1982.
81. Burch, P.G., and Stanski, D.R.: The role of metabolism and protein binding in thiopental anesthesia. Anesthesiology, 58:146, 1983.
82. Ghoneim, M.M., and Pandya, H.B.: Plasma protein binding of thiopental in patients with impaired renal or hepatic function. Anesthesiology, 42:545, 1975.
83. Becker, K.E., Jr.: Gas chromatographic assay for free and total plasma levels of thiopental. Anesthesiology, 45:656, 1976.
84. Csogor, S.I., and Kerek, S.F.: Enhancement of thiopental anesthesia by sulphafurazole. Br. J. Anaesth., 42:988, 1970.
85. Burch, P.G., and Stanski, D.R.: Thiopental pharmacokinetics in renal failure. Anesthesiology, 55:A7176, 1981.
86. Jung, D., Mayersohn, M., Perrier, D., Calkins, J., and Saunders, R.: Thiopental disposition as function of age in female patients undergoing surgery. Anesthesiology, 56:263, 1982.
87. Patrick, R.T., and Faulconer, A.: Respiratory studies during anesthesia with ether and with pentothal sodium. Anaesthesiology, 13:252, 1952.
88. Hirshman, C.A., McCullough, B.S., Cohen, P.J., and Weil, J.V.: Hypoxic ventilatory drive in dogs during thiopental, ketamine, or pentobarbital anesthesia. Anesthesiology, 43:628, 1975.
89. Gross, J.B., Zebrowski, M.E., Care., W.D., Gardner, S., and Smith, T.C.: Time course of ventilatory depression after thiopental and midazolam in normal subjects and patients with chronic obstructive pulmonary disease. Anesthesiology, 58:540, 1983.
90. Bellville, J.W., and Seed, J.C.: The effect of drugs on the respiratory response to carbon dioxide. Anesthesiology, 21:727, 1960.
91. Tovell, R.M., Anderson, C.C., Sadove, M.S., Artusio, J.F., Papper, E.M., Coakley, C.S., Hudon, F., Smith, S.M., and Thomas, G.J.: A comparative clinical and statistical study of thiopental and thiamylal in human anesthesia. Anesthesiology, 16:910, 1955.
92. Wyant, G.M., Dobkin, A.B., and Aasheim, G.M.: Comparison of seven intravenous anaesthetic agents in man. Br. J. Anaesth., 29:194, 1957.
93. Seltzer, J.L., Gerson, J.I., and Allen, F.B.: Comparison of the cardiovascular effects of bolus iv. incremental administration of thiopentone. Br. J. Anaesth., 52:527, 1980.
94. Sonntag, H., Hellberg, K., Schenk, H.D., Donath, U., Regensburger, D., Kettler, D., Duchanova,

H., and Larsen, R.: Effects of thiopental (Trapanal) on coronary blood flow and myocardial metabolism in man. Acta Anaesthesiol. Scand., *19*:69, 1975.

95. Filner, B.E., and Karliner, J.S.: Alterations of normal left ventricular performance by general anesthesia. Anesthesiology, *45*:610, 1976.

96. White, P.F.: Comparative evaluation of intravenous agents for rapid sequence induction—thiopental, ketamine and midazolam. Anesthesiology, *57*:279, 1982.

97. Flickinger, H., Fraimow, W., Cathcart, R.T., and Nealon, T.F., Jr.: Effect of thiopental induction on cardiac output in man. Anesth. Analg., *40*:694, 1961.

98. Nauta, J., Stanley, T.H., deLange, S., Koopman, D., Spierdijk, J., and van Kleef, J.: Anaesthetic induction with alfentanil: comparison with thiopental, midazolam, and etomidate. Can. Anaesth. Soc. J., *30*:53, 1983.

99. Christensen, J.H., Andreasen, F., and Kristoffersen, M.B.: Comparison of the anaesthetic haemodynamic effects of chlormethiazole and thiopentone. Br. J. Anaesth., *55*:391, 1983.

100. Lebowitz, P.W., Cote, M.E., Daniels, A.L., Ramsey, F.M., Martyn, J.A.J., Teplick, R.S., and Davidson, J.K.: Comparative cardiovascular effects of midazolam and thiopental in healthy patients. Anesth. Analg., *61*:771, 1982.

101. Reiz, S., Balfors, E., Friedman, A., Haeggmark, S., and Peter, T.: Effects of thiopentone on cardiac performance, coronary hemodynamics, and myocardial oxygen consumption in chronic ischemic heart disease. Acta Anaesthesiol. Scand., *25*:103, 1981.

102. Lyons, S.M., and Clarke, R.S.J.: A comparison of different drugs for anaesthesia in cardiac surgical patients. Br. J. Anaesth., *44*:575, 1972.

103. Tarabadkar, S., Kopriva, C.J., Sreenivasan, N., Lescovich, F., and Barash, P.B.: Hemodynamic impact of induction in patients with decreased cardiac reserve. Anesthesiology, *53*:S43, 1980.

104. Fischler, M., Dubois, C., Brodaty, D., Schlumberger, S., Melchior, J.C., Guilmet, D., and Vourc'h, G.: Circulatory response to thiopentone and tracheal intubation in patients with coronary artery disease. Br. J. Anaesth., *57*:493, 1985.

105. Tarnow, J., Hess, W., and Klein, W.: Etomidate, althesin and thiopentone as induction agents for coronary artery surgery. Can. Anaesth. Soc. J., *27*:338, 1980.

106. Milocco, I., Loef, B.A., William-Olsson, G., and Appelgren, L.K.: Haemodynamic stability during anaesthesia induction and sternotomy in patients with ischaemic heart disease. Acta Anaesthesiol. Scand., *29*:465, 1985.

107. Frankl, W.S., and Poole-Wilson, P.A.: Effects of thiopental on tension development, action potential, and exchange of calcium and potassium in rabbit ventricualr myocardium. J. Cardiovasc. Pharmacol., *3*:554, 1981.

108. Eckstein, J.W., Hamilton, W.K., and McCammond, J.M.: The effect of thiopental on peripheral venous tone. Anesthesiology, *22*:525, 1961.

109. Conway, C.M., and Ellis, D.B.: The haemodynamic effects of short-acting barbiturates. Br. J. Anaesth., *41*:534, 1969.

110. Skovsted, P., Price, M.L., and Price, H.L.: The effects of short-acting barbiturates on arterial pressure, preganglionic sympathetic activity and barostatic reflexes. Anesthesiology, *33*:10, 1970.

111. Kissin, I., Motomura, S., Aultman, D.F., and Reves, J.G.: Inotropic and anesthetic potencies of etomidate and thiopental in dogs. Anesth. Analg., *62*:961, 1983.

112. Komai, H., and Rusy, B.F.: Differences in the myocardial depressant action of thiopental and halothane. Anesth. Analg., *63*:313, 1984.

113. Todd, M., Drummond, J.C., and U, H.S.: The hemodynamic consequences of high-dose thiopental anesthesia. Anesth. Analg., *64*681, 1985.

114. Nussmeier, N.A., Arlund, C., and Slogoff, S.: Neuropsychiatric complications after cardiopulmonary bypass: cerebral protection by a barbiturate. Anesthesiology, *64*:165, 1986.

115. Dundee, J.W., and Moore, J.: Thiopentone and methohexital: a comparison as main anesthetic agents for a standard operation. Anaesthesia, *16*:50, 1961.

116. King, E.: The treatment of army casualties in Hawaii. Army Med. Bull., *61*:18, 1942.

117. Knapp, R.B., and Dubow, H.S.: Diazepam as an induction agent for patients with cardiopulmonary disease. South Med. J., *63*:1451, 1970.

118. Knapp, R.B., and Dubow, H.: Comparison of diazepam with thiopental as an induction agent in cardiopulmonary disease. Anesth. Analg., *49*:722, 1970.

119. Crawford, M.E., Carl, P., Andersen, R.S. and Mikkelsen, B.O.: Comparison between midazolam and thiopentone-based balanced anaesthesia for day-care surgery. Br. J. Anaesth., *56*:165, 1984.

120. Reves, J.G., Vinik, R., Hirschfield, A.M., Holcomb, C., and Strong, S.: Midazolam compared with thiopentone as a hypnotic component in balanced anaesthesia: a randomized, double-blind study. Can. Anaesth. Soc. J., *26*:42, 1979.

121. Hoff, J.T., Smith, A.L., Hankinson, H.L., and Nielsen, S.L.: Barbiturate protection from cerebral infarction in primates. Stroke, *6*:28, 1975.

122. Michenfelder, J.D., and Milde, J.H.: Influence of anesthetics on metabolic, functional and pathologic responses to regional cerebral ischemia. Stroke, *6*:405, 1975.

123. Moseley, J.I., Laurent, J.P., and Molinari, G.F.: Barbiturate attenuation of the clinical course and pathological lesions in primate stroke model. Neurology, 25:870, 1975.

124. Smith, A.L., Hoff, J.T., Nielsen, S.L., and Larson, C.P.: Barbiturate protection in acute focal cerebral ischemia. Stroke, 5:1, 1974.

125. Steen, P.A., and Michenfelder, J.D.: Cerebral protection with barbiturates: relation to anesthetic effect. Stroke, 9:140, 1978.

126. Steen, P.A., and Michenfelder, J.D.: Barbiturate protection in tolerant and nontolerant hypoxic mice: comparison with hypothermic protection. Anesthesiology, 50:404, 1979.

127. Wilhljelm, B.J., and Arnfred, I.: Protective action of some anaesthetics against anoxia. Acta Pharmacol. Toxicol. (Copenh.), 22:93, 1965.

128. Christensen, J.H., and Andreasen, F.: Individual variation in response to thiopental. Acta Anaesthesiol. Scand., 22:303, 1978.

129. Brodie, B.B., Mark, L.C., Lief, P.A., Bernstein E., and Papper, E.M.: Acute tolerance to thiopental. J. Pharmacol. Exp. Ther., 102:215, 1978.

130. Stone, H.H., and Donnelly, C.C.: The accidental intraarterial injection of thiopental. Anesthesiology, 22:995, 1961.

131. Thomas, E.T.: The relative potencies of methohexitone and thiopentone. Anaesthesia, 22:16, 1967.

132. Clarke, R.S.J., Dundee, J.W., Barron, D.W., and McArdle, L.: Clinical studies of induction agents. XXVI: The relative potencies of thiopentone, methohexitone and propanidid. Br. J. Anaesth., 40:593, 1968.

133. Whitwam, J.G.: Editorial: Methohexitone. Br. J. Anaesth., 48:617, 1976.

134. Breimer, D.D.: Pharmacokinetics of methohexitone following intravenous infusion in humans. Br. J. Anaesth., 48:643, 1976.

135. Hudson, R.J., Stanski, D.R., and Burch, P.G.: Pharmacokinetics of methohexital and thiopental in surgical patients. Anesthesiology, 59:215, 1983.

136. Lui, L.M.P., Gaudreault, P., Friedman, P.A., Goudsouzian, N.G., and Liu, P.L.: Methohexital plasma concentrations in children following rectal administration. Anesthesiology, 62:567, 1985.

137. Korttila, K., Linnoila, M., Ertama, P., and Hakkinen, S.: Recovery and simulated driving after intravenous anesthesia with thiopental, methohexital, propanidid, or alphadione. Anesthesiology, 43:291, 1975.

138. Green R., Long, H.A., Elliott, C.J.R., and Howells, T.H.: A method of studying recovery after anaesthesia. Anaesthesia, 18:189, 1963.

139. Korttila, K., Ghoneim, M.M., Jacobs, L., and Lakes, R.S.: Evaluation of instrumented force platform as a test to measure residual effects of anesthetics. Anesthesiology, 55:625, 1981.

140. Choi, S.D., Spaulding, B.C., Gross, J.B., and Apfelbaum, J.L.: Comparison of the ventilatory effects of etomidate and methohexital. Anesthesiology, 62:442, 1985.

141. Hirshman, C.A., Edelstein, R.A., Ebertz, J.M., and Hanifin, J.M.: Thiobarbiturate-induced histamine release in human skin mast cells. Anesthesiology, 63:353, 1985.

142. Lamalle, D.: Cardiovascular effects of various anesthetics in man. Four short-acting intravenous anesthetics: althesin, etomidate, methohexital and propanidid. Acta Anaesthesiol. Belg., 27:208, 1976.

143. Prys-Roberts, C., Greene, L.T., Meloche, R., and Foex, P.: Studies of anaesthesia in relation to hypertension. II. Haemodynamic consequences of induction and endotracheal intubation. Br. J. Anaesth., 43:532, 1971.

144. Todd, M.M., Drummond, J.C., and U, H.S.: The hemodynamic consequences of high-dose methohexital anesthesia in humans. Anesthesiology, 61:495, 1984.

145. Dundee, J.W.: Intravenous anaesthetic agents. *In* Current Topics in Anaesthesia. Vol. 1. London, Edward, Arnold, 1979.

146. Verma, R., Ramasubramanian, R., and Sachar, R.M.: Anesthesia for termination of pregnancy: midazolam compared with methohexital. Anesth. Analg., 64:792, 1985.

147. Prys-Roberts, C.: Practical and pharmacological implications of continuous intravenous anesthesia. Acta Anaesthesiol. Belg., 3:225, 1980.

148. Doenicke, A., Kugler, J., Kalmar, L., Bezecny, H., Laub, M., Schmidinger, K., and Slavik, B.: Klinisch experimentelle, Untersuchungen mit Propanidid. Anaesthesist, 22:255, 1973.

149. Bernhoff, A., Eklund, B., and Kaijser, L.: Cardiovascular effects of short-term anaesthesia with methohexitone and propanidid in normal subjects. Br. J. Anaesth., 44:2, 1972.

Chapter 7

DISSOCIATIVE ANESTHESIA

HISTORY

Corssen and Domino introduced the concept of "dissociative anesthesia," a peculiar state of unconsciousness in which the patient is in a cataleptic state, "disconnected" from the surroundings and able to undergo surgery in comfort and without recall.[1] The first agent to achieve these goals was phencyclidine [1-(1-phenylcyclohexylpiperidine], also known as CI-395, PCP, Sernyl, and Sernylan (Fig. 7–1). Sernyl was synthesized by Maddox, and after basic studies by Chen, et al., the drug was introduced clinically by Greifenstein, et al. and Johnstone, et al.[2–5] Unfortunately, an unacceptably high incidence of post-anesthetic hallucinations and delirium reactions precluded further use of the drug in the operating room. Curiously, these side-effects seem minimal in young children, elderly patients, and animals. Sernyl is used successfully in veterinary anesthesia. The drug is also widely distributed as a street drug of abuse (PCP and Angel Dust).

Cyclohexamine or CI-400 (Fig. 7–2), a congener of phencyclidine (N-ethyl-1-phenylcyclohexylamine), was then studied clinically by Lear, et al.[6] When compared to PCP, cyclohexamine was less effective in producing satisfactory anal-

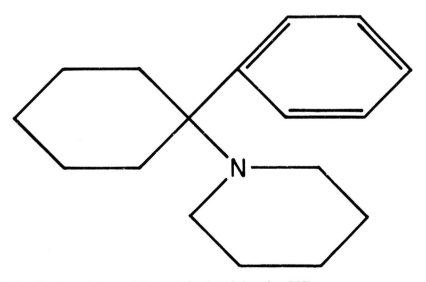

Fig. 7–1. Structure of phencyclidine (CI-395, Sernyl, Sernylan, PCP).

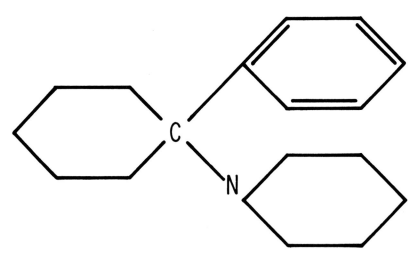

Fig. 7–2. Structure of cyclohexamine (CI-400).

gesia; the emergence delirium and other psychic disturbances were at least as serious as with PCP. The use of cyclohexamine too has been discontinued.

The next dissociative agent was ketamine (2-(*o*-chlorophenyl)-2-(methylamino)cyclohexanone), another of more than 200 congeners of phencyclidine, also known as CI-581, Ketalar, and Ketaject (Fig. 7–3). After preliminary studies in animals were conducted by McCarthy, et al., Chang, et al., and Chen, et al., Domino, Chodoff, and Corssen explored the pharmacologic effects of ketamine in humans;[7–10] Corssen, et al., first administered the drug clinically.[1] Since then, ketamine has been critically evaluated by anesthesiologists and other scientists around the world and a vast body of literature has been accumulated describing this drug as a new, "different," and possibly safer anesthetic agent.

Because ketamine is an optically active drug currently supplied as a racemic mixture (i.e., equal parts) of its component stereoisomers (Fig. 7–4), it seemed worthwhile to compare the effects of the separate isomers in animals and in

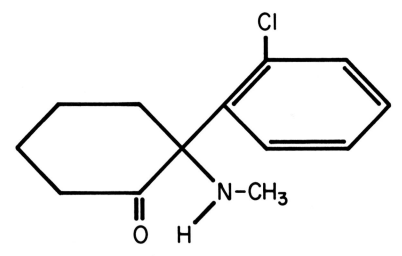

Fig. 7–3. Structure of ketamine (CI-581, Ketalar, Ketaject).

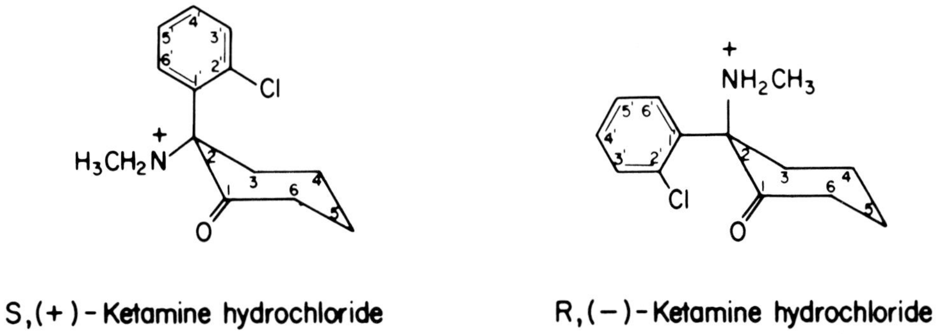

S,(+)-Ketamine hydrochloride   **R,(−)-Ketamine hydrochloride**

Fig. 7–4. Stereoisomers of ketamine.

man.[11-16] The S(+)-ketamine isomer seems to share most of the physical and pharmacologic properties of racemic ketamine, including water solubility, compatibility with human tissues, and rapid onset of action, and causing blood pressure elevation, minimal respiratory depression, analgesia, and anesthesia. When compared to both the parent racemate and the R(-) isomer, however, the S(+) isomer causes less spontaneous motor activity and tachycardia during anesthesia, is more potent, and is followed by fewer psychic emergence reactions without excitement or delirium.[16] The incidence of postoperative pain is minimal and the level of patient acceptability is maximal with S(+)-ketamine.[16] Parallelism of the plasma decay curves of racemic ketamine and its two stereoisomers, as well as similarities in the patterns of appearance and excretion of the ketamine metabolites for all these preparations, suggest that the differences between the isomers are due to pharmacodynamic factors rather than to pharmacokinetic variations. Whether these findings will affect future clinical practice remains to be seen.[17]

Finally, the chemically different dissociative agent CL-1848C (etoxadrol; (+)-2-(2-ethyl-2-phenyl-1,3-dioxolan-4-yl)-piperidine) (Fig. 7–5) was studied clinically by Wilson, et al., Traber, et al., and Kelly, et al., who found the drug more potent, less toxic, and longer acting than ketamine.[18-20] In addition, these authors

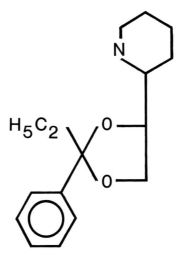

Fig. 7–5. Structure of etoxadrol.

observed that etoxadrol relaxes smooth muscles and causes less random movements; however, because this agent is not yet available for widespread clinical use, its relative merit vis-a-vis clinical anesthesia has still to be established.

DISSOCIATIVE ANESTHESIA AND KETAMINE

Chemistry, Physical Properties, and Available Preparations

Ketamine, with a molecular weight of 238 and a pKa of 7.5, is a white, crystalline salt and is soluble in water up to 20%. The solution is clear, colorless, and stable at room temperature. Available pharmaceutic preparations are slightly acidic (pH 3.5 to 5.5), and are formulated for intravenous or intramuscular injection in concentrations containing the equivalent of 10, 50, or 100 mg of ketamine base per milliliter, with phemerol (benzethonium chloride) (1:10,000) used as a preservative. The 10 mg/ml solution is made isotonic with sodium chloride.

Tissue Compatibility

Results of local toleration studies in various animal species revealed that concentrations of ketamine intended for intravenous or intramuscular administration were well tolerated by arteries, veins, and muscles.[21] In human volunteers and in clinical patients, neither venous complications, such as thrombophlebitis or phlebothrombosis with intravenous administration, nor local irritation or induration with intramuscular injections of ketamine were encountered.

PHARMACOKINETIC

Uptake and Distribution

Peak plasma levels of ketamine are reached immediately after intravenous administration and within 5 minutes of intramuscular injection.[22] Because of its high lipid solubility, ketamine, as with thiopental, initially floods into the brain and other highly perfused organs, being distributed more slowly to less well-perfused tissues.[23] Ten minutes after ketamine was delivered intravenously to rats, nearly 70% of the total amount of the drug was found in skeletal muscle, gut, liver, and skin.[24] Fat and other vessel-poor tissues are the last to equilibrate with the falling plasma level.[25] The $t\frac{1}{2}$ α, or distribution phase, of ketamine in man is approximately 11 minutes, whereas the $t\frac{1}{2}$ β, or elimination phase, may range from $2\frac{1}{2}$ to 4 hours or more.[26,27] Redistribution of ketamine from the brain and other vital organs to more poorly vascularized tissues, as with thiopental, is undoubtedly the key factor in terminating its central nervous system (CNS) depression; speed of biotransformation is of secondary importance.[23] Duration of hypnosis is not affected by either induction or inhibition of the enzymes involved.[23,24]

Placental Transfer

Although results of studies in animals (dogs and monkeys) show appreciable concentrations of ketamine in fetal blood and tissues 50 to 90 minutes after its administration to the mother, placental transfer of this highly lipid-soluble drug is actually much swifter.[28–30] Indeed, there is no barrier to the free passage of ketamine across the human placenta; rapid fetal uptake and excessive depression of the neonate were noted after full doses of ketamine (2.0 to 2.2 mg/kg intravenously) were delivered to mothers in preparation for vaginal or cesarean delivery.[31–33] Predictably, as with thiopental, the fetus is protected from adverse effects of lesser doses of ketamine (0.2 to 1.0 mg/kg intravenously) given to its mother during labor by a combination of factors: rapid decline in maternal drug levels, uterine contractions, cord compression, nonhomogeneity of blood in the intervillous space, extraction by the fetal liver, and progressive dilution and shunting in the fetal circulation.[34]

Metabolism

Microsomal enzymes residing in the endoplasmic reticulum of the liver mediate the biotransformation of ketamine in several stages (Fig. 7–6).[35] The first step is *N*-demethylation to form norketamine (metabolite I; Fig. 7–6). Norketamine is then hydroxylated at either of two positions in the cyclohexanone ring to form the hydroxy-norketamine metabolites III and IV. These metabolites are then either conjugated with glucuronic acid (not shown in Fig. 7–6) or dehydrated to form a cyclohexene derivative (metabolite II). Ketamine itself may also undergo ring hydroxylation directly, i.e., without prior *N*-demethylation (also not shown). The potency of norketamine (metabolite I) is reportedly 10 to 33% that of ketamine and metabolite II, and 1% that of ketamine, neither contributing significantly to the pharmacologic effects of the parent drug.[28]

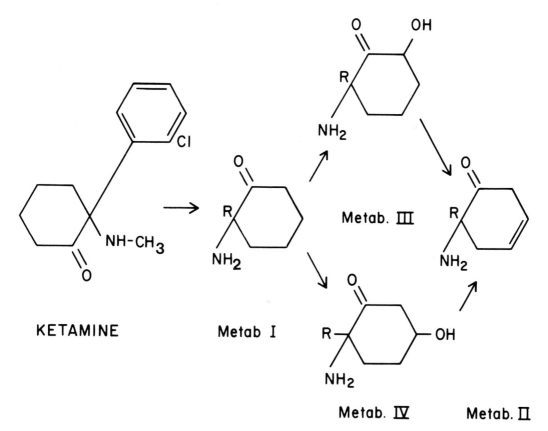

Fig. 7–6. Biotransformation of ketamine. (Modified from Chang, T., and Glazko, A.J.: Biotransformation and disposition of ketamine. Int. Anesthesiol. Clin., *12*:157, 1974.)

As with many drugs, ketamine induces its own metabolism by stimulating the enzymes involved, but, as noted previously, this ability does not alter its duration of action.[23,24] Indeed, because induction requires maintenance of an adequate concentration of the inducing agent in the liver cells for a minimum period of time, a short-acting drug (e.g., ketamine) causes induction in man only after repeated administration.[36] Thus, an acute tolerance to ketamine, noted in animals and attributed to enzyme induction, has not been found in man.

Halothane slows the distribution and redistribution of ketamine and, less importantly, also inhibits its metabolic breakdown; its action is thereby prolonged.[37] Conversely, even at subhypnotic dose levels, ketamine increases the amount of halothane required for anesthesia.[23] Similarly, equipotent doses of other sedatives (diazepam, hydroxyzine, and secobarbital) cause identical prolongation of sleep time after ketamine because of prolongation of its elimination half-life.[38] Presumably, the actions of these drugs are pharmacologically additive.

Excretion

Although results of balance studies in rats receiving tritium-labeled ketamine demonstrate that most of the radioactivity was traced to the urine and feces, the measurements do not discriminate between the parent drug and its metabolites, and hence are moot.[28] Also inconclusive are the findings of prolonged sleep time with ketamine and elevated plasma levels of ketamine and its N-demethylated metabolite after ligation of the common bile duct in rats, invalidating excretion as a major mechanism in man.[39] One must be wary of species differences. Indeed, in rhesus monkeys receiving tritium-labeled ketamine, 94 to 96% of the radioactivity appeared in the urine within 24 hours of injection; fecal excretion accounted for less than 2% of the dose. Even in one monkey with a bile fistula, only 8.6% of the radioactivity was retrieved in the bile within 24 hours, whereas more than 90% appeared in the urine.[36] These findings are not compatible with a biliary mechanism, whatever the identity of the molecules recovered.

PHARMACOLOGY

Central Nervous System (CNS)

The onset of anesthesia is somewhat slower with ketamine than with the ultra-short-acting barbiturates. The end point of onset of sleep is not clearly defined with ketamine. As the patient enters the dissociative state, the eyes open widely and horizontal or vertical nystagmus appears. The eyeballs then become centered in a fixed gaze as the patient enters a state of pharmacologic isolation. The characteristic facial expression is that of being "disconnected" from the surroundings, rather than of being asleep (Fig. 7–7). With full doses of ketamine (1 to 2 mg/kg intravenously), there is a latent period of 15 to 30 seconds, occasionally as many as 50 to 60 seconds, before consciousness is lost and analgesia begins.

In the dissociative state, the pupils, moderately dilated, react promptly to light. The corneal reflex is intact; lacrimation, eye blinking, and salivation are common. Laryngeal, pharyngeal, and other protective reflexes, such as coughing, sneezing, and swallowing, are active, even enhanced. The patellar and Achilles reflexes are hyperactive. Muscle tone is usually increased in the neck, the extremities, the muscles of mastication, and the intraoral musculature, particularly the

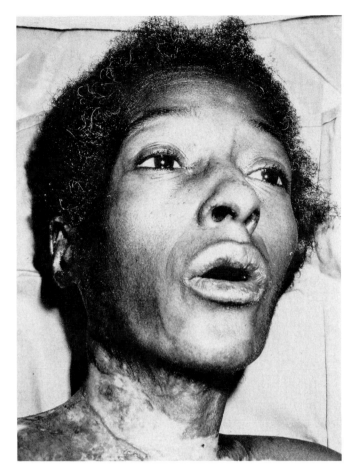

Fig. 7-7. Facial expression as dissociation is achieved.

tongue, which invariably shows distinct fibrillatory activity. Purposeless movements of the extremities that are unrelated to painful stimuli may occur. Respiration may be slightly depressed, but ventilatory assistance is rarely needed; manual support of the chin is occasionally needed to maintain a patent airway.

ANALGESIA

Ketamine produces excellent analgesia of skin, bones, and joints. For reasons that remain unclear, however, this agent is only partially effective in controlling pain from mucous membranes and viscera. Its usefulness as the sole anesthetic in operations involving body cavities, the tracheobronchial tree, or the genito-urinary system is thus limited. In these instances, adequate visceral analgesia usually requires supplementary use of conventional anesthetics (e.g., nitrous oxide). Analgesia precedes loss of consciousness, as first noted in a volunteer who, while still awake, was unaware of being pinched with a towel clip. Other investigators have since confirmed that at certain dosage levels of ketamine, analgesia may occur independent of loss of consciousness.[40–42]

Correspondingly, analgesia usually outlasts return of consciousness, as in burn patients who are alert but pain-free after recovering from ketamine anesthesia.[43–46]

Ketamine thus differs from the barbiturates in not causing analgesia at very low plasma levels.[41] When comparing the duration of postoperative analgesia caused by ketamine and fentanyl when these two drugs were used as intraoperative supplements for nitrous oxide-oxygen relaxant anesthesia, postoperative analgesia in the group of patients given ketamine lasted 282 minutes, whereas those patients receiving fentanyl experienced 177 minutes of postoperative analgesia.[47]

The discrepancy between analgesia and anesthesia correlates well with plasma levels of ketamine, analgesia being associated with concentrations of 100 to 150 μg/ml and anesthesia with 640 to 1000 μg/ml.[48]

DURATION OF ANESTHESIA

Ketamine is a relatively short-acting agent, the effects of which are, of course, dose dependent. An intravenous injection of 0.1 mg/kg causes no significant

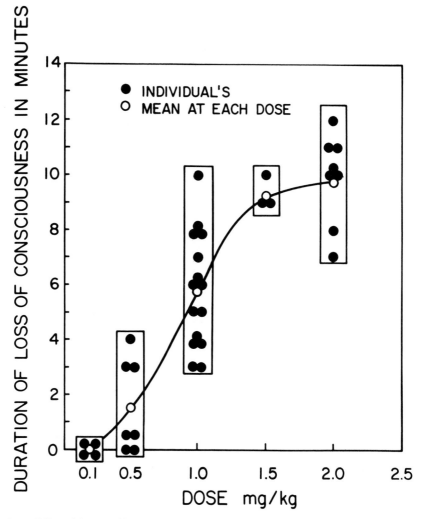

Fig. 7–8.   Effect of dosage of ketamine on duration of coma. (From Domino, E.F., Chodoff, P., and Corssen, G.: Pharmacologic effects of CI-581, a new dissociative anesthetic in man. Clin. Pharmacol. Ther., 6:279, 1965.)

alteration of sensorium (Fig. 7–8). It seems that 0.5 mg/kg (intravenous dose) is a threshold dose at which 50% of the patient population become unconscious. At a dose of 1 mg/kg, unconsciousness lasts 3 to 10 minutes, with a mean of 5.8 minutes, whereas at 2 mg/kg, the mean duration is about 10 minutes (Fig. 7–8). Duration can be extended for more prolonged procedures with additional injections of one half or less of the initial dosage.[10]

When injected intramuscularly, higher doses (5 to 10 mg/kg) of ketamine are required; onset of anesthesia is delayed 1½ to 3 minutes as the drug is absorbed from the intramuscular depot. To hasten absorption and the onset of dissociative anesthesia, one half of the dose may be injected into each deltoid or gluteus muscle. This action will ordinarily provide 20 to 40 minutes of anesthesia; again, more prolonged loss of consciousness and analgesia require supplemental intramuscular injections at one half or less of the initial intramuscular dose. Neither acute tolerance nor tachyphylaxis is encountered; each successive injection produces approximately the same period of anesthesia.

Recovery may, however, be delayed by the administration of supplemental doses, suggesting some cumulative effect. Chronic tolerance may develop, requiring some increase in dosage after repeated administrations, as noted in patients undergoing multiple sessions of radiotherapy requiring immobilization or innumerable dressing changes for extensive burns.[46,49–51]

RECOVERY

During awakening, the patient initially appears detached and unaware of the surroundings, and tends to relapse repeatedly into superficial sleep periods. In a peaceful environment, if the patient is left undisturbed by the attending personnel, emergence from the dissociative state to full alertness is usually uneventful. Consciousness returns within approximately 10 to 15 minutes after a single dose of ketamine (2 mg/kg intravenously). Spontaneous closing of the eyes usually heralds the return to consciousness; shortly thereafter, the patient can respond to questions. Analgesia and some slurred speech continue for a few minutes after verbal contact has been re-established. Orientation as to person, time, and place returns within 15 to 30 minutes after administration of the single dose.[52,53]

The time required for full recovery depends on several factors: route of administration; intravenous technique (continuous drip or intermittent injections); type of preanesthetic medication (sedatives, hypnotics, tranquilizers, and narcotic-analgesics); other concurrent medication, including concomitant use of various anesthetic agents; and the patient's age and physical status. Full recovery is itself subject to interpretation.[10] Ketamine has consequently been classified as both long and short acting.[54,55] Ketamine can be truly short acting when effective doses are given intravenously in only one or two injections, and the use of adjunctive agents is avoided or kept to a minimum, as in anesthesia for outpatient surgery (see subsequent discussion). Thus, full recovery, permitting discharge of outpatients accompanied by a responsible adult or return of hospital patients to their ward or private room, usually occurs within 1 hour, although a delay of 2 hours or more may follow repeated doses or the administration of adjunctive drugs. Children and young to middle-aged adults tend to recover more rapidly than elderly patients. Pediatric outpatients can often be discharged within 30 to 60 minutes of completion of the procedure, because restoration of full equilibrium and visual acuity is not essential prior to the release of the child in the care of a responsible adult.[56] Blurring of vision and inability to focus may persist for several hours before complete return of visual function and restoration of equilibrium.[54,57,58] Some patients feel fatigued and want to rest, even bluntly stating they wish to be left alone. Re-establishment of alpha rhythm in the electroencephalogram (EEG) may require 30 to 60 minutes.[9,10]

EEG EFFECTS

The sequence of EEG changes produced by ketamine differs sharply from the well-known progression of EEG effects noted with the use of thiopental and inhaled anesthetics. With all of the latter preparations, the random EEG activity at rest changes to fast-wave activity (10 to 30 Hz) of moderate amplitude (75 to 80 μV) while the patient is still awake, to high voltage (100 to 200 μV), slow (2 to 6 Hz) waves with some interspersed alpha activity (10 Hz) as consciousness is lost, to periods of burst suppression or electric silence (i.e., flattening of the EEG tracing) of increasingly longer duration as depression deepens.

The EEG changes after introduction of ketamine are different.[9,10,59] In anesthetic doses, its characteristic effect is to induce "theta" activity in the EEG, i.e., slow (4 to 7 Hz) waves of moderate to high amplitude (50 to 150 μV) (Figs. 7–9 to 7–11). Figure 7–9 is an illustration of the transition to theta waves that appeared within 30 to 40 seconds of the beginning of a 2.2 mg/kg intravenous injection of ketamine in a 10-year-old child; loss of consciousness and absence of response to painful stimuli coincided with this transition. Although theta rhythm was recorded from all leads, the frontal and central regions of the cerebral cortex in children seem to be affected earlier and more intensely than the parietal and posterior cortical areas. Thus, 2 minutes later, theta activity was still predominant in the frontal and central cortex (Fig. 7–10). Curiously, adult responses seem somewhat different. In Figure 7–11, the upper left panel shows EEG tracings recorded from the frontal, central, parietal, and occipital cortex. The upper right panel shows theta rhythm in an adult volunteer noted 6 minutes after delivery of an effective sleep dose of ketamine (1.5 mg/kg intravenously). This activity, present in all leads, was somewhat more prominent in the parietal area. Four minutes later (lower left panel), with recovery of consciousness but persistence of analgesia, theta waves were replaced by low voltage, fast-wave activity, but no alpha waves. Indeed, even after analgesia disappeared and the subject was fully awake, alpha rhythm did not return, nor was it re-established until at least 30 to 60 minutes after drug injection (Fig. 7–11, lower right panel). Other studies of EEG alterations during dissociative anesthesia with ketamine in children showed theta waves decreased in amplitude and interspersed with waves of faster frequency as the patients began to respond to painful stimuli. Apparently with ketamine, theta waves signal the presence of full analgesia, and alpha waves indicate its absence. Similarly, theta activity and analgesia persist together in the early recovery period after cyclopropane anesthesia, thus validating the correlation.[60–62]

Another interesting difference, related to age, but unrelated to ketamine, was apparent in the EEG. During the control period, the adult volunteers, presumably mentally relaxed, invariably displayed alpha rhythm in all leads, especially in the occipital area. During the same period, most of the pediatric patients exhibited low-voltage, fast-wave activity, with minimal alpha rhythm.

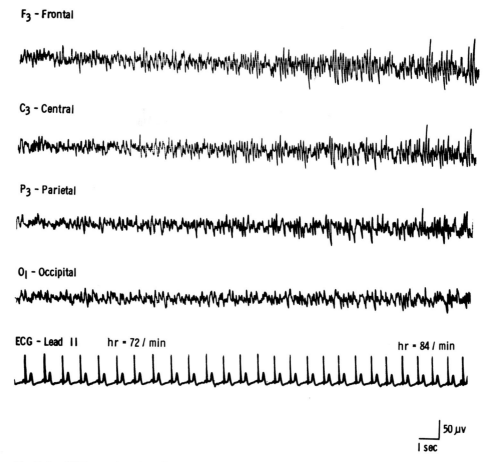

F₃ - Frontal

C₃ - Central

P₃ - Parietal

O₁ - Occipital

ECG - Lead II   hr = 72 / min   hr = 84 / min

50 μv
1 sec

Fig. 7–9. EEG recording from frontal, central (temporal), parietal, and occipital cortex of a 10-year-old boy 20 seconds after ketamine delivery (2.2 mg/kg intravenously). Note transition from low-voltage, fast-wave activity to theta waves, especially in frontal and temporal cortex. (From Corssen, G., Hayward, J.R., Gunter, J.W., and Groves, E.H.: A new parenteral anesthetic for oral surgery. J. Oral Maxillofac. Surg., 27:627, 1969.)

EVOKED RESPONSES

A light flashed into the eyes produces electric activity in the CNS called the visually evoked response (VER). By using computer programs to average background "noise" in the EEG from the occipital region, the VER can then be identified as a series of waves (numbered 1 to 6).[63] In the "control" portion of Figure 7–12, note especially the highest peak (no. 3) and the deepest trough (no. 4), followed by an afterdischarge, the frequency of which resembles alpha rhythm (10 Hz).

The effects of a sleep dose of ketamine on the VER (Fig. 7–12) resemble those previously observed with the use of secobarbital: flattening of wave 3, deepening and broadening of wave 4, and abolition of the afterdischarge, in keeping with the disappearance of alpha waves from the EEG.[64] At awakening, waves 3 and 4 are present but are somewhat depressed, and the afterdischarge is still absent; full recovery requires at least 1 hour. Ketamine similarly affects acoustic evoked responses, as demonstrated by Giesen, et al., in a study in children.[65] In contrast,

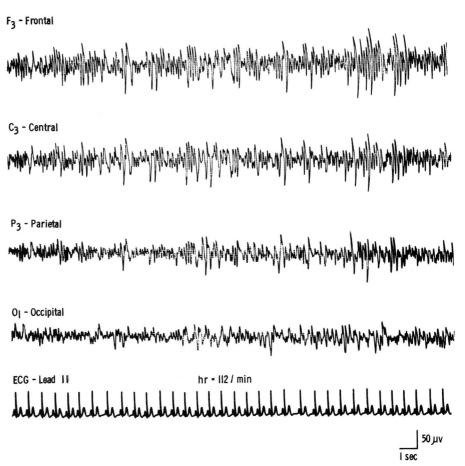

Fig. 7–10. Same as in Fig. 7–9, 2 minutes after ketamine. Theta waves predominate in frontal and temporal cortex.

the somatosensory evoked response (SER) recorded from the post-Rolandic region during electric stimulation of the contralateral median nerve shows enhancement of all components and little effect on afterdischarge after delivery of the same sleep dose of ketamine (Fig. 7–13).[10] This finding is interesting, in view of the ability of the drug to produce subjective numbness without impairment of touch sensation.[10] Thirty minutes to 2 hours after injection are required for the SER to return to a normal level.

NERVE CONDUCTION

Ketamine alters sodium conductance in giant squid axons, causing a marked rise in intracellular sodium levels.[66] The resultant depolarizing action, blocking of nerve conduction, may contribute to the central effects of ketamine.[66]

MECHANISMS OF KETAMINE ANESTHESIA

The diffuse thalamo-neocortical projection system (corresponding to the upper "extralemniscal" pathways) is a primary site of action of ketamine.[67] During induction of anesthesia, this drug differs uniquely from classic anesthetics in its

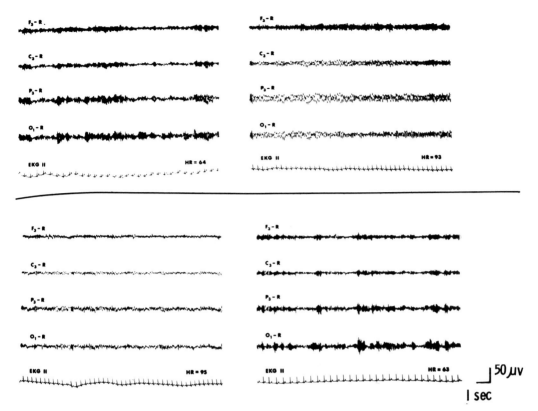

Fig. 7–11. EEG effects of ketamine (1.5 mg/kg intravenously) in an adult volunteer. Key: F_3-R = frontal; C_3-R = central; P_3-R = parietal; O_1-R = occipital; left upper panel-pre-injection (control); right upper panel-6 minutes post-injection (unresponsive); left lower panel-10 minutes post-injection (conscious, analgesic); right lower panel-42 minutes post-injection (fully recovered). (From Domino, E.F., Chodoff, P., and Corssen, G.: Pharmacologic effects of CI-581, a new dissociative anesthetic in man. Clin. Pharmacol. Ther., 6:279, 1965.)

ability to depress parts of the cortex (especially association areas) and thalamus, while simultaneously activating parts of the limbic system, including the hippocampus, in a functional disorganization of nonspecific pathways in midbrain and thalamic areas.[68,69] This dissociation between the thalamo-neocortical and the limbic systems also appears prominently during emergence from ketamine anesthesia. Dissociative effects even occur within the neocortical regions, with delta wave activity prominent in the somatosensory and association areas, but not in the auditory and visual cortex.[67,70] Again, VERs are unaffected in the visual cortex when they are significantly suppressed in the centromedial thalamus.[70]

Similarly, VERs and SERs from tooth-pulp stimulation indicate that anesthetic doses of ketamine do not impair afferent signals presumably traveling via spinoreticular tracts to cortical areas (lower "extralemniscal" pathways) concerned with the affective-emotional components of pain perception. This finding suggests that "sensory isolation" during ketamine anesthesia is produced within the brain, presumably through depression of cortical association areas: afferent impulses reach the cortex but are not interpreted and hence do not trigger the appropriate responses to visual, auditory, or painful stimuli.[10] The ability to localize somatic pain stimulus, however, seems relatively unimpaired by subanesthetic, analgesic doses of ketamine, in keeping with the highly selective depressant action of

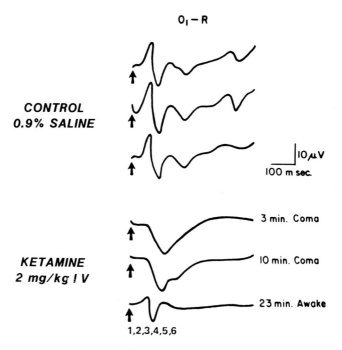

Fig. 7–12.   Effects of ketamine on visually evoked response (VER). (From Domino, E.F., Chodoff, P., and Corssen, G.: Pharmacologic effects of CI-581, a new dissociative anesthetic in man. Clin. Pharmacol. Ther., 6:279, 1965.)

ketamine observed on the medullary reticular formation, a known relay station for transmission of affective-emotional components of nociception from the spinal cord to the cerebral cortex.[71]

Other selective effects of ketamine include a demonstrated greater sensitivity of auditory evoked responses than of VERs to ketamine, which corresponds to findings of significant depression by ketamine of regional glucose utilization in the medial geniculate and inferior colliculus (primary auditory nuclei), but not in the lateral geniculate or superior colliculus (visual relay nuclei).[72–74] Elsewhere, e.g., in the limbic system (especially the hippocampus and cingulate gyrus), local cerebral glucose utilization is sharply increased with ketamine use, corresponding to reports of strong stimulation of this system by this drug.[52,67]

All of these findings are in accord with the peculiar state of dissociation induced by ketamine, characterized by auditory and somatosensory deprivation superimposed on a metabolically disorganized but still active CNS. In fact, the intense activity of the hippocampus may account in part for the excitatory manifestations, even seizures associated with ketamine, which in turn inhibit auditory, visual, and other sensory systems.[75,76] Thus, loss of consciousness during ketamine anesthesia and during petit mal seizures may result from the same mechanism.[76]

It seems overly simplistic to label ketamine as a cataleptic CNS excitant (along with nitrous oxide, enflurane, and γ-hydroxybutyrate), as opposed to a CNS depressant (such as halothane, thiopental, and ether).[77–79] This two-category classification of anesthetic agents ignores the fact that (1) numerous mechanisms exist to regulate the delicate balance between excitatory and inhibitory neurons; (2) CNS excitation can result indirectly from drug-induced depression of inhib-

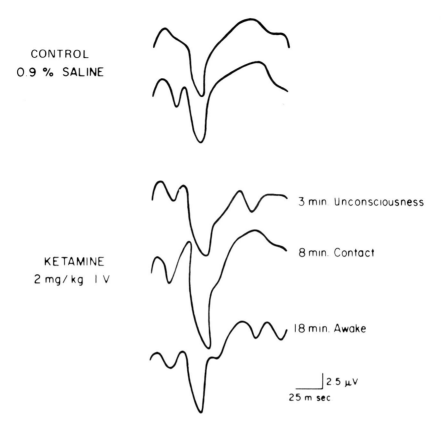

CONTROL
0.9 % SALINE

KETAMINE
2 mg/kg I V

3 min. Unconsciousness

8 min. Contact

18 min. Awake

25 µV
25 m sec

Fig. 7–13. Effects of ketamine on somatosensory evoked response (SER). (From Domino, E.F., Chodoff, P., and Corssen, G.: Pharmacologic effects of CI-581, a new dissociative anesthetic in man. Clin. Pharmacol. Ther., 6:279, 1965.)

itory mechanisms; and (3) CNS "depressant" anesthetics are all capable of excitation or activation of CNS function as manifested by spikelike EEG activity that resembles seizure discharges, especially during light anesthesia with the brain at a critical level of depression.[80]

Validation of the hypothesis that ketamine produces anesthesia by dissociating the cerebral cortex from the limbic system requires that there be an intact, functioning cortex. This requirement can explain reports of failure to produce analgesia with ketamine in patients with congenital or acquired cortical defects.[81,82] On the other hand, successful anesthesia with ketamine in a hydranencephalic infant with no cortex suggests that seizure-like activity in the brainstem alone, as with petit mal seizures, might contribute to alterations in level of consciousness and response to pain in normal individuals.[83] Lower sites in the spinal cord may also be involved in the analgesic action of ketamine. The drug suppresses neuronal unit activity in laminae I and V of the dorsal horn, which respond to noxious stimuli, but not in laminae IV and VI;[84,85] the response of these neurons to innocuous tactile stimuli was unaffected.[85]

Another intriguing explanation of the analgesic action of ketamine, even in subhypnotic doses, is that it acts as an agonist of opiate receptors in the brain and spinal cord.[86–88] This action, antagonized by naloxone, may also be caused by a release of endorphins, but researchers who conducted various binding studies confirmed a direct interaction of ketamine with opiate receptors.[86–88] The descending inhibitory neuronal pathway from the periaqueductal pathway to the spinal cord does not contribute to its antinociceptive action.[89] Another possibility is based on the observation that ketamine inhibits acetylcholinesterase activity in mammalian brain.[90] Reduction of acetylcholine turnover rates in subcortical structures, such as the caudate nucleus and the hippocampus, during ketamine anesthesia suggests that acetylcholine utilization may be related to anesthetic-induced electrophysiologic changes in these regions of the brain.[91] Conversely, prejunctional release of acetylcholine in the CNS, induced by the curare antagonist 4-aminopyridine, may be the mechanism by which this drug terminates the CNS-depressant effects of ketamine.[92] Both 4-aminopyridine and physostigmine can significantly shorten post-anesthetic recovery without psychologic upset or impairment of analgesia.[93–98]

Cardiovascular System

Almost unique among anesthetics (except for the now outmoded cyclopropane and diethyl ether), ketamine is a cardiovascular stimulant that causes increases in heart rate, blood pressure, cardiac output, and central venous pressure.[1,10,54,55,99] These effects are clearly mediated by activation of the sympathetic nervous system, the inactivation of which, by total epidural blockade or by ganglionic blockade with hexamethonium, not only abolishes the ketamine-induced pressor effect but also produces a depressor response.[100–102] The role of central stimulation is also verified when ketamine is injected directly into the cerebral circulation by an intracarotid route with resultant prompt increases in blood pressure, heart rate, and cardiac output; peripheral depression of baroceptors, however, may be an alternate mechanism.[103,104] Ketamine also inhibits the re-uptake of norepinephrine in isolated, perfused animal hearts, thereby contributing to its sympathomimetic action in vivo.[105]

Findings from other studies of central adrenergic effects show that ketamine itself, like thiopental, exerts a direct, dose-related depressant action on the isolated heart muscle or the intact heart in vitro.[102,104,106–115] Indeed, this direct depressant effect may account for the biphasic action of ketamine sometimes encountered in vivo with a transient initial decrease in blood pressure (not blocked by atropine) preceding the more usual sustained increase (Fig. 7–14).[7,116] Note that reversal of ketamine-induced arterial hypertension (but not tachycardia) in man by the calcium antagonist verapamil suggests that ketamine stimulates the myocardium by increasing the availability of calcium across myocardial and Purkinje cell membranes.[117] Despite this supposition, direct infusion of ketamine into the left main coronary artery in a concentration similar to the peak level, subsequent to a bolus intravenous injection, produces a negative inotropic effect that recovers fully upon termination of the infusion.[113]

Coincident with the direct myocardial depressant effect of ketamine, an anti-arrhythmic effect was demonstrated against epinephrine-induced arrhythmias during halothane anesthesia in dogs (Fig. 7–15) and in surgical patients (Fig. 7–16).[104,118] Ketamine has also been proved effective in reversing arrhythmias caused by digitalis toxicity.[119] Curiously, larger intravenous doses of ketamine (e.g., 6 mg/kg in dogs) may render the myocardium sensitive to catechol-

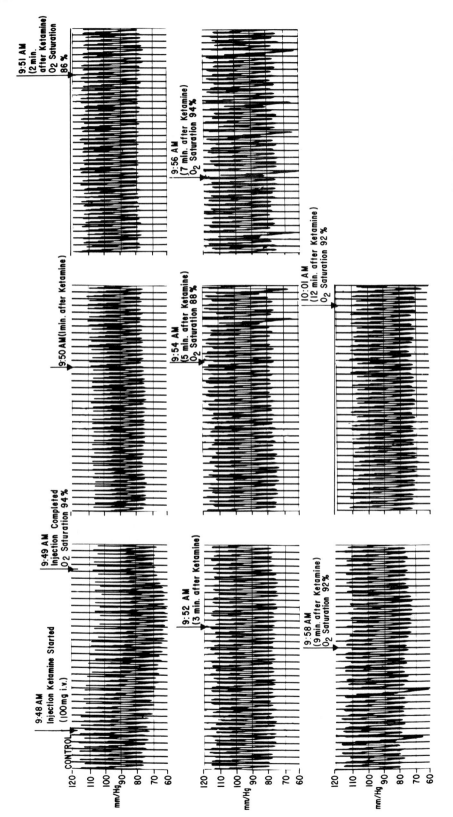

Fig. 7–14. Biphasic action of ketamine on blood pressure: transient initial decline followed by sustained rise (G. Corssen, unpublished data).

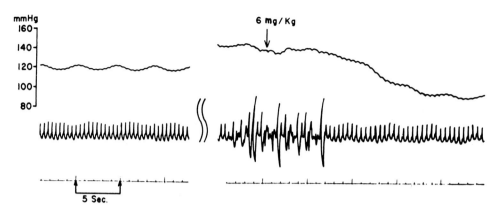

Fig. 7–15. Antiarrhythmic effect of ketamine (6 mg/kg intravenously) on halothane-epinephrine ventricular arrhythmia in a dog. Top-mean femoral arterial pressure; middle-EKG; bottom-time in seconds. (From Dowdy, E.G., and Kaya, K.: Studies of the mechanism of cardiovascular response to CI-581. Anesthesiology, 29:931, 1968.)

amines.[120,121] The arrhythmogenic effect is transient, lasting only 10 to 12 minutes after a bolus intravenous injection of ketamine.

The cardiovascular stimulant effect of ketamine administered peripherally increases the work of the heart, hence myocardial oxygen consumption rises. This rise is connected with a parallel increase in coronary blood flow, although earlier reports claimed that the augmented supply of oxygen to the heart may be insufficient to meet the metabolic demands of the myocardium caused by the ketamine-induced increase of the rate-pressure product and cardiac work.[122–127]

PERIPHERAL CIRCULATION

As with the heart, a dual action occurs in the peripheral vascular beds. Direct local dilatation is countered by sympathetically mediated vasoconstriction, so systemic vascular resistance is essentially unchanged or is slightly decreased.[112,128–130] Cerebral vascular resistance is unchanged or is decreased.[112,130–132]

CEREBRAL CIRCULATION

Ketamine increases cerebral blood flow (CBF) by as much as 62 to 80%, with return to normal values after 20 to 30 minutes, pari passu with the changes in arterial blood pressure.[133,134] Early findings to the contrary from studies in dogs may be related to methodology, whereas other researchers reported a slight decrease in CBF after ketamine injection during nitrous oxide-halothane anesthesia.[135–137] In any case, it is generally agreed that CBF does increase with ketamine use.[138–150] The rise has been attributed both to cerebral vasodilatation, with decreased cerebral vascular resistance, and to increased cerebral oxygen consumption ($CMRO_2$) but the role of each has been questioned.[133,134] Marked variability in regional CBF (rCBF) was observed in neurologic patients with the aid of [133]xenon; some individuals showed sharp rises in the frontotemporal region, whereas others showed these changes in the parieto-occipital regions.[141]

These observations are incompatible with the knowledge of a direct, general vasodilating effect of ketamine; therefore it is possible that ketamine increases global CBF indirectly by stimulating regional neuronal activity, which in turn

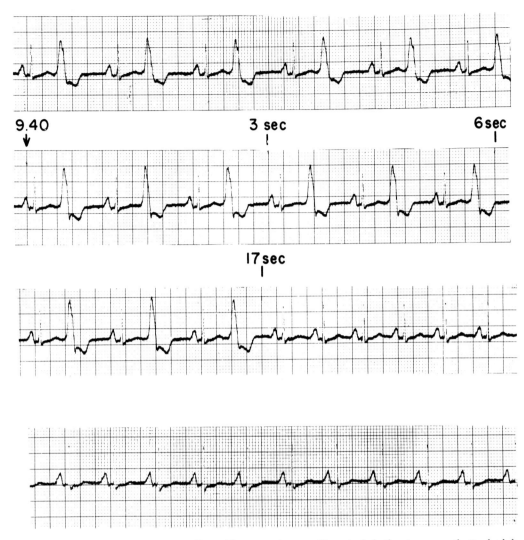

Fig. 7–16. Antiarrhythmic effect of ketamine in man. Bigeminal rhythm in unanesthetized adult patient abolished by ketamine (2.0 mg/kg intravenously) starting at arrow; 17 seconds later, after one half of the dose is received, sinus rhythm is restored.

increases regional $CMRO_2$ and regional CBF.[141] Concomitant elevation of CSF pressure can be reversed by hyperventilation, which indicates that the cerebral vessels remain responsive to changes in $Paco_2$ during ketamine anesthesia.[151] Another group of investigators found no significant change with ketamine use in man in any of three measured indices of cerebral metabolism: $CMRO_2$, CMR glucose, and CMR lactate.[133] Other researchers reported findings in dogs that included a 16% increase in $CMRO_2$, data hardly adequate to explain a concomitant 80% rise in CBF.[134] In addition, results of studies of local CMR glucose levels in rats anesthetized with ketamine by using the $2[^{14}C]$-deoxyglucose method showed sharp increases (70%) in the cingulate gyrus and hippocampus; moderate increases (20 to 40%) in the extrapyramidal system and corpus callosum, coupled with reductions (40%) in sensorimotor and auditory cortex, medial geniculate, and inferior colliculus; and no significant changes in 22 other structures that were monitored (Table 7–1).[73,74] Although these data may explain both the sensory deprivation (inhibition of auditory and sensorimotor areas) and the excitatory manifestations (limbic and extrapyramidal systems and the corpus callosum), on balance a metabolic basis for the global rise in CBF seems unlikely.[73,74]

Whether measured directly or indirectly in the lumbar area, intracranial pressure (ICP) increases with ketamine in a fashion commensurate and contemporary with the alterations in CBF. The rise in ICP seems more marked in patients with

Table 7–1. Cerebral Regional Glucose Utilization During Ketamine Anesthesia in Rats

REGION	CONTROL	KETAMINE
Auditory System		
Cortex	128 $\pm$ 4	105 $\pm$ 8*
Medial geniculate	100 $\pm$ 3	87 $\pm$ 8
Inferior colliculus	166 $\pm$ 5	109 $\pm$ 9
Visual System		
Cortex	94 $\pm$ 3	116 $\pm$ 10
Lateral geniculate	78 $\pm$ 2	84 $\pm$ 7
Superior colliculus	76 $\pm$ 3	84 $\pm$ 7
Limbic System		
Cingulate gyrus	73 $\pm$ 7	127 $\pm$ 8**
Hippocampus	73 $\pm$ 2	119 $\pm$ 8**
Mammillary body	97 $\pm$ 3	140 $\pm$ 12*
Interpeduncular nucleus	89 $\pm$ 7	113 $\pm$ 3*

Dose: 10 mg/kg IV
Values in mmol/100 g/min; means $\pm$ S.E.
* P <0.05
† P <0.01
(Note: P <0.05 for hippocampus, medial geniculate, and inferior colliculus in another similar study.[73])
(Adapted from Crosby, G., Crane, A.M., and Sokoloff, L.: Local changes in cerebral glucose utilization during ketamine anesthesia. Anesthesiology, 52:330, 1980.)

already elevated levels resulting from pre-existing disease, including an intracranial space-occupying lesion.[145,152] A ketamine-induced elevation in ICP can be prevented by prior administration of thiopental or, once manifest, can be reversed with either or both thiopental and passive hyperventilation.[134,146,152]

PULMONARY CIRCULATION

Ketamine increases pulmonary artery pressure in animals and man, together with elevated right ventricular stroke work and minute work of the heart secondary to increased pulmonary vascular resistance.[130,153–155] These changes are associated with a transient increase in intrapulmonary shunt.[130] Changes in pulmonary hemodynamics recorded in children and infants after the administration of ketamine are probably secondary to increased cardiac output rather than to primary pulmonary vasoconstriction; these changes can be mostly counteracted by prior administration of an alpha-adrenergic blocking agent, such as droperidol.[156]

RENAL CIRCULATION

Renal blood flow may be reduced transiently in passive response to the initial decrease in systemic arterial pressure occasionally encountered with ketamine.[157] The drug does not appear to affect the renal circulation directly.

UTEROPLACENTAL CIRCULATION

Uterine blood flow is increased concomitant with the rise in maternal arterial pressure produced by ketamine.[29]

CLINICAL OBSERVATIONS

In healthy, unpremedicated subjects, ketamine increases the level of arterial blood pressure and pulse rate even at subanesthetic intravenous doses (as small an amount as 0.1 mg/kg causes a rise in blood pressure of approximately 25 mm Hg systolic and 16 mm Hg diastolic), together with a lesser increase in heart rate.[1,10,99] With increasing dosage, the blood pressure level continues to rise until a total dose of about 1.0 to 1.5 mg/kg is reached, after which the circulatory responses seem to plateau. Figure 7–17 illustrates the effects of two successive intravenous doses of ketamine (1 mg/kg) given to an unpremedicated subject.[10]

Cardiovascular stimulation was maximal 3 to 5 minutes after the start of injection. After return of consciousness, repeat doses produced approximately the same duration of unconsciousness, with no further rise in blood pressure level or heart rate. These values gradually returned to control levels, unrelated to the recovery from unconsciousness. Thus, about 10 to 20 minutes after partial recovery, with the subject now clearly in contact with the environment, the blood pressure level was still slightly elevated, returning to a normal level only after about 1 hour. Interestingly, successive doses of ketamine seem to cause successive increases in blood pressure values only if the rise from the prior dose is receding.[54] The degree of elevation seems related, in part, to the mode of administration of ketamine, the greatest increases noted after rapid intravenous injection; the incidence and degree of rise are reduced with slower intravenous injection or intramuscular administration.[1] Ketamine-induced changes in blood pressure seem less pronounced in children than in adults, but there is no clear relationship between the age of the patient and the hypertensive response.[1]

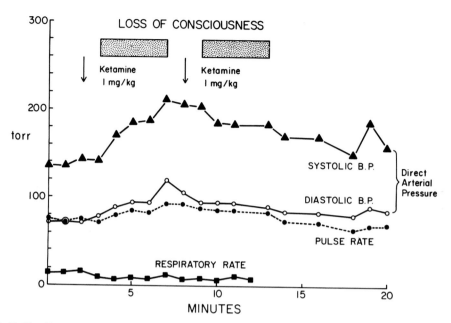

Fig. 7–17. Vasopressor response to ketamine in man. (From Domino, E.F., Chodoff, P., and Corssen, G.: Pharmacologic effects of CI-581, a new dissociative anesthetic in man. Clin. Pharmacol. Ther., 6:279, 1965.)

Conversely, the initial, short-lasting depression of cardiovascular function shown in Figure 7–14 may not always be a transient phenomenon, but may cause a precipitous fall in blood pressure level during induction of anesthesia with ketamine in elderly patients suffering from congestive heart failure or who are critically ill or acutely traumatized.[158] Cautious administration of restricted doses minimizes the incidence and severity of this complication.

The initial blood pressure determination does not seem to have any bearing on the degree of hypertension produced by ketamine, despite earlier findings of greatest or least elevations in hypertensive patients.[99,159,160]

ATTENUATION OF CARDIOSTIMULATORY EFFECTS

Excessive cardiac stimulation may be undesirable, especially during induction of anesthesia for open-heart surgery. These responses attributable to an increase in plasma catecholamines can be attenuated by prior treatment with CNS depressants, such as thiopental, thiamylal, and, in particular, the benzodiazepines, diazepam, lorazepam, flunitrazepam, and midazolam.[161–175] In one technique termed "ataract analgesia," diazepam (0.2 mg/kg intravenously) administered 3 to 5 minutes before intravenous ketamine injection (2 mg/kg) causes significant reduction in systolic blood pressure and heart rate without respiratory depression or airway obstruction.[171] The combination of pancuronium and ketamine-nitrous oxide anesthesia is also effective in preventing a rise in the level of plasma norepinephrine and in reducing arterial blood pressure and pulse rate. Therefore, the combination of ketamine and pancuronium may be employed safely in patients in whom marked circulatory changes should be avoided, although other investigators caution against combining ketamine and pancuronium, considering blood pressure elevation and tachycardia encountered with this technique unacceptable.[172,176,177] Droperidol is ineffective in significantly reducing ketamine-induced cardiostimulatory effects.[178]

HEMORRHAGIC SHOCK

The sympathomimetic action of ketamine, with sustained increases in both systolic and diastolic blood pressure levels, improves survival rates in experimental animals exposed to hemorrhagic or septic shock, especially when combined with droperidol or phenoxybenzamine.[179–182] In patients with hypovolemic or traumatic shock, the temporary circulatory stimulation induced by ketamine restores perfusion of tissues, including the kidneys.[183,184] This restoration may offer a false sense of security unless perfusion is sustained by appropriate blood and fluid replacement.[180]

Respiratory System

Anesthetic doses of ketamine may result in slight, transitory depression of respiratory function (Fig. 7–18) that starts soon after completion of the injection and lasts 1 to 3 minutes.[10,55,185,186] The depression, if present, is most marked within the first minute. The tidal volume tends to decrease more than the respiratory rate. Arterial P_{O_2}, P_{CO_2}, and pH remain within physiologic limits. Although a mild, transient reduction in Pa_{O_2} may occur, responses to CO_2 challenge are not significantly altered.[150] Respiratory support is usually not needed, but accidental doubling or tripling of the usual dose of ketamine may depress respiration, possibly causing apnea.[187]

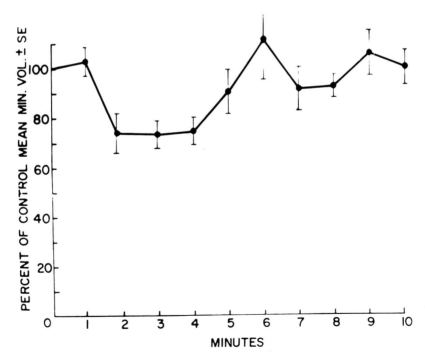

Fig. 7–18. Transient respiratory depression after ketamine (0.45 mg/kg intravenously) in man. (From Domino, E.F., Chodoff, P., and Corssen, G.: Pharmacologic effects of CI-581, a new dissociative anesthetic in man. Clin. Pharmacol. Ther., 6:279, 1965.)

These depressant effects are attributable to peripheral pharmacologic deafferentation involving the pulmonary stretch receptors, and are directly related to the dose and speed of administration.[188] Thus, after delivery of a bolus of ketamine (2 mg/kg) injected rapidly intravenously or with rapid intravenous infusion, significant reduction in PaO_2 may occur, lasting 5 to 10 minutes.[189] Characteristic changes in respiratory pattern may follow intravenous doses of ketamine that exceed 2 mg/kg with increased respiratory rate, decreased tidal volume, and apneic phases that last 15 to 30 seconds, often followed by deep sighs with breath holding for 3 to 5 seconds at the peak of inspiration. Premedication with tranquilizing drugs or narcotics may cause a transient but significant respiratory depression, even to the point of apnea.[55,190]

Infants and small children are more susceptible to these respiratory depressant effects of ketamine administration than are older children or adults.[191] An inversely dose-related stimulation, rather than depression, of respiration, however, was observed with ketamine use in one series of acutely burned and postburn children undergoing reconstructive surgery.[192] Three minutes after ketamine administration (1 mg/kg intravenously), 4 mg/kg of the drug were delivered intramuscularly (instead of more usual doses of 2 mg/kg intravenously and 5 to 10 mg intramuscularly). All respiratory parameters were increased: the rate, by a mean of 11 breaths per minute; minute volume, by about 250%: tidal volume, by 100%: and PaO_2, to a mean maximal rise of 8 mm Hg; the exception, of course, was $PaCO_2$, which increased to a mean maximum of 14 mm Hg. Presumably, larger, more appropriate doses of ketamine would have blocked these responses to external stimuli, e.g., obtaining arterial blood gas samples or merely applying the equipment for measuring ventilatory function.

Ketamine plays a role in the relaxation of tracheal and bronchial smooth muscle, antagonizes the spasmogenic effects of carbachol and histamine, and potentiates the antispasmodic effects of epinephrine.[1,193-198] Curiously, use of the drug does not lessen respiratory resistance that is artificially increased by ultrasonic aerosols, but ketamine is as effective as halothane and enflurane in preventing experimentally induced bronchospasm in dogs.[196,198] Not surprisingly, airway resistance is decreased (Fig. 7–19) and pulmonary compliance is increased when ketamine is chosen for use in the patient with asthma. Consequently, in most asthmatic patients, bronchospasm noted before induction of anesthesia promptly disappears or markedly abates upon administration of ketamine, although airway resistance is not significantly altered by ketamine delivery in patients free of pulmonary disease.[199,200] The effect can be most dramatic in status asthmaticus, as illustrated by a reported case study.[200]

A 5-year-old girl weighing 11.25 kg with severe generalized epidermolysis bullosa dystrophica had conjunctival adhesions in both eyes. Attempts to operate on the eyes under local anesthesia had failed because of difficulty of controlling the child's movements. General anesthesia with ketamine was planned to obviate placement of a face mask and an endotracheal tube. On arrival in the examination room, the child was severely dyspneic and cyanotic, with loud wheezes audible over both lungs, markedly prolonged exhalation, and distended jugular veins. Anesthesia was induced with ketamine (25 mg IV). Upon completion of the injection, bronchospasm abruptly disappeared, her respiratory exchange improved significantly, and cyanosis subsided. Eight minutes later, as the ophthalmologist was cutting the conjunctival adhesions, bronchospasm gradually returned. Ketamine (15 mg IV) again relieved the symptoms. Over the next 20 minutes, three additional IV increments of ketamine (10, 10, and 15 mg) were administered as bronchospasm recurred. A total of 75 mg of ketamine was given during the 30-minute procedure.

About 15 minutes after completion of the operation, as the patient gradually awakened, bronchospasm reappeared, but seemed less intense, and cyanosis was not as marked as pre-operatively,

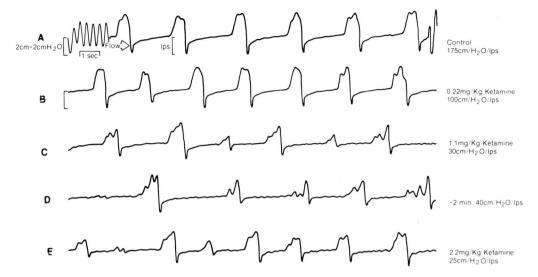

Fig. 7–19. Effect of ketamine on airway resistance in obstructive lung disease in man. (From Huber, F.C., Reves, J.G., Gutierrez, J., and Corssen, G.: Ketamine: its effect on airway resistance in man. South. Med. J., 65:1176, 1972.)

although auscultation revealed wheezing in both lungs. She was discharged 90 minutes later, complaining of being hungry.

In this child the reappearance of wheezing during lighter planes of anesthesia and its clearing upon deepening the dissociative state are consistent with observations that a ketamine-induced increase in airway patency begins approximately 1 to 1½ minutes after drug administration and diminishes within 6 to 8 minutes.[199]

The most dramatic improvement in airway patency occurred in a 45-year-old man with chronic obstructive lung disease who developed acute bronchospasm prior to induction of anesthesia. The effect of ketamine medication on the airway resistance of this patient when the method of "forced oscillation" was employed is demonstrated in Figure 7–19. Tracing A (control) shows airway resistance of 175 cm H_2O/L/second before ketamine administration. In tracing B, reduction in airway resistance to 100 cm/H_2O/L/second after the intravenous administration of ketamine (0.22 mg/kg) is demonstrated. An additional intravenous dose of 1.0 mg/kg of ketamine reduced airway resistance to 30 cm/H_2O/L/second (tracing C). Tracing D shows an increase in airway resistance to 40 cm/H_2O/L/second recorded 2 minutes after the peak drug effect. Tracing E reflects further reduction in airway resistance to 25 cm/H_2O/L/second after a 2.2-mg/kg dose of ketamine. The mechanism responsible for the bronchodilator action of ketamine is probably a combination of a direct action on bronchial smooth muscle, an increase in circulating endogenous catecholamines, and perhaps a vagolytic action. It appears that ketamine acts at sites other than beta receptors, because propranolol blocks the smooth muscle relaxant effect of epinephrine but not of ketamine. Bronchospasm should not be confused with paroxysmal coughing, which may be precipitated when ketamine is delivered to patients suffering from an upper respiratory tract infection.[52] In this case, additional ketamine may worsen rather than stop the coughing, with concomitant cyanosis and hypoxia.

AIRWAY REFLEXES

The triggering of protective pharyngeal and laryngeal reflexes is not suppressed by ketamine; muscle tone is retained in the tongue and jaw. Consequently, although coughing, sneezing, gagging, or swallowing may occur in response to intra-airway stimulation by a foreign body, the risk of airway obstruction is small. Patent air passages are the rule, and the need to support the jaw or to insert an oropharyngeal or endotracheal airway is exceptional with ketamine use. Nevertheless, the anesthesiologist must remain alert to the possibility of mechanically supporting the airway whenever necessary. Overconfidence in the ability of ketamine to guarantee airway patency even under the most challenging conditions (e.g., emergency surgery without an endotracheal tube in an unpremedicated patient with a full stomach) can have dire consequences.[201,202] The competence of the laryngeal closure reflex under the effect of ketamine has been carefully assessed by various investigators. In several studies, silent pulmonary aspiration of radiopaque material (propyliodone; Dionosil) that was deposited over the base of the tongue was demonstrated in all (7 of 7), few (1 of 10), or none (0 of 8) of the subjects.[203–206] Four individuals in the last group developed laryngospasm, a reminder that, because of retained activity of protective reflexes, laryngospasm can also be provoked by pharyngeal accumulation of secretions, blood, or regurgitated gastric contents. Ketamine stimulates salivation, and therefore, it is important to include an antisialagogue in the preanesthetic medication. A marked increase in salivation, especially in children with small air passages, can cause severe respiratory obstruction.[207,208]

Musculoskeletal

In humans, the resting tone of the muscles of the neck and extremities tends to increase after the administration of ketamine. As a rule, however, this fact is clinically unimportant. It is noteworthy that increased muscle tone may occasionally lead to generalized extensor spasm or opisthotonus.[209] Although the abdominal muscles remain relaxed and reduced skeletal muscle tone was reported to have occurred during ketamine anesthesia, the drug itself has no muscle relaxant property.[210,211]

The muscles in the eyelid merit special attention. With the onset of dissociative anesthesia, the eyes tend to open (see Fig. 7–7) and remain open until the effects of ketamine begin to dissipate. During prolonged surgery, prophylactic taping of the eyelids so they remain closed and the optional use of a bland eye ointment will prevent corneal damage.

Extrapyramidal muscle activity, fasciculations, purposeless movements, and minor clonic spasms of the extremities may occur during ketamine anesthesia without corresponding changes in the EEG. Such activity, undesirable during delicate operations, e.g., in the eye or middle ear, can usually be suppressed by a small dose of diazepam (1 to 5 mg given intravenously, depending on the age and weight of the patient).

Ketamine appears to augment the effects of both depolarizing and non-depolarizing muscle relaxants, perhaps by interfering with calcium binding and thereby reducing the requirements of these agents for adequate muscle relaxation during dissociative anesthesia.[212–215] Ketamine causes a slight fall in serum potassium levels, resulting in a decrease in the incidence and severity of muscle fasciculations induced by succinylcholine.[216,217]

Gastrointestinal System

Vomiting occurs infrequently after ketamine anesthesia, e.g., in only 1.8% of 1500 patients in one series.[52] Other researchers reported a slightly higher incidence of nausea and vomiting after minor operations with ketamine than with methohexital, but not after major operations.

Hepatic System

Ketamine does not significantly alter hepatic enzyme activity (SGOT and SGPT), alkaline phosphatase levels, thymol turbidity, or lipometabolism.[10,218]

Genitourinary System

Ketamine does not significantly affect renal function.[10,219] In elderly patients with impaired kidney function, a slight, statistically insignificant reduction in the glomerular filtration rate and urinary flow may occur, with no change in effective renal plasma flow.[220]

Ketamine (2.2 mg/kg intravenously) exerts a detumescent action on the penis, preventing or reversing erections caused by manipulation of this organ during genitourinary operations: lesser doses seem ineffective.[221,222] The mechanism of this unique action is unknown.

Uterine tone is not depressed by the administration of clinical doses of ketamine.[31,223] The drug in fact increases uterine tone and the frequency and intensity of uterine contractions.[224–227] The contractile pattern is unaffected by low doses (25 mg intravenously) of ketamine, responding only to larger doses (75 to 100 mg intravenously).[227] The resultant increase in frequency and intensity of contractions resembles that seen after one "physiologic" dose of oxytocin (8 to 10 mU/minute), but there is no associated rise in uterine resting pressure.[227] Uterine blood flow is increased concomitant with the rise in maternal arterial pressure produced by ketamine.[29]

Endocrine System

Ketamine may exert a slight antithyroid action, with reduction in serum levels of triiodothyronine (T_3) but not of thyroxine (T_4).[228] Urinary excretion of catecholamines is not altered by ketamine use, but the increased sympathetic activity causes a sharp rise in plasma levels of free norepinephrine.[186,229–232] Pressor responses to angiotensin I and II are accentuated, but plasma renin activity is unchanged.[233,234]

The pituitary-adrenal system in rats is activated by ketamine, causing a depletion of brain catecholamines and a rise in plasma ACTH levels.[235] These effects can be inhibited by effecting catecholaminergic blockade or by deepening the level of ketamine anesthesia.[235,236]

Metabolism

As with the use of most general anesthetics, body temperature decreases with ketamine anesthesia, probably from a combination of decreased heat production and increased heat loss facilitated by cutaneous vasodilation.[237]

Intraocular Pressure

Intraocular pressure is usually slightly increased, but may be unchanged during ketamine anesthesia.[54,238–248] Should the plan for the institution of anesthesia include endotracheal intubation, a significant but transient elevation in intraocular tension may result.[248] This change is unimportant if the eyeball is intact. In short, any elevation of intraocular pressure caused by ketamine use is clinically unimportant, and thus does not preclude its use in patients with glaucoma.

The mechanism responsible for this mild elevation in intraocular tension remains obscure. A transient imbalance in tone of extraocular muscles has been implicated.[240] In another theory, its effects on intraocular pressure are mediated in a manner analogous to the cardiovascular effects of ketamine, e.g., stimulation of the sympathetic nervous system, with concomitant rise in plasma norepinephrine levels.[54] There is, however, no detectable correlation between the effects of ketamine on intraocular pressure and those on arterial pressure, nor do any observed increases in intraocular tension with ketamine seem to be dose related.

Miscellaneous Effects

LACRIMATION

Increased lacrimation may occur during anesthesia with ketamine.[249] As with the use of any general anesthetic, this sign indicates that the level of anesthesia is decreasing.

IMMUNE RESPONSE

Unlike most general anesthetic agents, ketamine does not suppress the human immune responses.[250,251] Human lymphocyte transformation stimulated by phytohemagglutinin in vitro is not significantly inhibited by the use of clinically employed concentrations of ketamine.[252] This property of ketamine may be advantageous in the anesthetic management of burn patients and other individuals at risk because of a lowered resistance to pathogenic bacteria.

COMPLICATIONS

Emergence Reactions

Recovery from ketamine anesthesia may be complicated by restlessness, agitation, and even delirium. Vivid dreams or hallucinations may be associated with excitement, confusion, euphoria, sensations of bodily detachment, and floating. A case of transient (25 minutes) blindness was reported.[253] In a group of unpremedicated prison volunteers recovering from ketamine anesthesia, some subjects were completely oriented in time and place, whereas other subjects showed marked alterations in mood and affect, becoming apprehensive, aggressive, withdrawn, or deliriant.[10] Most volunteers felt entirely numb; several subjects stated they had no arms or legs or were dead, but they could recognize being touched or moved. All individuals exhibited horizontal, vertical, or rotatory nystagmus and ataxia with diminished visual acuity and blurred vision. Queries elicited occasional feelings of estrangement, isolation, negativism, hostility, apathy, dizziness, drowsiness, or inebriation. Some subjects had vivid, dreamlike recall of television programs or motion pictures seen a few days before, and others imagined being at home with relatives or floating in outer space. The experiences were so real that some subjects were later uncertain as to whether they had actually occurred. These psychologic aberrations usually subsided completely within about 30 minutes.

One investigator, who administered a continuous infusion of ketamine intravenously to himself, described the feeling of weightlessness as comparable to the experiences of astronauts in outer space.[254] The illusionary and hallucinatory reactions take place exclusively between the times of first response to verbal contact and complete reorientation to person, time, and place; only rarely do they continue beyond this period. Although dreams, proprioceptive and confusional illusions, and other psychic aberrations may occur after the use of any general anesthetic, their occurrence is undoubtedly more frequent with ketamine.[255,256] Adults who received ketamine, however, experienced the same frequency of post-anesthetic anxiety as did those individuals who received thiopental, nitrous oxide, and halothane.[256]

MECHANISM

The aforementioned emergence phenomena are mostly attributable to the dissociative state induced by ketamine. Results of studies of cerebral regional utilization of glucose in animals verify the stimulation of the hippocampus and other components of the limbic system, with corresponding inhibition of auditory and sensorimotor areas.[73,74] This occurrence leads to misperception and misinterpretation of stimuli from these areas, e.g., loss of tactile and proprioceptive responses from the skin and the musculoskeletal system facilitates development of specific illusions, such as splitting the body image, depersonalization, and traveling to the moon in a spaceship.[257,258] The case of transient blindness reported previously was attributed to ketamine-induced derangement of cerebral components of the visual system (lateral geniculate, optic radiation, and visual cortex), but this theory has not been substantiated by studies in cerebral regional glucose utilization.[74,253] An hysterical origin cannot be excluded.

INCIDENCE

The reported incidence of psychic phenomena after ketamine ranges from 3 to more than 30%, and is related to the dosage and technique of administration; the nature of the operation; and the age, gender, and personality of the patient.[31,32,52,99,259] The use of preanesthetic and adjuvant medication can modify or eliminate the occurrence of psychic phenomena.

Dose. Large doses of ketamine (exceeding 2.2 mg/kg intravenously) or rapid intravenous bolus injections are usually associated with a higher incidence of post-anesthetic sequelae. For this reason, adjustment of the induction dose according to lean body mass has been recommended.[260] Emergence reactions may follow subanesthetic doses of ketamine, but this occurrence is unusual.[261]

Age. Ketamine-induced psychotomimetic activity occurs more frequently in adolescents older than 16 years of age and in adults (24 to 34% incidence of emergence reactions and unsatisfactory anesthesia) than in patients younger than 16 years of age (under 10%).[262] Because children rarely experience undesirable reactions or dreams during recovery from ketamine anesthesia, they generally recall this type of anesthesia as a pleasant event and do not object to its repetition.[49,263–266] Indeed, a "ketamine acceptance test" used in children after repeated ketamine administration showed improved acceptance with successive exposure to the drug.[259,266]

The very low incidence of reactions to ketamine in infants and young children cannot be dismissed as involving a communication gap. Children may indeed have brief periods of vivid dreaming when emerging from ketamine anesthesia; however, they usually do not undergo the psychomotor agitation and unpleasant dreaming experienced by adults. One possible explanation is that children have fewer life experiences and less psychologic trauma in their memory stores. Alternatively, they may have less need to understand and control their mental status; hence, unlike adults, children are not threatened by dissociation from self or their inability to interpret external stimuli. In any case, most children avoid severe psychic reactions to ketamine, which is a major reason for its preferential use in young patients.

Sex. Women are more likely than men to suffer unpleasant sequelae after the use of ketamine.[267,268] Only 29% of female patients receiving ketamine anesthesia for minor operations would choose it again.[99,269] Indeed, it has been our experience that psychotic reactions occur most often after ketamine anesthesia in patients undergoing dilatation and curettage to terminate pregnancy.

Nature of the Operation. Postanesthetic psychic upset is less severe after long operations that involve the body surface than after minor operations, and it is to a still lesser degree after abdominal surgery of 60 to 80 minutes' duration.[213]

Personality Disposition. The personality of the patient will influence the incidence of emergence phenomena after ketamine anesthesia. By employing Eysenck's Personality Inventory, it can be predicted that persons with a high score in "extraversion" usually experience a pleasant recovery from ketamine, whereas individuals with a high score in "psychotism" show a negative response to ketamine.[270] Patients who dream during ketamine anesthesia normally dream at home.[271]

Shielding from the Environment. Whether covering the eyes during the induction and recovery phases of ketamine anesthesia or allowing the patient to emerge from anesthesia in a quiet and shielded area (almost equivalent to sensory deprivation) significantly reduces the incidence of emergence phenomena is still controversial. It seems reasonable to request that recovery room personnel not attempt to arouse any patient who is unable to see, hear, or properly interpret the environment. Violation of this fundamental rule can initiate a chain of anxiety reactions ultimately leading to severe psychomotor outbreaks and irrational behavior.

PREANESTHETIC AND ADJUVANT MEDICATION

Many drugs, including belladonna derivatives, sedative-hypnotics, narcotic-analgesics, and general anesthetics, have been studied in an attempt to identify a compound that could eliminate the incidence of psychic disturbances during recovery from ketamine anesthesia.

Belladonna Drugs. Although atropine usefully controls increased salivation that often accompanies ketamine use, it has been reported to increase the frequency of unpleasant dreams.[213,272] Scopolamine is less suitable as a premedicant in adults because of a higher incidence of unpleasant sequelae;[99] in most infants and children, however, scopolamine provides optimal drying effects and satisfactory sedation without psychic alterations during emergence.[118] Recently, glycopyrrolate (Robinul), a most effective anticholinergic agent, was employed as a substitute for atropine because its highly polar quaternary ammonium group limits its passage across the blood-brain barrier.

Droperidol. Droperidol reportedly aids in providing preanesthetic tranquility and reduces the incidence of unpleasant dreams and other emergence reactions, although this contention has been disputed.[52,99,213,273–276] In addition, although droperidol also reduces the total dose of ketamine needed for adequate anesthesia, its use does prolong the recovery period.[277] Such an effect, of course, is undesirable after outpatient surgery because it delays the release of the patient. On the other hand, droperidol (2.5 to 5 mg intravenously) promptly terminates an acute psychomotor emergence reaction. Indeed, the injection of droperidol (5 mg intravenously) at the end of the operation may reduce ketamine-induced delirium reactions.[278]

Benzodiazepines. Diazepam (Valium) (0.15 to 0.3 mg/kg intravenously) administered before induction minimizes psychic emergence reactions after ketamine anesthesia.[99,279–281] Equally satisfactory results are observed when diazepam (e.g., 5 mg intravenously) is delivered at the termination of a surgical procedure.[99,281–283] When administered postoperatively, diazepam (20 mg intramuscularly) also decreases the occurrence of distressing mental phenomena, especially when lack of speech control and visual distortion renders patients unable to communicate their fears to the nursing staff.[258] Apparently, "floating" sensations and dreaming are not fully suppressed by diazepam during awakening after ketamine anesthesia.[283] A combination of diazepam and droperidol delivered intravenously immediately prior to ketamine administration can be efficacious.[284]

The diazepam congeners, lorazepam (Ativan), flunitrazepam (Rohypnol), and midazolam (Dobralam), seem to be superior to diazepam in "taming" ketamine.[174,285–289] These agents minimize not only emergence phenomena but also, unlike diazepam, recall of unpleasant dreams; all of these drugs surpass diazepam in amnesic potency. Lorazepam (2 to 4 mg) is equally effective by oral or intramuscular administration. The use of flunitrazepam (0.03 mg/kg intravenously) is beneficial, but the drug is not yet available in the United States.[174,287,288] Application for its release in the United States is pending. Midazolam (0.07 mg/kg intravenously) appears to be the agent that is closest to the ideal benzodiazepine.[289] The drug is uniquely water soluble, unlike all other benzodiazepines, which when supplied are dissolved in highly irritating organic solvents, prone to causing venous complications. Some other benzodiazepines also have long elimination half-lives and hence tend to prolong recovery from ketamine anesthesia.

Ultra-Short-Acting Barbiturates, Morphine, and General Anesthesia. By combining ketamine with thiopental or general anesthetic agents, the incidence of post-anesthetic emergence phenomena may be significantly reduced.[290,291] Thiopental (150 mg intravenously) delivered after minor gynecologic procedures reduced the incidence of ketamine-induced emergence reactions from 36% in the control group (without thiopental) to 6% in the thiopental-treated group.[292] Similarly, administration of nitrous oxide-oxygen mixtures at the termination of an operation reduces unpleasant experiences during recovery from ketamine anesthesia. Morphine combined with ketamine also effectively reduces psychotomimetic effects after anesthesia with ketamine.[293,294]

Tetrahydroaminacrine and Chlormetiazole. Tetrahydroaminacrine is a potent cholinesterase inhibitor, capable of reversing psychotic reactions precipitated by anticholinergic psychotomimetic agents. Chlormetiazole is a sedative hypnotic with anticonvulsive properties. Both drugs can modify or terminate psychotomimetic effects during recovery from ketamine anesthesia, tetrahydroaminacrine in laboratory animals and chlormetiazole in man.[255,295] Neither is medically available in the United States.

Can Ketamine Cause Permanent Psychotic Alterations?

The possibilities of hallucinatory recurrences and permanent psychotic alteration after ketamine anesthesia have been considered.[257] Long-term (6 months or more) clinical and experimental studies, with repeated interviews and psychologic testing after ketamine anesthesia, elicited no long-lasting psychic effects or impairment of personality functioning.[296,297] This finding was true even after repeated exposure to the drug.

Amnesia

Preoperative retrograde amnesia with ketamine is negligible, except with the use of heavy preanesthetic medication. Memory of events occurring hours after apparent recovery from the ketamine effect may be impaired, however, in proportion to the total dose of ketamine administered.

Can Ketamine Induce Epileptic Seizures?

Observations of opisthotonus in two infants, convulsions in a healthy adult woman, focal motor seizures in two of eight brain-damaged epileptic patients during ketamine anesthesia, and a grand mal seizure that occurred in one other of the eight epileptic subjects during recovery suggest a seizure potential for the drug.[209,298,299] In two epileptic patients awaiting pneumoencephalography, however, ketamine suppressed tonic-clonic convulsions, with reappearance of seizure activity as the ketamine effect waned. This apparent anti-epileptic effect has since been confirmed by successful use of ketamine to treat convulsions refractory to conventional therapy.[52,300] The findings from two prospective studies of epilepsy are confirmatory.[301,302] In one study, ketamine anesthesia did not induce EEG seizure activity in nonepileptic patients or in epileptic patients with normal EEG findings.[301] Although the EEG findings of a patient may become more severe during ketamine anesthesia, this is uncommon. Ketamine also did not precipitate generalized convulsions, even in epileptic patients with abnormal EEG findings. On the contrary, ketamine suppressed EEG seizure discharges in epileptic patients, as illustrated in Figure 7–20. In the second study, patients with focal or generalized epilepsy were observed during hyperventilation or photic stimulation, while awake, during sleep (after 18 to 24 hours of sleep deprivation), and during and after having received ketamine intravenously.[302] In these patients, sleep was found to be a more potent stimulator of seizure activity than was ketamine. Thus it seems unlikely that ketamine would precipitate convulsions in patients with epilepsy or other seizure disorders. Nevertheless, caution is required, as with any other general anesthetic, with ketamine use in these patients.

ILLICIT USE

The consumption of ketamine as a psychedelic drug is of concern because its congener, phencyclidine, is a major component of street drugs sold as PCP, "Angel Dust," "Green" (taken from its green crystalline appearance), and "1980 Supergrass" (when combined with marijuana).[303] Ketamine itself, known as "K," "Super Acid," "Purple," "Mauve," "Special L.A. Coke," and "Super C," is ingested orally or intranasally ("snorting").[304] Its abuse has become particularly prevalent in the

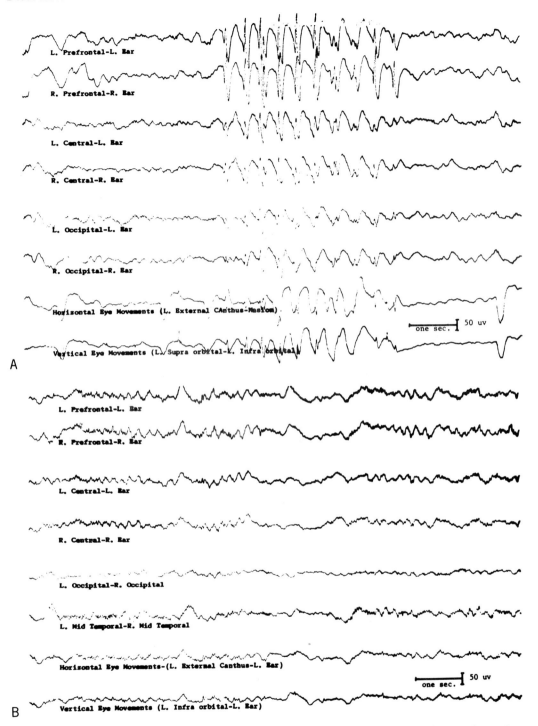

Fig. 7–20. *A*, anti-epileptic effect of ketamine. EEG of 19-year-old boy, weighing 68 kg, with a history of idiopathic petit mal and grand mal epilepsy since childhood, obtained prior to ketamine administration (control). Note short (subclinical) discharge of type that accompanied clinical ("absence") seizures. *B*, EEG of same patient 228 seconds after ketamine (2.2 mg/kg) given intravenously. Note that previous frequent 3-sec wave and spike discharges have almost completely disappeared. (From Corssen, G., Little, S.G., and Tavakoli, M.: Ketamine and epilepsy. Anesth. Analg., 53:319, 1974.)

western United States. A major attraction of ketamine to street users is the rapid onset and relatively short duration of its psychedelic action, which apparently includes antidepressant effects. The abuse problem is compounded by the relative ease with which this drug can be manufactured in underground laboratories. Although self-inflicted injuries during ketamine abuse are rare, serious injuries and even suicides have been reported with phencyclidine use.[305]

The characteristic eye signs and symptoms of ketamine intoxication in street users are diplopia associated with uncoordinated eye movements and coarse horizontal nystagmus; the eyes usually remain wide open, even in unresponsive individuals.[304] Hypertension is common with phencyclidine poisoning and, if unrecognized and untreated, can lead to death.[306]

CLINICAL CONSIDERATIONS

Preoperative Visit

During the usual preanesthetic discussion with the patient who is to receive ketamine, the possibility of intraoperative dreaming should be mentioned, together with the positive suggestion that he or she concentrate on some enjoyable activity immediately prior to the induction of anesthesia. This practice should sharply reduce the incidence of unpleasant, even frightening psychic experiences during and after the dissociative anesthetic state. The minimal frequency of such disturbances in obstetric patients receiving ketamine reinforces the importance of the preanesthetic psychologic "set."[31]

Preanesthetic Medication

Various combinations of opiates, hypnotics, tranquilizers, and belladonna drugs may be used to minimize or eliminate any undesirable effect of ketamine, including excessive salivation, hypertension, tachycardia, lacrimation, diaphoresis, musculoskeletal rigidity, involuntary muscle movements, and, in particular, agitation and delirium during emergence from anesthesia. Most of these drugs tend to prolong the duration of anesthesia or the recovery period, thereby negating the benefit of the short-acting nature of ketamine to varying degrees. In infants and children, if prompt recovery is desired (e.g., after outpatient surgery), scopolamine alone may be given intramuscularly in slightly higher (e.g., 0.1 mg more) than usual dosage, according to age and weight, 30 minutes to 1 hour before induction of anesthesia. This relatively simple medication usually achieves sedation and tranquility, with minimal incidence of excessive salivation during anesthesia. A barbiturate (pentobarbital or secobarbital) or other hypnotic provides additional sedation, but at the cost of some prolongation of post-anesthetic recovery.

Ketamine itself, together with a belladonna drug, can constitute useful premedication in pediatric patients.[307–309] A dose of 2.5 mg/kg intramuscularly given 15 to 25 minutes before induction of anesthesia usually produces a dissociative anesthetic state in which the patient has no memory of the transfer from the ward to the operating room. Induction must be started 15 to 25 minutes after such premedication. If induction begins sooner than 10 minutes after injection, the belladonna drug will not have achieved peak efficacy against ketamine-induced increased salivation, permitting copious secretions to interfere with airway patency. If induction occurs after more than 25 minutes, the optimal depressant effect of ketamine has passed; hence, induction may be less than satisfactory. This technique of "stealing" the patient from the ward may be of special benefit to poor-risk pediatric patients, e.g., those with complex congenital heart anomalies in whom marked excitation could be extremely deleterious. In adults, short-acting hypnotics (e.g., pentobarbital) not only provide optimal sedation prior to induction of anesthesia but also are effective in reducing the incidence and severity of ketamine-induced emergence reactions.[310] Atropine or glycopyrrolate are effective drying agents.

Although droperidol in adult patients exerts reliable antipsychotic effects, it can markedly prolong the awakening phase. Recently, various diazepines were found to be effective: 20 to 30 mg of diazepam (Valium) or 2 to 5 mg of lorazepam (Ativan) given orally 60 to 90 minutes before anesthesia, smaller intravenous doses of these drugs given 5 to 10 minutes before anesthesia, or 0.07 mg/kg of midazolam given 30 minutes before induction of anesthesia. Midazolam produces hypnotic, amnesic, and anxiolytic effects within 15 minutes of its intravenous injection.[311]

Diazepam (5 to 10 mg) or lorazepam (2 to 3 mg) may also be administered intravenously just before the end of a surgical procedure.[268] Pretreatment with flunitrazepam (0.015 mg/kg intravenously) effectively controls undesirable cardiovascular and psychotomimetic effects of ketamine in surgical patients; however, this drug is not currently available in the United States.[173]

Monitoring

EEG

The means to evaluate the effectiveness of anesthesia with ketamine differ markedly from those used to evaluate other general anesthetics.[312] EEG recording is probably the most reliable, but is not always a readily available method for assessing the depth of the dissociative anesthetic state (see previous section, "EEG Effects"). Ketamine induces theta (5 to 7 Hz) activity as consciousness is lost and analgesia is established. Theta waves seem to be correlated with analgesia: during ketamine anesthesia patients do not respond to painful stimuli as long as theta activity is present. With waning of anesthesia and the initial return of pain perception, the theta activity changes to waves of lower amplitude interspersed with waves of faster frequency.[59]

BLOOD PRESSURE AND HEART RATE

Changes in cardiovascular activity are closely associated with the depth of the dissociative state. Slight to moderate elevation of systolic and diastolic blood pressure determinations and pulse rate usually indicate establishment of dissociative anesthesia or, with supplemental injections to prolong anesthesia, adequate maintenance of the anesthetic state. Further increases in blood pressure or heart rate in response to surgical manipulation may signal lightening of the dissociative state and the need to administer additional ketamine.

EYE SIGNS

The pupils tend to be moderately dilated and remain so throughout anesthesia with ketamine. Transient horizontal or vertical nystagmus is most characteristic, occurring when the patient lapses into the dissociative state and recurring during emergence from anesthesia. The presence of nystagmus is a reliable signal to recovery room personnel that the patient is still under the effect of ketamine. Note, however, that nystagmus may be diminished or absent when droperidol, benzodiazepines, or other CNS depressants are included in the preanesthetic medication.

MUSCLE ACTIVITY

Purposeless movements should not be interpreted as responses to surgical stimulation. The movements are drug-induced, usually extrapyramidal in origin, and respond to small intravenous doses of diazepam or antiparkinsonian drugs, such as benztropine (Cogentin). Small doses of thiopental are also effective. Purposeful muscle movements, however, usually indicate lightening of anesthesia and the need for supplemental doses of ketamine. The anesthesiologist must constantly correlate the relationship between any motion of the patient and any painful stimuli. The addition of adjunctive agents to inhibit such undesirable movements may be desirable, although these agents may eliminate some of the unique advantages of ketamine, e.g., preservation of pharyngeal and laryngeal reflexes, maintenance of adequate respiration, and short duration of action.[294]

Dosage

Ketamine is supplied as the hydrochloride in vials containing 1% (10 mg/ml), 5% (50 mg/ml), and 10% (100 mg/ml) forms. The 1% concentration is preferred for intravenous administration, whereas the 5 and 10% forms are administered intramuscularly.

INTRAVENOUS ADMINISTRATION

Dose Calculations. Despite reasonable predictability of effects, individual variations in drug response preclude rigid standardization of ketamine dosage. Doses should therefore be adjusted to the requirements and response of each patient. Whether the dosage chosen for the induction of anesthesia should be calculated according to total body weight (the author's preference) or to lean body mass may be of more academic than clinical interest (except in the very obese patient in whom lean body mass is a more appropriate criterion).[260]

Technique. Ketamine may be administered intravenously in fractional increments or by continuous infusion. In the fractional injection technique, the initial dose that is effective for most patients is 1.0 to 2.2 mg/kg, administered over 15 to 30 seconds to avoid an excessive pressor effect and to minimize respiratory depression. This amount of ketamine normally produces 6 to 10 minutes of dissociation. To prolong anesthesia, additional doses, usually not exceeding one half of the initial dose (i.e., 0.5 to 1.0 mg/kg or less), may be given at intervals of 8 to 15 minutes or whenever the patient begins to show signs of responding to surgical stimulation. Intravenous doses of ketamine (less than 1 mg/kg) may be employed for use during procedures that are expected to last only a few minutes. For example, intravenous doses as small as 0.25 mg/kg usually produce about 3 minutes of dissociative anesthesia in pediatric oral surgery outpatients, which is an adequate amount of time to extract one or two teeth or to remove intraoral sutures after cleft palate repair. Recovery time under these circumstances is less than 15 minutes.

The continuous infusion technique permits close titration of ketamine with regard to depth of anesthesia desired, thereby reducing the total dose administered. With this technique, ketamine is usually administered in solutions of 0.1 or 0.2% (1 or 2 mg/ml). An initial drip rate of 120 to 150 drops/minute is recommended, with the solution delivered either gravitationally or with the aid of a sigmamotor microhead infusion pump.[170] The drip is continued until loss of consciousness ensues. The drip is resumed at a rate that is sufficient to titrate an anesthesia-analgesia level that is usually accomplished by infusing 1 to 2 mg/kg/hour of ketamine. Muscle relaxation, if needed, is provided by an intravenous drip of succinylcholine (0.1%). Some clinicians recommend the use of a 0.2% ketamine solution; anesthesia is induced by the administration of 10 ml/minute of the solution.[274,275] The intravenous infusion technique with ketamine may be initiated with a bolus of 1 mg/kg of ketamine. Diazepam (0.2 mg/kg intravenously) may be included in the preanesthetic medication.[313]

When ketamine is administered by continuous intravenous infusion, it may be used in combination with diazepam.[314] A 1.5 mg/kg amount of diazepam is given within the first 3 minutes of induction; at the beginning of each minute lapse, 5 mg of diazepam is added to the infusion for a total of 15 mg. During the second minute, 0.5 mg/kg of d-tubocurare is delivered intravenously in a bolus, and an endotracheal tube is placed during the fourth minute after induction. Nitrous oxide-oxygen (1:1) is administered with ventilation being controlled manually. Anesthesia is maintained with intravenous doses of 0.2 mg/kg of ketamine and intermittent increments of diazepam (5 mg every 30 minutes). During the second and subsequent hours, the ketamine dose is reduced to 0.1 mg/kg, and that of diazepam is reduced to 2.5 mg given every 30 minutes. d-Tubocurare is given intermittently at appropriate doses to sustain adequate muscle relaxation. With the marked reduction of the dosage of ketamine and the combination of ketamine and diazepam, the incidence of post-anesthetic psychotomimetic phenomena may be markedly reduced or completely eliminated. In addition, the sympathetic stimulatory effects of ketamine may be ameliorated. With the use of this low-dose ketamine-diazepam technique, ketamine may be not only "tamed" but also "trimmed."

Although the administration of ketamine by continuous infusion may be a somewhat more cumbersome technique than the single injection method, the possible disadvantage of a more taxing technique is outweighed by the advantage of reducing the total dose of ketamine, which results in fewer side-effects and a more rapid return to the awake state. As discussed subsequently, the method appears particularly effective when employed in combination with other anesthetics or adjunctive agents, in the anesthetic management of high-risk and geriatric patients, in outpatient dentistry, in obstetric anesthesia, and in post-operative pain relief in elderly and debilitated patients.

INTRAMUSCULAR ADMINISTRATION

Ketamine is absorbed fairly promptly from intramuscular sites of injection, thus rendering this route clinically useful. Effective intramuscular doses are three to five times larger than comparable intravenous doses, so the initial dose of ketamine given intramuscularly may range from 5 to 10 mg/kg. The drug should be injected deeply into the deltoid, gluteal, or vastus lateralis muscle. Anesthesia is established within 2 to 3 minutes and lasts approximately 12 to 25 minutes. As the effects begin to wane, supplemental intraoperative intramuscular injections of 2.5 to 5.0 mg/kg will each prolong anesthesia for an additional 15 to 20 minutes. Lesser doses (e.g., 0.44 mg/kg) of ketamine can be administered intramuscularly to produce analgesia without loss of consciousness.[40] The onset of analgesia is more rapid and its duration is substantially shorter than with meperidine (0.5 to 1.0 mg/kg intramuscularly). These analgesic but subanesthetic doses of ketamine can be useful for short manipulative procedures with or without supplementation by other anesthetics, or as substitutes for narcotic analgesics in high-risk patients in whom respiratory and circulatory depression could be detrimental.[40] For reasons unknown, psychic reactions to these subdissociative doses of ketamine are predominantly pleasant; agitation phenomena are virtually absent.

RECTAL ADMINISTRATION

Ketamine (8 to 10 mg/kg to a maximum of 150 mg) delivered rectally can facilitate induction of anesthesia in the frightened or hostile child.[315] Concentrations of 1% are appropriate for infants and small children (weighing less than 15 kg), and a 5% solution is optimal for children weighing over 15 kg. When adequate dissociation is achieved, anesthesia may be continued with the chosen general anesthetic.

Supplementary Agents

When indicated, ketamine anesthesia may be usefully augmented by general and local anesthetics and muscle relaxants. Supplementation with nitrous oxide-oxygen mixtures seems most helpful with visceral pain; ketamine dosage can be markedly reduced and recovery time is shortened by over 50%.[316] When used with halothane, ketamine, even in subanesthetic doses, decreases the amount of halothane needed to maintain anesthesia; however, recovery may be prolonged by as much as 3 hours because of halothane-induced inhibition of the biotransformation of ketamine.[37,118,317] The action of the benzodiazepines augments that of ketamine in the induction and maintenance of anesthesia, especially with ketamine infusions. The combination of the two agents prevents a ketamine-induced rise in the rate-pressure product and significantly reduces unpleasant emergence reactions, but the disadvantage of prolonged post-anesthetic recovery is introduced.

Ketamine potentiates the effects of some muscle relaxants, thereby reducing the doses needed. This augmentative action applies to d-tubocurare and to decamethonium, but not to pancuronium.[215] The neuromuscular blocking action of succinylcholine is thought not to be affected, but this observation has been questioned.[214,215]

SPECIFIC CLINICAL APPLICATIONS

Burns

Ketamine offers distinct advantages in the anesthetic management of severe burns, especially in children; outstanding results have been achieved.[1,46,52,53,187,318–327] Having survived the initial injury, these patients face a series of surgical procedures requiring debridement, skin grafting, dressing changes, and, in many instances, extensive reconstructive surgery. Severely burned patients may suffer from "chronic shock," characterized by toxemia, dehydration, anemia, oliguria, protein deficiency, and severe impairment of homeostatic reflex mechanisms. The nutritional status may be further impaired by the persistent anorexia often noted after repeated administration of conventional anesthetics.

Anesthetic considerations for such high-risk patients include avoidance of further circulatory depression, maintenance of airway patency under trying conditions (e.g., the prone position), and early postoperative return to normal activities, including nutritional intake. In addition, with burns involving the face, neck, or oral cavity, the placement of an endotracheal tube may be technically difficult or inadvisable because of the danger of introducing pathogenic organisms into the upper respiratory tract. Ketamine in intravenous doses of 1.5 to 2.2 mg/kg frequently suffices as the sole anesthetic. This dosage provides rapid onset of anesthetic action and satisfactory operating conditions for 8 to 10 minutes, during which time skin grafts are obtained (the most painful phase of the procedure). Subsequent placement of the grafts is not painful. A light state of dissociation is therefore maintained with smaller increments of ketamine (one fourth to one third of the initial dose) given every 20 to 30 minutes. With ketamine so administered, relatively rapid post-anesthetic recovery is assured. A degree of tolerance may develop in some patients after six to eight exposures to ketamine, so that gradually increased doses may be needed thereafter.[46]

In the absence of suitable veins, ketamine may also be administered intramuscularly (doses of 4 to 10 mg/kg). With this route of administration, however, recovery may be somewhat delayed, especially in adult patients.

The use of ketamine intravenously or intramuscularly obviates the placement of a face mask on freshly burned or grafted facial areas. Plate I depicts a 5-year-old boy with third-degree gasoline burns over 40% of his body surface. The photo on the right shows the patient after $3\frac{3}{4}$ hours of ketamine anesthesia during which the burn areas were covered with skin from the lower part of his body. Tracheal intubation was not needed to maintain a patent airway. Ketamine was the sole anesthetic used during six subsequent operations. The boy was discharged in good physical condition 63 days after the burn injury.

Preservation of protective pharyngeal and laryngeal reflexes during ketamine anesthesia facilitates maintenance of free air passages without mechanical appliances, distinctly advantageous in procedures for burn patients, especially when positional changes are needed. Although airway obstruction can occur even with ketamine use (requiring that the anesthesiologist remain alert to this eventuality and prepared to act promptly whenever necessary), this problem rarely occurs, even in such challenging situations as contracture of the neck. In this instance, visualization of the larynx may be impossible and endotracheal intubation to correct airway obstruction may be extremely difficult.[325] Anesthesia with ketamine allows for relatively easy and safe airway management, as evidenced by the case of a 28-year-old woman with third-degree grease burns over 55% of her body (head, neck, and upper chest) who developed a large scar between the chin and sternum (Plate II, top).[46] During anesthesia with ketamine, the scar was excised and a metal bar was driven through the mandible to allow extension of the head (Plate II, middle). The large defect between her chin and sternum was covered with skin from the lower part of her body (Plate II, bottom). Tracheal intubation was not required.

Other advantages of ketamine use for severely burned patients of any age are its lack of cumulative toxicity to any vital organ system and the absence of anorexia, nausea, or vomiting; the former enables repeated use of ketamine (e.g., as many as 18 times with impunity); the latter enables the majority of the burn patients receiving ketamine to take liquids by mouth shortly after regaining consciousness.[46] Consequently, good nutritional status can be achieved in these frequently debilitated individuals.

Elderly Individuals

In elderly patients with minimal compensatory reserves, the combination of ketamine with nitrous oxide and muscle relaxants, especially pancuronium, offers cardiovascular support with few side-effects and post-anesthetic complications.[328–339] Pancuronium seems the preferred relaxant because it too increases heart rate, cardiac output, and arterial pressure with no change in peripheral resistance. A useful preoperative sequence consists of preanesthetic medication with either droperidol (2.5 to 5 mg intramuscularly) or a benzodiazepine, preferably lorazepam (2 to 4 mg orally), 30 to 60 minutes before induction of anesthesia with ketamine (1 to 1.5 mg/kg intravenously) limited to a maximum of 150 mg. Two successive increments are administered; the first, not to exceed 100 mg, is injected slowly over 30 to 40 seconds and is followed 30 seconds later by the second dose of no more than 50 mg. Muscle relaxation as needed is achieved by the administration of pancuronium (0.08 to 0.1 mg/kg intravenously), and anesthesia is maintained with nitrous oxide-oxygen together with additional small (25 mg) doses of ketamine given intravenously whenever vital signs indicate lightening of the dissociative anesthetic state. These doses of ketamine seem adequate, although the use of somewhat larger initial doses (200 mg intravenously) followed by increments of 30 mg given intravenously has been recommended.[338,339] Indeed, even smaller doses of ketamine (0.75 mg/kg intravenously) combined with the imminently available benzodiazepine, midazolam (in doses of 0.14 mg/kg intravenously), have been suggested for rapid-sequence induction of general anesthesia for emergency operations.[175]

Most patients are responsive before leaving the operating room, without subsequent recall of either dreams or the operation. An important subgroup of patients in this category, those in early acute hemorrhagic shock, also benefit from the use of ketamine.[183,340] Figure 7–21 shows the cardiovascular effects of ketamine in patients in hemorrhagic shock for whom operative intervention was urgently needed for survival.[183] Prior to induction of anesthesia, all patients received appropriate fluid or blood replacement, with some improvement in arterial blood pressure level. Five minutes after ketamine delivery (2 mg/kg intravenously), mean systolic blood pressure values had risen by 17% and heart rate showed an increase of 3% over the preinduction values. The subsequent nitrous oxide-relaxant anesthetic was supplemented by small increments of ketamine (25 mg intravenously) as needed. Blood pressure, heart rate, and urinary output determinations all remained slightly elevated throughout the operation.

Note that the modest increases in blood pressure level and heart rate with ketamine use in patients in hemorrhagic shock (Fig. 7–21) contrast with the marked pressor response commonly observed in normotensive patients because of the ketamine-induced increase in plasma catecholamines.[229,230] Pancuronium exerts different actions in these two groups. The vasopressor effects of ketamine are attenuated in normovolemic persons but are enhanced in individuals in hemorrhagic shock.[341,342] The value of ketamine administration to persons in hem-

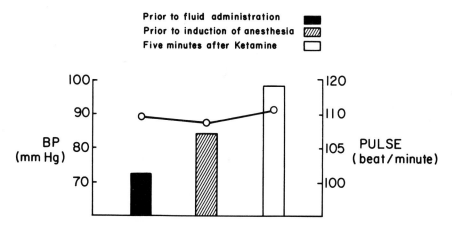

Fig. 7–21. Cardiovascular effects of ketamine in hemorrhagic shock. (From Corssen, G., Reves, J.G., and Carter, J.R.: Neuroleptanesthesia, dissociative anesthesia and hemorrhage. Int. Anesthesiol. Clin., *12*:145, 1974.)

orrhagic shock has been questioned, however, on the basis of findings of shorter survival times of myocardial tissue in laboratory animals who received ketamine when compared to those who underwent barbiturate and halothane anesthesia.[343]

The situation of patients in chronic shock is different. In persons stressed by several days of hypotension, the cardiovascular stimulatory action of ketamine may be reduced and its myocardial depressant action may be unmasked.[17] Decreased ventricular contractility and cardiac output then result.[158]

Orthopedic Emergencies

Ketamine is well suited for pain control during orthopedic emergencies, such as fractures requiring closed reduction and application of plaster casts.[344–351] In shocklike states, the sympathomimetic properties of the drug may help to sustain arterial blood pressure until concomitant intravenous fluid replacement becomes fully effective. Because the drug does not provide muscle relaxation and may even increase muscle tone, the administration of short-acting muscle relaxants may be required before orthopedic manipulations. During the ensuing neuromuscular blockade, respiration may be controlled with a face mask, with or without intubation of the trachea, as needed.

Cardiothoracic Surgery

Ketamine is a suitable anesthetic for use during open-heart surgery (and closed valvotomy), especially in infants and small children with congenital heart defects or great vessel anomalies, with or without induced hypothermia.[352–364] The cardiovascular-stimulating properties of the drug are potentially useful in desperately ill patients with minimal cardiac reserve who are unable to tolerate further depression of myocardial function produced by conventional anesthetic substances.[358] The same stimulation may, however, be deleterious if the increased myocardial oxygen demand cannot be met because of impaired coronary artery blood flow.[365] The ketamine-induced rise in pulmonary vascular resistance is undesirable in patients with valvular heart disease, especially if associated with tachyarrhythmias and in patients with limited right ventricular functional reserve, as in pulmonary hypertension or pulmonary embolism.[155,352] Another contraindication is implantation of a permanent cardiac pacemaker; ketamine may cause a marked increase in afterload, which might cause myocardial failure in patients with limited cardiac reserve.[366] Fortunately, however, the range of usefulness of ketamine in patients with impaired myocardial function can be extended by using diazepam and pancuronium to prevent the elevation of plasma catecholamines produced by ketamine.[163,165,177]

High doses of diazepam (0.3 to 0.5 mg/kg intravenously) can attenuate the cardiovascular stimulatory action of ketamine that is so undesirable in these patients.[163,165,269,367–369] In one example of such use in open-heart surgery, anesthesia was induced with diazepam (0.3 to 0.5 mg/kg) administered intravenously in 5-mg increments, followed by an initial dose of ketamine (1 mg/kg), a "microminidrip" of diazepam (5 to 15 mg), and ketamine (150 mg) in 150 ml of glucose 5% in water.[370] Initial doses of d-tubocurare (0.2 mg/kg) or pancuronium (0.04 mg/kg) were followed by additional doses as needed. This sequence allows maintenance of relatively constant and adequate plasma levels of ketamine and diazepam, with minimal cardiovascular disturbance and no post-anesthetic emergence reactions. Similarly, in patients receiving coronary artery bypass grafts, ketamine-nitrous oxide anesthesia produces greater mean maximal increases in systolic blood pressure and rate-pressure product than does morphine-diazepam-nitrous oxide anesthesia, although the difference can be eliminated by the addition of diazepam to the ketamine-nitrous oxide combination.[371] Indeed, administration of high doses of diazepam (0.5 mg/kg intravenously) combined with ketamine (1 to 2 mg/kg intravenously) for induction and 15 to 30 mg/kg/minute for maintenance is a viable alternative to morphine-nitrous oxide anesthesia for patients undergoing coronary bypass or heart-valve replacement.[369] In patients with cardiac tamponade or constrictive pericarditis, ketamine seems superior to other general anesthetics, even though it may increase pulmonary vascular resistance; the sympathetic stimulating action of the drug, although limited in duration, does maintain cardiovascular homeostasis.[372]

The combined use of ketamine and diazepam may be superior to conventional anesthetics for use in one-lung anesthesia, producing lower pulmonary shunt fractions and higher PaO_2 values than those obtained with halothane anesthesia, with no change in oxygen consumption.[168,373]

Cardiac Catheterization in Children

Ketamine is an effective anesthetic agent to use during cardiac catheterization and angiography in children, including those with severe cardiovascular impairment.[374–380] It meets the requirement of a general anesthetic in providing a steady state of cardiovascular parameters, even in such exaggerated postures as the so-called hepatoclavicular position (Fig. 7–22).[380,381] An added advantage of the drug is its antiarrhythmic action, resulting in fewer catheter-associated arrhythmias than are noted with other general anesthetics.[104]

In one technique, which has been highly effective in 3500 infants and children over a period of 9 years, patients are premedicated with pentobarbital (5 to 6 mg/kg), meperidine (1 mg/kg), and scopolamine (0.01 to 0.02 mg/kg intramuscularly) 45 to 60 minutes before transfer to the catheterization laboratory.[380] Such "heavy" preanesthetic medication prevents agitation or crying and is well tolerated even by infants and children with low pulmonary blood flow and cyanotic heart disease.

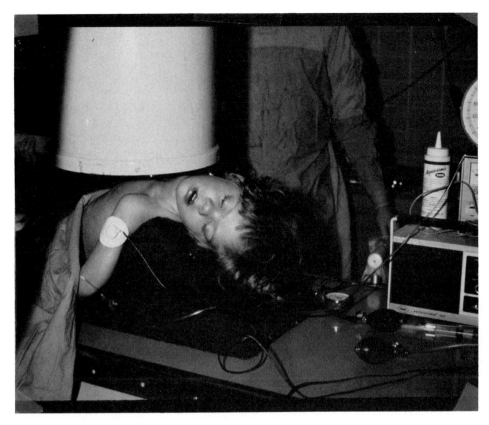

Fig. 7–22. Use of ketamine during cardiac catheterization and angiography in children. (From Samuelson, P.N.: Anesthesia for pediatric cardiac catheterisation. Symposium of Pediatric Cardiac Anesthesia, American Academy of Pediatrics. Maui, Hawaii, March, 1982.)

Ketamine (4 mg/kg intramuscularly) may be used if needed to facilitate venous cannulation. Anesthesia is induced with ketamine (0.5 to 1.0 mg/kg intravenously); this dose is repeated in intervals as required. Infants and children usually tolerate these highly unphysiologic positions well; only occasionally is it necessary to assist breathing with use of a face mask in neonates and young infants. Intubation through the trachea and controlled ventilation are ordinarily reserved for use in infants who are less than 1 month old, who weigh less than 3 kg, or who are extremely ill. Recovery is usually uneventful.

Ketamine should be used with caution in patients with decreased pulmonary blood flow because of its tendency to increase pulmonary vascular resistance. This increase, often associated with infundibular contraction, results in increased right ventricular pressures and directional shunt flow.[380] Unexpectedly, infants and children with decreased pulmonary blood flow become less cyanotic after ketamine administration. Improvement in skin color may be due to increased peripheral vascular resistance, resulting in a decrease in the right to left shunt frequently present. Improvement may also be attributable to either or both increased cardiac output and decreased oxygen utilization.[380]

Bronchospastic Disease

Because ketamine reduces airway resistance and increases pulmonary compliance, it protects against precipitation of bronchospasm in asymptomatic asthmatic patients and ameliorates or eliminates wheezing present at the start of anesthesia.[199] Ketamine also effectively counters bronchospasm that occurs with the use of other anesthetic agents, including halothane.[200] Usual doses (1 to 2.2 mg/kg intravenously) are safe when used for rapid induction of anesthesia in patients of any age with reactive airway disease. Subanesthetic doses also effectively lower increased airway resistance, e.g., in refractory status asthmaticus and other kinds of bronchospasm and asthma, including the asthmatic parturient.[200,382–385]

The drug may be preferred for use in severely anemic asthmatic patients and in other individuals requiring high inspired-oxygen concentrations, because it can be administered with 100% oxygen. Curiously, ketamine seems ineffective against airway resistance increased by ultrasonic aerosols.[198] In summary, ketamine is a welcome alternative to halothane, enflurane, or isoflurane in patients with reactive airway disease; at times, its use may even be preferable.

Obstetrics

Ketamine enables the anesthesiologist to offer the parturient (1) excellent analgesia, with (2) prompt and pleasant onset; (3) high maternal inspired oxygen concentrations; (4) cardiovascular support; (5) minimal effect on uterine contractions; and (6) minimal neonatal depression. These benefits can be realized within the limitations imposed by the pharmacodynamics and pharmacokinetics of ketamine. For example, uterine blood flow is increased concomitant with the rise in systemic arterial pressure.[29] Ordinarily advantageous, this increase would be undesirable in the face of impending rupture of the uterus. Again, unlike other anesthetics, which especially in large doses tend to depress uterine tone and contractions, large doses of ketamine (75 to 100 mg intravenously) increase both frequency and intensity of contractions (but not in smaller doses, e.g., 25 mg intravenously).[227] Its relatively small molecular size and high lipid solubility permit rapid transfer of ketamine across the placenta into the fetus.[30] Nevertheless, small doses of ketamine (0.2 to 1.0 mg/kg intravenously) to the mother are prevented from achieving depressant concentrations in the fetus by a succession of events, including rapid decline in maternal drug levels, uterine contractions, cord compression, non-homogeneity of blood in the intervillous space, extraction by the fetal liver, and progressive dilution and shunting in the fetal circulation.[29] Alas, this protection is only relative: larger doses of ketamine (2.0 to 2.2 mg/kg) readily result in depressed infants with low Apgar scores.[31–34,277]

Vaginal Delivery

Pain control during labor and delivery is rapidly achieved with subanesthetic doses of ketamine (0.2 to 0.5 mg/kg intravenously).[386–390] The initial dose of ketamine (12.5 to 25 mg) is administered when the baby's head crowns. Because uterine contractions during labor interpose an intermittent obstruction to perfusion of the placenta, the injection should be timed to coincide with the onset of a contraction, allowing the initial rapid decline in maternal plasma concentrations of ketamine to occur while access to the placenta is temporarily denied. By the time perfusion returns to a normal level, the concentration gradient of ketamine across the placenta will have been greatly reduced, minimizing fetal exposure to the drug. Additional increments of ketamine are given as needed, similarly at the onset of subsequent contractions. The total dose of ketamine should not exceed 100 mg. The administration of oxygen by face mask should be instituted immediately upon completion of the initial injection of ketamine and continued until delivery is completed.[391] Note that this low-dose ketamine technique is recommended only for speedy, uneventful vaginal delivery. If any complication is anticipated, slightly higher doses of ketamine (as much as 1 mg/kg intravenously) are preferred, supplemented with 50% nitrous oxide and 50% oxygen by an endotracheal tube to safeguard against aspiration of gastric contents. With this technique, there is virtually no recall of discomfort; dreaming may occur in 20% of the mothers, but it is usually pleasant and acceptance by patients is excellent.[387]

CESAREAN SECTION

For use during cesarean section, after approximately 3 minutes of oxygen breathing through a face mask, ketamine (1 mg/kg intravenously) is administered over a period of 30 seconds followed by succinylcholine (1 mg/kg intravenously) to facilitate the insertion of a cuffed endotracheal tube; cricoid pressure is applied concurrently to prevent regurgitation of acid gastric contents.[392] Analgesia is maintained with ketamine in increments of 0.25 mg/kg intravenously every 8 to 10 minutes or whenever movements of the head or extremities of the mother indicate lightening of anesthesia. Alternatively, nitrous oxide and oxygen (50:50) may be added, in which case no further ketamine is administered until the baby is delivered and the umbilical cord is clamped. Additional doses of succinylcholine (0.5 mg/kg intravenously) or pancuronium (0.05 mg/kg intravenously) may be given as needed to maintain adequate abdominal muscle relaxation. If pancuronium is used, the neuromuscular block should be reversed with delivery of an anticholinesterase preparation at the end of the procedure.

The once usual administration of nitrous oxide-oxygen (70:30) during anesthesia for cesarean section is no longer acceptable because of possible deleterious effects on the fetus and newborn.[393] This change has led to the widespread adoption of the use of higher concentrations (50% or more) of oxygen, with resultant increased incidence of awareness during operation.[394] Ketamine offers the advantage of virtually eliminating intraoperative awareness, while simultaneously contributing importantly as an analgesic agent.[395,396] When compared with thiopental, the incidence of undesirable emergence reactions is low and significantly different from those noted with ketamine. Although few studies in humans have been conducted, ketamine causes no ill effects on fetal acid-base status in sheep.[29] Neonatal blood pressure is less depressed with ketamine than with thiopental.[397] In one study of the use of ketamine as the sole anesthetic for cesarean section, the fetal mortality rate was less than one-half that recorded with the use of other general anesthetics.[398]

DELIVERY IN THE PRESENCE OF MEDICAL COMPLICATIONS

Ketamine anesthesia for vaginal delivery or cesarean section may be indicated for patients with bronchospastic disease, including asthma; when bleeding results in hypovolemia or shocklike states; in patients with retained placenta that requires manual removal, especially in developing countries where anemia may be common but blood transfusion facilities are not, or, because of its antiepileptic action, in the anesthetic management of pre-eclamptic and eclamptic patients.[277,399-403] Ketamine use may be preferred in the termination of pregnancy for medical reasons.[404]

Neurobehavioral Studies in Neonates

Newly developed tests for assessing alterations in the neurobehavioral function of neonates, attributable to the anesthetic used, were applied on the first and second days of life after anesthesia with regional block, thiopental-nitrous oxide, or ketamine-nitrous oxide for vaginal delivery or cesarean section.[405,406] Not surprisingly, neurobehavioral scores were highest in the neonates after regional anesthesia; scores were intermediate with ketamine-nitrous oxide, but were not significantly higher than those recorded after thiopental-nitrous oxide. The full implications of such relatively new testing procedures are still to be established. Clearly, drugs that depress tone, rooting, and sucking may not significantly affect healthy infants, but they may tip the balance against neonates at risk.

Outpatient Surgery

PEDIATRIC PATIENTS

Ketamine at doses of 0.5 to 1.5 mg/kg intravenously or 2 to 4 mg/kg intramuscularly is suitable for use in children for all kinds of brief diagnostic and therapeutic procedures. The intravenous route is preferred for use in outpatient procedures because of its shorter recovery period. The intramuscular route is reserved for uncooperative children or those for whom intravenous access is difficult. Increased salivation is usually slow to develop, presenting no problem for the first 10 to 15 minutes of anesthesia. Hence, preanesthetic medication with antisialogogues may be omitted for procedures of 15 minutes or less in duration. For longer operations, scopolamine in dosage according to age and weight may be administered intramuscularly 30 minutes prior to induction of anesthesia. All procedures should be completed within approximately 30 minutes; only rarely is deviation from this rule permitted. Complications in umpremedicated patients include undesirable cardiovascular stimulation and partial airway obstruction.[407]

Minor Surgery. Ketamine is optimal, when used for many types of minor pediatric surgery, especially procedures involving the head and face for which endotracheal anesthesia may impair sterility and interfere with the performance of the operation.[272,321,408-422] If there is any doubt about airway patency, however, placement of an endotracheal tube is mandatory.

Ophthalmologic Surgery. The value of ketamine when used during ophthalmologic procedures reflects its usefulness for pediatric outpatients. Fundoscopy, tonometry, goniotomy, dacryocystorhinostomy, and removal of corneal sutures are some ophthalmologic procedures for which ketamine is particularly valuable.[423] Here, the absence of masks, tubes, and other anesthetic appliances, permitting unencumbered access to the operative field, is a distinct advantage.[409,424-428] A single intravenous injection of ketamine usually provides anesthesia of adequate duration for diagnostic and brief therapeutic procedures. Ketamine is not appropriate for use during longer corrective ophthalmic operations in an outpatient setting because recovery is prolonged and discharge of the patient is delayed.

Ketamine produces a mild but statistically significant rise in intraocular pressure, unrelated to age or blood pressure changes and insufficient in magnitude to contraindicate its use in individuals with glaucoma.[54,237–243] For complete ocular examinations, particularly when the presence of glaucoma is suspected, the temporary, slight increase in intraocular tension during ketamine anesthesia (unlike the decrease with most anesthetics) may be advantageous in that it provides the ophthalmologist with more meaningful diagnostic values. Although the fine ocular movements observed in some children during ketamine anesthesia do not interfere with extraocular operations, occasional gross movements of the head may cause problems.[246,423] The need for skilled airway management without an endotracheal tube and the difficulties in ensuring a quiet undisturbed term of recovery are disadvantages related to ketamine anesthesia in ophthalmologic practice.[424]

Oral Surgery, Maxillofacial Surgery, and Dentistry. Ketamine is particularly appropriate for use during tooth extractions and other brief surgical procedures in and around the mouth and jaw in an outpatient setting. Pharyngeal and laryngeal reflexes are not obtunded and the muscles of the tongue and jaw are not relaxed; the airway therefore usually remains patent without artificial support, facilitating access to the surgical field. The placement of a bite-blocking wedge and removal by the assistant of blood, pus, or dental material is essential. Pulmonary aspiration or other respiratory compromise is thus unlikely. Postural hypotension related to the sitting of semirecumbent position is virtually eliminated by ketamine anesthesia because of the concomitant cardiovascular stimulation. In most children, removal of orthodontic appliances and other minor intraoral manipulations are feasible with a single injection of ketamine (1.0 to 1.5 mg/kg intravenously); even lower doses (0.5 to 1.0 mg/kg intravenously or 1 to 3 mg/kg intramuscularly) are adequate.[429–435] Indeed, for procedures lasting no more than 3 minutes, e.g., removal of several incisor or premolar teeth, the dose may be reduced to as small an amount as 0.25 mg/kg intravenously. It is advisable to wait 60 to 90 seconds to establish adequate dissociation before starting to operate; the recovery period is shortened to under 15 minutes.

In the general practice of dentistry, ketamine may be employed concomitant with local anesthesia.[436] To provide 15 minutes of operating time, one should administer weight-scaled doses of ketamine as follows[437]: for patients who weigh less than 22.5 kg, approximately 1.5 mg/kg administered intravenously; for those who weigh 22.5 to 45 kg, no more than 2.2 mg/kg administered intravenously; and for patients who weigh more than 45 kg, as much as 3 mg/kg administered intravenously. For as much as 30 minutes of dental conservation in children, ketamine (1 mg/kg intravenously) may be administered with supplemental doses in increments of 10 mg intravenously as needed.[438] Unmanageable or apprehensive children can be made completely cooperative with ketamine (4 mg/kg intramuscularly), whereas in severely mentally retarded children, subanesthetic doses (2 to 3 mg/kg intramuscularly) permit tooth extraction and conservation procedures not feasible with local anesthesia.[434,439] Ketamine given intramuscularly is also useful in infants and small children for removal of sutures after cleft lip or palate repair.[440] Note that nitrous oxide-oxygen mixtures administered through a nose piece reduce the requirement for additional doses of ketamine and also decrease the incidence and severity of side-effects. Pain-relieving medication is rarely required postoperatively because ketamine-induced analgesia seems to extend well into the early recovery phase.[264]

Ear, Nose, and Throat Surgery. Ketamine (1 to 1.5 mg/kg intravenously) use in children readily permits the performance of ear examinations; myringotomies, including insertion of plastic tubes; and procedures to remove foreign bodies from the ear canal.[441] Because additional injections of the anesthetic are rarely needed, recovery is prompt, especially if preanesthetic medication is omitted. During such delicate manipulations, the head should be steadied by the anesthesiologist to avoid interference from involuntary head movements. Although ketamine has been utilized as the sole anesthetic for adenotonsillectomy, such practice is not recommended, even with an unusually skilled surgeon who can reduce operating time to a minimum.[442–444] Gagging, retching, and coughing may interfere with the proper conduct of surgery, but more importantly, pulmonary aspiration may occur despite active laryngeal reflexes. Ketamine can be used safely for this procedure, however, when combined with the use of other general anesthetics and tracheal intubation, although it may not offer particular advantages over other agents.[265,445]

The risk of pulmonary aspiration should not be overlooked during ketamine anesthesia for intranasal and intraoral operations.[446] Obviously, the patient should be intubated through the trachea whenever the possibility exists. If the continued presence of an endotracheal tube is required to ensure airway patency (e.g., in acute epiglottitis), proper use of sedatives or tranquilizers to control restlessness or excitement during emergence from ketamine anesthesia can prevent accidental extubation.[447]

Bronchoscopy. Although ketamine anesthesia is safe for use during bronchoscopy in children without an endotracheal tube, it offers no unique advantage for this purpose.[448] Introduction of the bronchoscope may result in vigorous coughing unless the respiratory mucosa has first been thoroughly sprayed with a topical anesthetic, which may not be feasible with an uncooperative child. In addition, should a respiratory tract inflammation be present, coughing spells induced by foreign body stimulation of the airway could be exacerbated during ketamine anesthesia.

Immobilization for Radiotherapy. In infants and small children, such restraint usually necessitates the use of general anesthesia of short duration. With conventional anesthetics, endotracheal intubation is essential to ensure airway patency during the time of irradiation, when the patient is temporarily unattended. Use of ketamine is now widely accepted for this purpose because the airway can usually be secured without artificial support.[266,322,449–452] Other advantages include rapid induction, cardiovascular stability, and low toxicity with repeated administrations. One caveat: ketamine should be used with caution in children with increased intracranial pressure because the drug itself may temporarily exacerbate that increase.

For many anesthesiologists, dissociative anesthesia with ketamine is now the method of choice for immobilizing infants and small children for radiotherapy. Doses of 2 to 3 mg/kg intravenously or 3 to 5 mg/kg intramuscularly usually suffice for the first few sessions. Delivery of larger doses, 6 to 10 mg/kg intramuscularly, can achieve a longer effect.[453,454] Tolerance to ketamine may develop after repeated administrations, requiring some increase in dosage for further treatments.[50,51,450] As illustrated in Figure 7–23, a 6-year-old boy with inoperable intracerebral ependymoma was irradiated on 45 consecutive days. With ketamine anesthesia (2 mg/kg intravenously) the child was immobilized for an average of 7 minutes. No tolerance developed and no adverse toxic effects on vital organ systems, including the hemopoietic system, were encountered.

ADULT PATIENTS

Most gynecologic, urologic, orthopedic, and general surgical diagnostic or therapeutic procedures not exceeding 15 minutes can be safely conducted in adults with subanesthetic doses (0.2 to 0.5 mg/kg intravenously) of ketamine, with nitrous oxide added to control visceral pain or to produce unconsciousness if desired. Recovery from a full dissociative dose of ketamine (2.2 mg/kg intravenously or 10 mg/kg intramuscularly) sufficient to enable discharge of the patient in the care of another adult usually occurs within 1 hour, but delay may be considerable, especially with intramuscular administration of ketamine or with repeated doses to prolong anesthesia. Complete restoration of visual acuity and

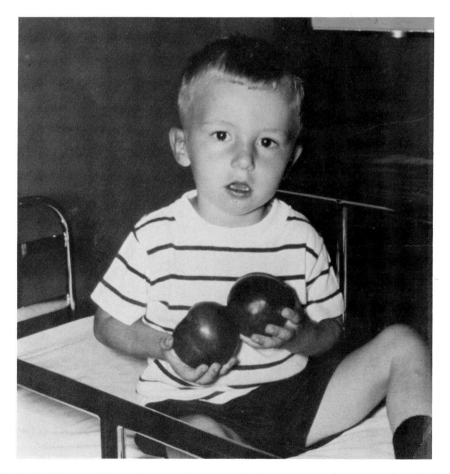

Fig. 7–23. Six-year-old boy with inoperable intracerebral ependymoma after recovery from the forty-fifth round of ketamine anesthesia. The boy was given two peaches as a reward for his continuous cooperative behavior throughout the 45-day radiation therapy period.

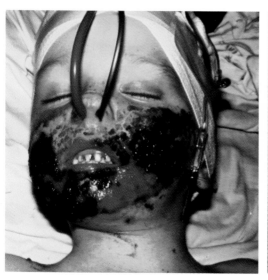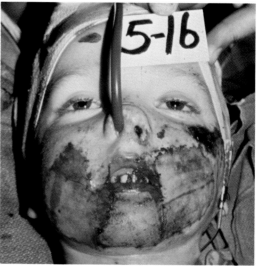

Plate I. Left, ketamine used for burn treatment. Five-year-old boy at start of operation. Right, same patient at end of operation. (From Corssen, G., and Oget, S.: Dissociative anesthesia for the severely burned child. Anesth. Analg., 50:95,1971.)

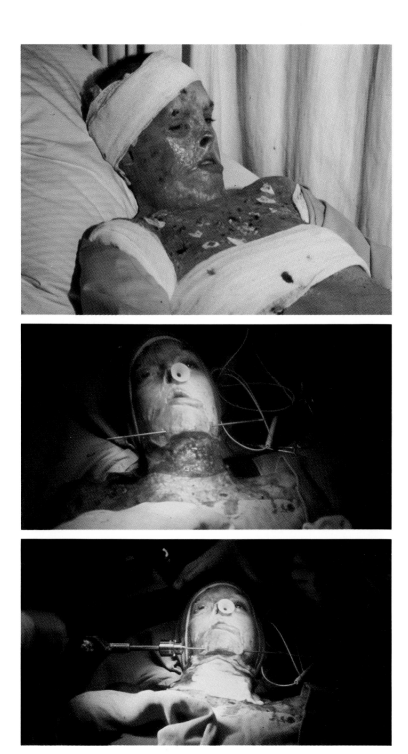

Plate II. Top, Ketamine used for burn treatment. Woman awaiting plastic surgical repair of extensive contracture of the neck. Middle, During ketamine anesthesia, scar is excised, and a rod transfixing the mandible is placed to facilitate extension of the head for skin grafting of neck. Bottom, Skin placement is completed. (From Bjarnesen, W., and Corssen, G.: CI-581: a new non-barbiturate short-acting anesthetic for surgery in burns. Mich. Med., 66:177, 1967.)

equilibrium may require several hours. Note too that benzodiazepines or other drugs added to reduce undesirable effects of ketamine prolong the recovery period.

Ketamine is singularly useful in subanesthetic dosage for gynecologic outpatients. Culdoscopy, laparoscopy, laparoscopic sterilization, and dilatation and curettage can be performed satisfactorily with the use of nitrous oxide to control visceral pain. For laparoscopic sterilization, ketamine in full dosage (2 to 2.2 mg/kg intravenously) may be used as the sole anesthetic, may be combined with other agents (e.g., diazepam or droperidol), or may be used in conjunction with conduction blocks in a 1-day surgery setting.[275,455–458] Ketamine anesthesia combined with paracervical block seems especially suitable for therapeutic abortions, because the ketamine-induced increase in uterine tone minimizes intra- and postoperative bleeding.[276] Because of the emotional implications of this procedure, preanesthetic medication adequate to reduce stress and anxiety is essential.[459] Any undesirable post-anesthetic sequelae may deter patient acceptance.[460]

Neurodiagnostic Procedures

The use of ketamine is advantageous in both children and adults undergoing pneumoencephalography, ventriculography, cerebral angiography, and myelography.[461–463] Concomitant intense discomfort and lack of cooperation, especially in infants and children, may be averted. Also the postural hypotension so often observed in patients under conventional anesthesia, related to the sitting position frequently required for these procedures (Fig. 7–24A), is rarely encountered because of the counterbalancing cardiovascular stimulatory effects of ketamine. The occasional episode of postural hypotension is readily reversed upon return to the recumbent position. Wrapping the lower extremities with bandages is a useful precaution. Airway management with changes and distortions of position (Fig. 7–24B) is facilitated because the tone of intraoral muscles is maintained. Vomiting occurs infrequently with ketamine anesthesia; should it result from the procedure itself, aspiration of vomitus is unlikely because of the persistent action of pharyngeal and laryngeal reflexes during ketamine anesthesia.

Adequate anesthesia is readily established in pediatric patients in this group with an initial dose of ketamine ranging from 0.5 to 1.5 mg/kg intravenously or (if venous access or the patient proves difficult) 5 to 10 mg/kg intramuscularly, and is maintained with small increments every 15 to 20 minutes as needed. Supplementation with nitrous oxide should, of course, be avoided because of the hazard of overdistention of the ventricular system. Ketamine has been administered to adults undergoing carotid arteriography and in small doses (10 to 20 mg intravenously) with diazepam (2.5 to 5.0 mg intravenously) and droperidol (2.5 mg intravenously) to persons undergoing pneumoencephalography, without adverse cardiovascular or respiratory effects.[464]

Ketamine increases cerebral blood flow (CBF), which tends to raise intracranial pressure (ICP). Ketamine is thus not recommended for use in patients with elevated ICP. In normal individuals, ICP should be monitored, and rapid decompression, if needed, should be accomplished by removal of CSF, by injection of thiopental (100 mg intravenously), or by hyperventilation to lower Pa_{CO_2}.[151,465] The removal of CSF is the least desirable method, because it could result in herniation of brain tissue at the tentorium or foramen magnum, with detrimental effects on cardiorespiratory function.

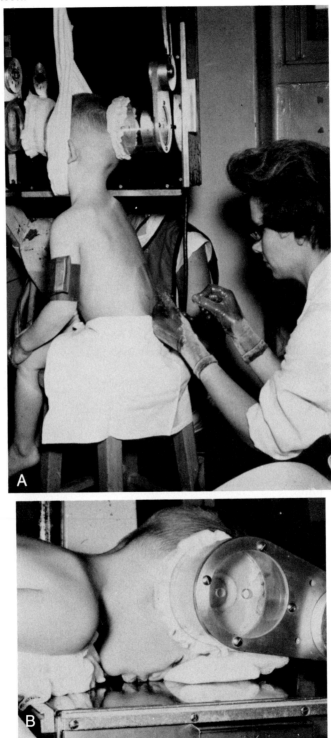

Fig. 7–24. *A*, Use of ketamine during pneumoencephalography in children. Child shown in sitting position for lumbar puncture 1 minute after ketamine administration (1.5 mg/kg intravenously). *B*, Same patient, in prone position for radiologic studies. (From Corssen, G., Groves, E.H., Gomez, S., and Allen, R.J.: Ketamine: its place in anesthesia for neurological diagnostic procedures. Anesth. Analg., *48*:181, 1969.)

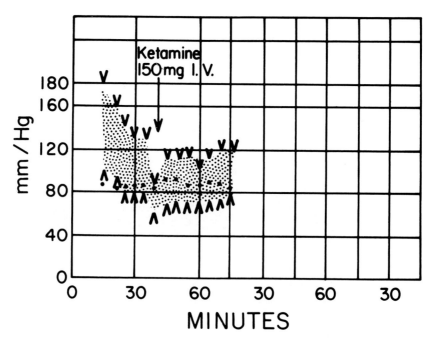

Fig. 7–25. Antihypotensive effect of ketamine during regional anesthesia. Hypotension occurs after epidural block for lumbar laminectomy in prone position. Normal pressures are promptly restored after ketamine (2 mg/kg intravenously) is used as an adjunct to the block. (From Erdemir, H.A., Huber, F.C., and Corssen, G.: Dissociative anesthesia with ketamine: a suitable adjunct to epidural anesthesia. Anesth. Analg., *49*:623, 1970.)

Adjunct to Local and Regional Anesthesia

Ketamine is useful as such an adjunct because it provides analgesia, sedation, and amnesia without respiratory depression. Unlike other sedative or analgesic supplements, ketamine stimulates cardiovascular function, thereby counteracting the hypotensive effects that can be encountered with the establishment of regional blocks (Fig. 7–25).[466–468] The antiarrhythmic effect of the drug also protects against side-effects related to excessive amounts of epinephrine that may be used for hemostasis during infiltration of local anesthetics. In addition, ketamine produces instant analgesia, eliminating the delay of waiting for the regional anesthesia to be complete before starting the operation. On the other hand, diminishing analgesia caused by a waning block can be adequately restored by additional small injections of ketamine (0.2 to 0.5 mg/kg intravenously). Similarly, if the initial analgesic effect is inadequate (e.g., if residual tissue damage from a previous laminectomy impedes diffusion of the local anesthetic through the epidural space), ketamine may remedy the deficit. The advantages of using ketamine as an adjunct to regional anesthesia are exemplified by a comparison with diazepam and Innovar for sedation and analgesia prior to intercostal nerve blocks.[469] More than 50% of the group of patients treated with diazepam and Innovar were inadequately sedated, whereas ketamine produced excellent results and patient acceptance (e.g., only 10% of the patient group had unpleasant dreams) was above average.

Plastic Surgery

The ketamine-diazepam combination is satisfactory for use during cosmetic surgical procedures.[118] More recently, the longer-acting substance diazepam is being replaced by lorazepam (2 to 4 mg intravenously or orally), which rapidly produces sedation and tranquility; ketamine (0.5 to 1.0 mg/kg intravenously) is then delivered 30 to 60 seconds later. The light dissociative state established lasts for approximately 15 minutes. During this period, the surgeon performs the most painful part of the procedure, e.g., grafting or excising skin, with the patient in a dreamlike, comfortable, and cooperative state. Subsequently, during the less painful period, e.g., placing and suturing skin, a superficial dissociative state may be maintained by the administration of supplemental doses of ketamine (0.5 mg/kg intravenously) every 15 to 20 minutes. Emergence reactions are negligible, and patient acceptance is excellent.[470]

Surgery in Developing Countries

Ketamine should not be administered by individuals not trained and equipped to handle any emergency that may arise in an unconscious patient.[471] A tentative exception to this rule might be the use of ketamine in developing countries, where physician-anesthesiologists and well-trained nurse anesthetists are scarce. Under these conditions, the disadvantageous properties of ketamine may be insignificant in view of the simplicity of its administration (syringe and needle) and its relative safety in a primitive environment where the practitioner is isolated or separated from the source of supply.[472] In somewhat more favorable circumstances, low doses of ketamine can usefully augment regional anesthetic techniques. Constant supervision by an individual familiar with anesthetic problems and their management, however, is still desirable.[471–473]

Disaster Victims

Profound analgesia combined with cardiovascular stimulation, the absence of significant respiratory depression, efficacy when delivered intravenously and intramuscularly, preservation of protective reflexes, and maintenance of an unobstructed airway commend the potential role of ketamine in the anesthetic management of disaster victims. On the battlefield or in disaster situations, the use of ketamine has a decided advantage in that it can be administered without complicated equipment, although ancillary items including self-inflating breathing bags of Ambu type, pharyngeal airways, laryngoscopes, endotracheal tubes, and emergency drugs should be available for immediate use if needed.[474–476]

Ketamine underwent its first real test as an anesthetic for mass casualties in Guatemala, where in February of 1976 a 15-second earthquake and series of aftershocks killed 23,000 people and injured more than 175,000.[477] Roy D. Wilson of Baylor College of Medicine was on the scene with another anesthesiologist and four orthopedic surgeons 24 hours after the disaster. During the next 36 hours, this team treated approximately 150 patients with major orthopedic injuries. Wilson's report is quoted verbatim.

"All patients were anesthetized utilizing the technique of administration of 10 mg of intravenous diazepam, followed by the intravenous administration of a single dose of 50 mg of ketamine. In most instances, the drug was injected into the jugular vein. Surgery commenced instantly and was usually completed within 30 minutes. Excellent anesthesia was provided by this technique. In only three of the individuals was it necessary to use a small intravenous dose of succinylcholine (20 mg). During the period of apnea, the patients' respiration was controlled with an Ambu-bag. Most injuries involved adults because most children did not survive the force of the quake.

Of the 12 operating rooms available, none had running water and few had electricity. Minimal quantities of oxygen were available, and supplies of nitrous oxide were rapidly exhausted. Patients were evacuated by helicopters and carried to the hospital by wheelbarrows. The patients came from altitudes of 7000 to 9000 feet, having lived their entire lives at these elevations. Most of the patients were of Indian origin and were stoic by nature. In none of these patients did we discern, by interpreter or by actions, any emergence phenomena nor did any of the patients require prolonged observation. The ketamine dose was not repeated, and operative procedures were tailored to be completed when the anesthesia wore off. Obviously, the other anesthesiologists and I spent a minimal amount of time monitoring the patients, obtaining only periodic blood pressure values and using visual senses to follow the status of these patients. These were, indeed, battlefield conditions in the truest sense and not something that I would ever wish to duplicate in the United States, with its malpractice problems.

A team of surgeons and anesthesiologists from Costa Rica's medical school in San Jose arrived at approximately the same time we did, but stayed considerably longer. They utilized exactly the same techniques with the same excellent degree of success in the management of these patients.

All of us, including the surgeons, agreed that ketamine served an invaluable place in our armamentarium, although we had carried with us equipment to perform other types of anesthesia. The simplicity of this technique and the logistics of supply and resupply were such that we could not have approached the ease and apparent safety with any other technique that I could think of."

Wilson closed his report by saying, "I spent about 3 years of Air Force time trying to develop anesthesia for mass casualty situations. Nothing in my wildest dreams of minimal equipment ever approached the simplicity and safety of the ketamine technique under these true test conditions."

Other investigators confirmed the value of ketamine when used as the sole anesthetic in combination with diazepam in disaster situations or in the anesthetic management of combat casualties.[463,478–481]

Uncommon Medical or Surgical Problems

The constellation of properties of ketamine detailed previously render its use beneficial in a variety of anesthetic problem situations. Juvenile rheumatoid arthritis (Still's disease) may render intubation of the trachea extremely difficult, if not impossible; repeated attempts to do so may even jeopardize the life of the patient.[482] Patent air passages can be maintained with only an oro- or nasopharyngeal airway during ketamine anesthesia for major surgical procedures, such as total hip or shoulder replacements and knee arthroplasties. Comparable airway problems in children with infantile cerebral palsy undergoing corrective orthopedic surgery have been successfully managed with a combination of ketamine and diazepam.[483]

Reconstructive surgery can present an extraordinary challenge to the anesthesiologist. As illustrated in Figure 7–26, a 48-year-old woman underwent facial reconstruction after radical resection of the right mandible. Ketamine alone served to induce and maintain anesthesia for three consecutive surgical procedures, with an endotracheal tube used for airway support and prevention of aspiration.

Correction of tracheal stenosis has been accomplished during ketamine anesthesia, as has emergency tracheostomy in acutely ill infants and children for whom rapid induction of anesthesia without cardiovascular impairment is vital.[484–486] In the surgical treatment of cardiac tamponade or constrictive pericarditis, the anesthetic of choice seems to be ketamine, supplemented with nitrous oxide (50%), morphine, and pancuronium.[372] Operations in patients with malignant carcinoid syndrome may be complicated by bronchospasm and marked circulatory changes caused by catecholamine release. The combination of ketamine, diazepam, and pancuronium provides suitable anesthesia for these patients,

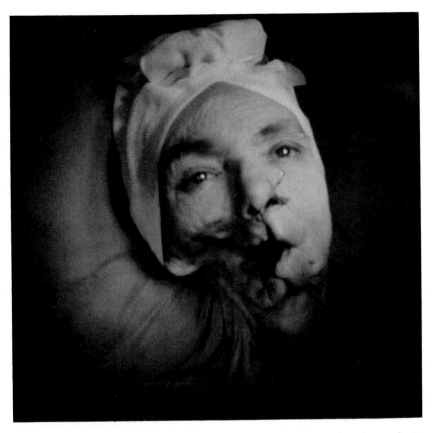

Fig. 7–26. Woman to undergo facial reconstruction receives ketamine as the sole anesthetic.

with ketamine controlling bronchospasm and both diazepam and pancuronium mitigating the catecholamine response to ketamine.[163,177,366]

Epidermolysis bullosa dystrophica is a rare skin condition characterized by the development of vesicles and bullae from even the slighest trauma to skin or mucous membranes. In these patients, physical contact during the delivery of anesthesia should be avoided, including even slight touching of the skin, e.g., elevation of the jaw to support the airway, and certainly the use of appliances, such as face mask, airways, and endotracheal tube. Ketamine anesthesia seems ideal for this purpose.[487,488]

Acute intermittent porphyria constitutes an absolute contraindication to the use of intravenous barbiturates, which stimulate hepatic production of the enzyme Δ-aminolevulinic acid synthetase ALA-S. Ketamine, like diazepam, droperidol, and propanidid, is a safe induction agent for such patients; these drugs do not induce ALA-S production, despite disproven evidence to the contrary.[489–493]

Penile turgescence induced by phallic manipulation during genitourinary procedures can be a distinct hindrance. Ketamine given intravenously can prevent or reverse an erection should it develop, as during hypospadia repair in young children; failure of ketamine to relieve priapism, however, has been reported.[221,222,494]

In patients with hemophilia and other bleeding diatheses, for whom regional anesthesia and other injections are contraindicated and tracheal intubation for general anesthesia may cause occult hemorrhage, ketamine offers a safe alternative.[495] In electroconvulsive therapy, ketamine affords no significant advantage over other anesthetic agents, execpt in patients with reactive airway disease.[496,497] Subanesthetic doses of ketamine played a role in relieving trigeminal neuralgia previously unresponsive to conventional analgesics.[498]

Uremic patients undergoing emergency operations tolerate ketamine well because of its lack of organ toxicity.[499] Similarly, when the use of multiple anesthetics is required, as with repeated bone marrow biopsies, ketamine appears to be the anesthetic agent of choice.[453,500]

Blind nasal intubation of the trachea in patients with serious airway problems, e.g., cervical trauma, neck contractures, micrognathia, maxillofacial injuries, oral tumors, and temporomandibular ankylosis, can be facilitated by dissociative anesthesia with ketamine, cocainization of the nostril and nasopharynx, and transtracheal injection of a topical anesthetic; the nasotracheal tube is readily inserted while the patient breathes spontaneously.[501] Patients who have experienced nasotracheal intubation both while awake but sedated and during dissociative anesthesia with ketamine invariably prefer the latter method.[501] Analgesia after major surgery can be provided by the administration of ketamine, either in single injections of 0.5 mg/kg intravenously or by continuous infusion (e.g., ketamine 0.1% in glucose 5%).[502,503] Especially after upper abdominal and thoracic surgery, with ventilatory "splinting" resulting from pain, ketamine in subanesthetic dosage can provide analgesia without the respiratory depression that invariably accompanies full analgesic doses of narcotics.

Hiccoughs that are refractory to other therapy and are potentially debilitating can be controlled by delivering ketamine in subanesthetic doses, perhaps because of the stimulatory effects of ketamine on subcortical regions.[504,505] Alternatively, ketamine-induced enhancement of protective gag, sneeze, and cough reflexes may mimic the reflex mechanism evoked by nasopharyngeal stimulation.[506] Delirium tremens can be controlled with ketamine use.[507] Diagnostic procedures performed in the dark, e.g., cardiac catheterization and certain ophthalmic diagnostic manipulations, can be made easier with the use of ketamine, recognizing that the administration of anesthesia under such adverse conditions can never be considered foolproof.[508,509]

In the "induced anxiety" technique of psychotherapy, in which the patient is aroused emotionally and physiologically, relaxation techniques are taught so the patient can reduce the arousal and thus learn to cope with the stresses of everyday life. The induced anxiety technique can be enhanced by ketamine use.[510] Minimal subanesthetic doses of ketamine (0.02 mg/kg intravenously) facilitate physiologic arousal during "affect induction," without inhibiting the subsequent relaxation. Although some individuals experienced momentary confusion and mild distortion of body image immediately after drug administration, the sessions on the whole seemed enjoyable.[510] These observations suggest that the use of ketamine at minimal intravenous dosage levels offers a valuable research tool to study emotional changes in response to stress and to elucidate some of the basic psychologic and biochemical mechanisms triggered by the dissociative state.[261]

CONTRAINDICATIONS AND CAUTIONS IN THE USE OF KETAMINE

The ease of administration of ketamine should not invite its casual use by unqualified individuals whenever a short-acting anesthetic is needed. Obviously, the physician or nurse anesthetist using ketamine should be fully equipped to handle any respiratory or cardiovascular emergency in the unconscious patient.

Because of its propensity toward stimulating the cardiovascular system, ketamine should not be given to patients with previous cerebrovascular accidents or poorly controlled hypertension, although mild to moderate hypertension does not contraindicate its use in geriatric patients.[331] The drug should be used with caution in patients with intracranial, thoracic, or abdominal aneurysms. Because ICP may increase after the administration of ketamine, especially if the level of ICP is already elevated as a result of craniocerebral trauma or disease, including tumor, aneurysm, or hemorrhage, the drug is not recommended for use in such patients.[145,146,299] In these conditions, usual doses of ketamine may prove inadequate because the main site of action of the drug is the neocortical-thalamic axis. The administration of excessive doses of ketamine to achieve satisfactory anesthesia can result in respiratory depression and apnea.[511]

Ketamine should be used with caution when intraocular pressure is increased, and not at all when open globe injury to the eye has occurred.[17] Caution also should be exercised with the use of ketamine anesthesia in patients with left ventricular insufficiency. Because ketamine increases pulmonary arterial pressure, causing elevated right ventricular stroke work, its use in patients with pulmonary hypertension is contraindicated. Although ketamine is suitable for performing minor diagnostic and surgical procedures, such as lumbar puncture, dressing changes, incision and drainage of abscesses, and superficial biopsies, the drug should not be used outside of the operating room unless all usual equipment to treat respiratory or cardiovascular complications is readily at hand.[415,416,512] Ketamine should not be employed as the sole anesthetic agent for otolaryngologic procedures, such as tonsillectomy and adenoidectomy, unless the airway is first secured with an endotracheal tube. Drug addicts and individuals afflicted with chronic alcoholism may require the use of excessive doses of ketamine, rendering them prone to such untoward reactions as respiratory depression.

Psychiatric disease does not preclude the use of ketamine, provided that, in the judgment of the anesthesiologist, ketamine is clearly the best alternative and that appropriate psychotropic agents are included in the preanesthetic medication.[513,514] The counsel of the psychiatric staff who monitor the care of psychotic patients is mandatory before ketamine is administered because the drug could exacerbate a psychotic condition.[515]

Ketamine may not be suitable for use in children under 1 year of age, especially those undergoing neurodiagnostic procedures for undetermined neurologic disorders. Even large doses of ketamine may fail to achieve an adequate dissociative state in these patients.[516] Ketamine is contraindicated as the sole anesthetic for bronchoscopy or other endoscopic procedures in children unless it is supplemented with adequate topical anesthesia.[448]

The role of ketamine use in preventing malignant hyperthermia in patients at risk has not been clearly established. When the drug was used as the sole anesthetic for parotidectomy in a patient with a family history of malignant hyperpyrexia, creatinine phosphokinase (CPK) levels decreased markedly during the 3½-hour operation.[517] Ketamine has also been reported to increase CPK levels.[518] Obviously, more data are needed.

Ketamine does not provide satisfactory operating conditions for intra-abdominal surgical procedures that involve the viscera unless it is supplemented with other anesthetics and muscle relaxants.[519–522] The use of ketamine should be avoided in patients being treated with L-dopa because of the possibility of an exaggerated sympathetic response.[523] Similarly, patients receiving thyroid replacement therapy may develop severe hypertension and tachycardia after the administration of ketamine.[524]

Ketamine is an unusually safe, rapid-acting parenteral anesthetic that produces unique sedation, amnesia, and profound somatoanalgesia without causing clinically significant respiratory depression. Side-effects include marked increases in blood pressure levels and heart rate; hypertonicity and involuntary movements of skeletal muscles; profuse salivation; and, most importantly, emergence reactions of agitation, delusions, illusions, and even hallucinations and delirium. Efforts to "tame" ketamine, eliminating or attenuating its undesirable effects with the administration of the benzodiazepines diazepam, flunitrazepam, and lorazepam, have been most effective; the still awaited water-soluble, short-acting midazolam promises to be closest to the ideal. By reducing the total dosage of ketamine administered by employing subanesthetic doses or continuous infusion technique, and by using the drug only for induction of anesthesia before longer operations, adverse effects have been further "tamed." As a result, dissociative anesthesia is being applied successfully for ambulatory and short-stay hospital patients, in children especially but also in adults; in patients requiring repeated operations for the surgical treatment of thermal injury; as an adjunct to conventional general anesthesia during cardiothoracic and other major surgery, especially when ventilatory problems affect the procedure; in the induction of anesthesia in geriatric and critically ill patients; and in obstetric emergencies, e.g., bronchospasm or asthma, during which it is used as a sedative and analgesic adjunct to local or regional anesthesia.

REFERENCES

1. Corssen, G., and Domino, E.F.: Dissociative anesthesia: further pharmacologic studies and first clinical experience with the phencyclidine derivative CI-581. Anesth. Analg., *45*:29, 1966
2. Maddox, V.H.: The historical development of Phencyclidin. *In* PCP (phencyclidine): Historical and Current Perspectives. Edited by E.F. Domino. Ann Arbor, NPP Books, 1981.
3. Chen, G., Ensor, C.R., Russel, D., and Bohner, B.: The pharmacology of 1-(1-phenylcyclohexyl) piperidine-HCL. J. Pharmacol. Exp. Ther., *127*:241, 1959.
4. Greifenstein, F.E., DeVault, M., Yoshitake, J., and Gajewski, J.R.: A study of a 1-aryl cyclo hexyl amine for anesthesia. Anesth. Analg., *37*:283, 1958.
5. Johnstone, M., Evans, V., and Baigel, S.: Sernyl (CI-395) in clinical anesthesia. Br. J. Anaesth., *31*:433, 1959.
6. Lear, E., Suntay, R., Pallin, I.M., and Chiron, A.E.: Cyclohexamine (CI-400): a new intravenous agent. Anesthesiology, *20*:330, 1959.
7. McCarthy, D.A., Chen, G., Kaump, D.H., and Ensor, C.: General anesthetic and other pharmacologic properties of 2-(*o*-chlorophenyl)-2-methylamino cyclohexanone HCl (CI-581). J. New Drugs, *5*:21, 1965.
8. Chang, T., Dill, W.A., and Glazko, A.J.: Metabolic disposition of 2-(*o*-chlorophenyl)-2-methylamino cyclohexanone HCl (CI-581) in laboratory animals and in man. Fed. Proc., *24*:268, 1965 (Abstr.).
9. Chen, G., Ensor, C.R., and Bohner, B.: The neuropharmacology of 2-*o*-chlorophenyl)-2-methylaminocyclohexanone hydrochloride. J. Pharmacol. Exp. Ther., *152*:332, 1966.
10. Domino, E.F., Chodoff, P., and Corssen, G.: Pharmacologic effects of CI-581, a new dissociative anesthetic in man. Clin. Pharmacol. Ther., *6*:279, 1965.
11. Trevor, A.J., Marietta, M.P., and Way, W.L.: The pharmacology of the optical isomers of ketamine. Pharmacologist, *18*:214, 1976.
12. Marietta, M.P., Way, W.L., Castagnoli, N., and Trevor, A.J.: On the pharmacology of the ketamine enantiomorphs in the rat. J. Pharmacol. Exp. Ther., *202*:165, 1977.

13. Ryder, S., Way, W.L., and Trevor, A.J.: Comparative pharmacology of the optical isomers of ketamine in mice. Eur. J. Pharmacol., *49*:15, 1978.
14. Meliska, C.J., and Trevor, A.J.: Differential effects of ketamine on scheduled-controlled responding and motility. Pharmacol. Biochem. Behav., *8*:679, 1978.
15. Meliska, C.J., Greenberg, A.J., and Trevor, A.J.: The effects of ketamine enantiomers on scheduled controlled behavior in the rat. J. Pharmacol. Exp. Ther., *212*:198, 1980.
16. White, P.F., Ham, J., Way, W.L. and Trevor, A.J.: Pharmacology of ketamine isomers in surgical patients. Anesthesiology, *52*:231, 1980.
17. White, P.F., Way, W.L., and Trevor, A.J.: Ketamine-its pharmacology and therapeutic uses. Anesthesiology, *56*:119, 1982.
18. Wilson, R.D., Traber, D.L., Barrat, E., Creson, T.L., Schmitt, R.C., and Allen, C.R.: An evaluation of CL-1848C, a new dissociative anesthetic in normal human volunteers. Anesth. Analg., *49*:236, 1970.
19. Traber, D.L., Priano, L.L., and Wilson, R.D.: Effects of CL-1848C, a new dissociative anesthetic on the cardiovascular and respiratory systems. J. Pharmacol. Exp. Ther., *175*:395, 1970.
20. Kelly, R.W., Wilson, R.D., Traber, D.L., and Priano, L.L.: Effects of two new anesthetic agents, ketamine and CL-1848C on the respiratory response to carbon dioxide. Anesth. Analg., *50*:262, 1971.
21. Kaump, D.H., Kurtz, S.M., Fisken, R.A., Schardein, J.L., Roll, D.E., and Reutner, T.F.: Toxicology of Ketamine. *In* Ketamine. Edited by H. Kreuscher. Berlin, Springer, 1969.
22. Cohen, M.L., Chan, S.L., Way, W.L., and Trevor, A.J.: Distribution in the brain and metabolism of ketamine in the rat after intravenous administration. Anesthesiology, *39*:370, 1973.
23. Cohen, M.L., and Trevor, A.J.: On the cerebral accumulation of ketamine and the relationship between metabolism of the drug and its pharmacological effects. J. Pharmacol. Exp. Ther., *189*:351, 1974.
24. Marietta, M.P., White, P.F., Pudwill, C.R., Way, W.L., and Trevor, A.J.: Biodisposition of ketamine in the rat: self-induction of metabolism. J. Pharmacol. Exp. Ther., *196*:536, 1976.
25. Korttila, K.: Pharmacokinetics of intravenous non-narcotic anesthetics. *In* Trends in Intravenous Anesthesia. Edited by J.A. Aldrete and T.H. Stanley. Miami, Symposia Specialists Inc., 1980.
26. Wieber, J., Gugler, R., Hengstmann, J.H., and Dengler, H.J.: Pharmacokinetics of ketamine in man. Anaesthesist, *24*:260, 1975.
27. Chang, T., Savory, A., Albin, M., Goulet, R., and Glazko, A.J.: Metabolic disposition of tritium-labeled ketamine (Ketalar: CI-581) in normal human subjects. Clin. Res., *18*:597, 1970.
28. Chen, G.: The pharmacology of ketamine. *In* Ketamine. Edited by H. Kreuscher. Berlin, Springer, 1969.
29. Levinson, G., Shnider, S.M., Gildea, J.E., and DeLorimier, A.A.: Maternal and foetal cardiovascular and acid-base changes during ketamine anaesthesia in pregnant ewes. Br. J. Anaesth., *45*:1111, 1973.
30. Ellingson, A., Haram, K., Sagen, N., and Solheim, E.: Transplacental passage of ketamine after intravenous administration. Acta Anaesthesiol., Scand., *21*:41, 1977.
31. Little, B., Chang, T., Chucot, L., Dill, W., Enrile, L.L., Glazko, A.J., Jassani, M., Kretchmer, H., and Sweet, A.Y.: Study of ketamine as an obstetric anesthesia agent. Am. J. Obstet. Gynecol., *113*:247, 1972.
32. Jackson, G.B., and Hickney, C.M.: Ketamine anesthesia for vaginal delivery. Presented at the annual meeting of the Southern Medical Society. Dallas, Nov. 17, 1970.
33. Downing, J.W., Mahomedy, D.E., and Allen, P.J.: Anaesthesia for caesarean section with ketamine. Anaesthesia, *31*:883, 1976.
34. Finster, M., and Mark, L.C.: Placental transfer of drugs and their distribution in fetal tissues. *In* Handbook of Experimental Pharmacology, Vol. 28. Concepts in Biochemical Pharmacology, Part I. Edited by B.B. Brodie and J.R. Gillette. Berlin, Springer, 1971.
35. Chang, T., and Glazko, A.J.: Biotransformation and disposition of ketamine. Int. Anesthesiol. Clin., *12*:157, 1974.
36. Percel, J.M., and Mark, L.C.: The interaction of anesthetic agents with hepatic microsomal enzymes. *In* Enzymes in Anesthesiology. Edited by F.F. Foldes, New York, Springer, 1978.
37. White, P.F., Marietta, M.P., Pudwill, C.R., Way, W.L., and Trevor, A.J.: Effects of halothane anesthesia on the biodisposition of ketamine in rats. J. Pharmacol. Exp. Ther., *106*:545, 1976.
38. Lo, J.N., and Cumming, J.F.: Interaction between sedative premedicants and ketamine in man and in isolated perfused rat livers. Anesthesiology, *43*:307, 1975.
39. Ireland, S.J., and Livingston, A.: Effect of biliary excretion on ketamine anesthesia in the rat. Br. J. Anaesth., *52*:23, 1980.
40. Sadove, M.S., Shulman, M., Hatano, S., and Fevold, N.: Analgesic effects of ketamine administered in subdissociative doses. Anesth. Analg., *50*:452, 1971.
41. Bovill, J.G., and Dundee, J.W.: Alterations in response to somatic pain associated with anesthesia-ketamine. Br. J. Anaesth., *43*:496, 1971.

42. Slogoff, S., Allen, G.W., Wessels, J.W., and Cheney, D.H.: Clinical experience with subanesthetic ketamine. Anesth. Analg., *53*:354, 1974.
43. Nolte, H., Teuteberg, H., Dudek, J., Muenchhoff, W., and Rumpf, K.: Vergleichende Untersuchungen ueber die Analgesie bei Kurznarkosen mit Ketamine, Thiopental und Propanidid. *In* Ketamin. Edited by H. Kreuscher. Berlin, Springer, 1969.
44. Teuteberg, H, and Nolte, H.: Ketamine. A new intravenous anesthetic with potent analgesic properties. Proceedings of the Brasilian-Portugese Congress of Anesthesiology. Lisbon, September, 1968.
45. Aguado-Matorras, A.: Experiencia personal de 300 casos de CI-581 (ketamina) en anestesiologia. Rev. Esp. Anestesiol. Reanim., *17*:302, 1970.
46. Bjarnesen, W., and Corssen, G.: CI-581: a new non-barbiturate short-acting anesthetic for surgery in burns. Mich. Med., *66*:177, 1967.
47. Benumof, J.L., Canada, E.D., Scanlon, T.S., and Herren, A.L.: Intravenous anesthesia and postoperative analgesia. Anesth. Analg., *60*:240, 1981.
48. Clements, J.A., and Nimmo, W.S.: Pharmacokinetics and analgesic effect of ketamine in man. Br. J. Anaesth., *53*:29, 1981.
49. Bennett, J.A., and Bullimore, J.A.: The use of ketamine hydrochloride anaesthesia for radiotherapy in young children. Br. J. Anaesth., *45*:197, 1973.
50. Byer, D.E., and Gould, A.B.: Development of tolerance to ketamine in an infant undergoing repeated anesthesia. Anesthesiology, *54*:255, 1981.
51. Amberg, H.L., and Gordon, G.: Low-dose intramuscular ketamine for pediatric radiotherapy: a case report. Anesth. Analg., *55*:92, 1976.
52. Corssen, G., Miyasaka, M., and Domino, E.F.: Changing concepts in pain control during surgery; dissociative anesthesia with CI-581: a progress report. Anesth. Analg., 47:746, 1968.
53. Corssen G., and Bjarnesen, W.: Recent advances in intravenous anesthesia. AANA J., *34*:416, 1966.
54. Langrehr, D., and Stolp, W.: Der Einfluss von Ketamine auf verschiedene Vitalfunktionen des Menschen (Experimentelle Untersuchungen und klinische Erfahrungen bei 1300 Faellen). *In* Ketamine. Edited by H. Kreuscher. Berlin, Springer, 1969.
55. Podlesch, I., and Zindler, M.: Erste Erfahrungen mit dem Phencyclidinederivat Ketamine (CI-581), einem neuen intravenoesen und intramuskularen Narkosemittel. Anaesthesist, *16*:299, 1967.
56. Corssen, G., Hayward, J.R., Gunter, J.W., and Groves, E.H.: A new parenteral anesthetic for oral surgery. J. Oral Maxillofac. Surg., *27*:627, 1969.
57. Kreuscher, H., Fuchs, S., and Bornemann, F.: Untersuchungen ueber die psycho-physische Leistungsfaehigkeit nach Ketamin. *In* Ketamin. Edited by H. Kreuscher. Berlin, Springer, 1969.
58. Doenicke, A., Kugler, J., Emmert, K., Laub, M., and Kleinert, H.: Ein Leistungsvergleich nach Ketamin und Methohexital. *In* Ketamin. Edited by H. Kreuscher. Berlin, Springer, 1969.
59. Corssen, G., Domino, E.F., and Bree, R.L.: Electroencephalographic effects of ketamine anesthesia in children. Anaesth. Analg., *48*:141, 1969.
60. Rubin, M.A., and Freeman, H.: Brain potential changes and skin temperature during cyclopropane anesthesia. Anesth. Analg., *20*:45, 1941.
61. Possati, S., Faulconer, A., Jr., Bickford, R.G., and Hunter, R.C.: Electroencephalographic patterns during anesthesia with cyclopropane: correlation with concentrations of cyclopropane in arterial blood. Anesth. Analg., *32*:130, 1953.
62. Brechner, V.L., Walter, R.D., and Dillon, J.B.: Practical electroencephalography for the Anesthesiologist. Springfield, IL, Charles C Thomas, 1962.
63. Ciganek, L.: The EEG response (evoked potential) to light stimulus in man. Electroencephalogr. Clin. Neurophysiol., *13*:165, 1961.
64. Corssen, G, and Domino, E.F.: Visually evoked responses in man. A method for measuring cerebral effects of preanesthetic medication. Anesthesiology, 25:330, 1964.
65. Giesen, M., Hoerkens, H., and Patschke, D.: Ketamin Auswirkungen auf das kindliche Audio-EEG. *In* Ketamin. Neue Ergebnisse in Forschung und Klinik. Edited by M. Gemperle, H. Kreuscher, and D. Langrehr. Berlin, Springer, 1973.
66. Shrivastav, B.B.: Mechanism of ketamine. Block of nerve conduction. J. Pharmacol. Exp. Ther., *201*:162, 1977.
67. Miyasaka, M. and Domino, E.F.: Neuronal mechanisms of ketamine-induced anesthesia. Int. J. Neuropharmacol., 7:557, 1968.
68. Sparkes, D.L., Corssen, G., Sides, J., Black, J., and Kholeif, A.: Ketamine-induced anesthesia: neural mechanisms in the rhesus monkey. Anesth. Analg., 52:288, 1973.
69. Sparkes, D.L., Corssen, G., Aizenman, B., and Black, J.: Further studies of the neural mechanisms of ketamine-induced anesthesia in the rhesus monkey. Anesth. Analg., *54*:189, 1975.
70. Massopust, L.C., Wolin, L.R., and Albin, M.S.: Electrophysiologic and behavioral responses to ketamine hydrochloride in the rhesus monkey. Anesth. Analg., *51*:329, 1972.
71. Ohtani, M., Kikuchi, H., Kitahata, L.M., Taub, A., Toyooka, H., Hanaoka, K., and Dohi, S.:

Effects of ketamine on nociceptive cells in the medial medullary reticular formation of the cat. Anesthesiology, *51*:414, 1979.

72. Dafny, N., and Rigor, B.M.: Dose effects of Ketamine on photic and acoustic field potentials. Neuropharmacology *17*:581, 1978.

73. Nelson, S.R., Howard, R.B., Cross, R.S., and Samson, F.: Ketamine-induced changes in regional glucose utilization in the rat brain. Anesthesiology, *52*:330, 1980.

74. Crosby, G., Crane, A.M., and Sokoloff, L.: Local changes in cerebral glucose utilization during ketamine anesthesia. Anesthesiology, *56*:437, 1982.

75. Mori, K., Kawamata, M., Mitani, H., Yamazaki, Y., and Fujita, M.A.: A neurophysiologic study of ketamine anesthesia in the cat. Anesthesiology, *35*:373, 1971.

76. Kayama, Y., and Iwama, K.: The EEG, evoked potentials, and single-unit activity during ketamine anesthesia in cats. Anesthesiology, *36*:316, 1972.

77. Winters, W.D., Mori, K., and Wallach, M.B.: Reticular multiple unit activity during a progression of states induced by CNS excitants, III. Electroencephalogr. Clin. Neurophysiol., *27*:514, 1969.

78. Winters, W.D., Ferrar-Allado, T., Guzman-Flores, C., and Alcaraz, M.: The cataleptic state induced by ketamine: a review of the pharmacology of anesthesia. Neuropharmacology, *11*:303, 1972.

79. Winters, W.: Epilepsy or anesthesia with ketamine. Anesthesiology, *36*:309, 1972.

80. Domino, E.F., and Ueki, S.: Differential effects of general anaesthetics on spontaneous electrical activity of neocortical rhinencephalic brain systems of the dog. J. Pharmacol. Exp. Ther., *127*:288, 1959.

81. Druray, W.L., and Clarke, L.C.: Ketamine failure in acute brain injury: a case report. Anesth. Analg., *49*:859, 1970.

82. Janis, K.M., and Wright, W.: Failure to produce analgesia with ketamine in two patients with cortical disease. Anesthesiology, *36*:405, 1972.

83. Morse, N., and Smith, P.C.: Ketamine anesthesia in a hydrancephalic infant. Anesthesiology, *40*:407, 1974.

84. Kitahata, L.M., Taub, A., and Dosaka, Y.: Lamina-specific suppression of dorsal-horn unit activity by ketamine hydrochloride. Anesthesiology, *38*:4, 1973.

85. Conseiller, C., Benoist, J.M., Hamann, K.F., Maillard, M.C., and Benson, J.M.: Effects of ketamine (CI-581) on cell responses to cutaneous stimulations in laminae IV and V in the cat's dorsal horn. Eur. J. Pharmacol., *18*:346, 1972.

86. Vincent, J.P., Cavey, D., Kamenka, J.M., Geneste, P., and Lazdunski, M.: Interaction of phencyclidines with the muscarinic and opiate receptors in the central nervous system. Brain Res., *152*:176, 1978.

87. Finck, A.D., and Ngai, S.H.: A possible mechanism of ketamine-induced analgesia. Anesthesiology, *51*:S34, 1979.

88. Smith, D.J., Westfall, D.P., and Adams, J.D.: Ketamine interacts with opiate receptors as an agonist. Anesthesiology, *53*:S5, 1980.

89. Smith, D.J., Perotti, J.M., Mansell, A.L., and Monroe, P.J.: Ketamine analgesia is not related to an opiate action in the periaqueductal grey region of the rat brain. Pain, *21*:253, 1985.

90. Cohen, M.L., Chan, S.L., Bhargava, H.N., and Trevor, A.J.: Inhibition of mammalian brain acetylcholinesterase by ketamine. Biochem. Pharmacol., *23*:1647, 1974.

91. Ngai, S.H., Cheney, D.L., and Finck, A.D.: Acetylcholine concentrations and turnover in rat brain structures during anesthesia with halothane, enflurane and ketamine. Anesthesiology, *48*:4, 1978.

92. Tung, A.S., Figallo, E.M., and Brandom, B.W.: Antagonism of ketamine by 4-aminopyridine and physostigmine. Br. J. Anaesth., *53*:191, 1981.

93. Agoston, S., Salt, P.J., Erdmann, W., Hilkemeijer, T., Bengini, A., and Langrehr, D.: Antagonism of ketamine-diazepam anaesthesia by 4-aminopyridine in human volunteers. Br. J. Anaesth., *53*:567, 1980.

94. Langrehr, D., Agoston, S., Erdmann, W., and Newton, D.: Pharmacodynamics and reversal of benzodiazepine-ketamine ataranalgesia. S. Afr. Med. J., *18*:425, 1981.

95. Balmer, H.G.R., and Wyte, S.R.: Antagonism of ketamine by physostigmine. Br. J. Anaesth., *49*:510, 1977.

96. Lawrence, D., and Livingston, A.: The effect of physostigmine on ketamine anaesthesia and analgesia. Br. J. Pharmacol., *67*:426, 1979.

97. Toro-Matos, A.: Physostigmine antagonizes ketamine. Anesth. Analg., *59*:764, 1980.

98. Houghton, A.: Antagonism of ketamine by physostigmine. Br. J. Anaesth., *50*:81, 1978.

99. Knox, J.W.D., Bovill, J.G., and Dundee, J.W.: Clinical studies of induction agents: ketamine. Br. J. Anaesth., *42*:875, 1970.

100. Traber, D.L., and Wilson, R.D.: Involvement of the sympathetic nervous system in the pressor response to ketamine. Anesth. Analg., *48*:248, 1969.

101. Traber, D.L., Wilson, R.D., and Priano, L.L.: Blockade of the hypertensive response to ketamine. Anesth. Analg., *49*:420, 1970.

102. Traber, D.L., Wilson, R.D., and Priano, L.L.: Differentiation of the cardiovascular effects of CI-581. Anesth. Analg., 47:769, 1968.
103. Ivankovich, A.D., Miletich, D.J., Reiman, C., Albrecht, R.F., and Zahed, B.: Cardiovascular effects of centrally administered ketamine in goats. Anesth. Analg., 53:924, 1974.
104. Dowdy, E.G., and Kaya, K.: Studies of the mechanism of cardiovascular responses to CI-581. Anesthesiology, 29:931, 1968.
105. Miletich, D.J., Ivankovich, A.D., Albrecht, R.F., Zahed, B., and Ilahi, A.A.: The effect of ketamine on catecholamine metabolism in the isolated perfused rat heart. Anesthesiology, 39:271, 1973.
106. Chodoff, P.: Evidence for central adrenergic action of ketamine. Anesth. Analg., 51:247, 1972.
107. Wong, D.H.W., and Jenkins, L.C.: An experimental study of the mechanism of action of ketamine on the central nervous system. Can. Anaesth. Soc. J., 21:57, 1974.
108. Goldberg, A.H., Deane, P.W., and Phear, W.P.C.: Effects of ketamine on contractile performance and excitability of isolated heart muscle. J. Pharmacol. Exp. Ther., 175:388, 1970.
109. Berry, D.G.: Effect of ketamine on the isolated chick embryo heart. Anesth. Analg., 53:919, 1974.
110. Davies, A.E., and McCane, J.L.: Effects of barbiturate anesthetics and ketamine on the force-frequency relation of cardiac muscle. Eur. J. Pharmacol., 26:65, 1979.
111. Fischer, K.: Experimentelle Untersuchungen zum Einfluss von Ketamin auf die myokardiale Kontraktilitaet. Proceed. 3rd Eur. Kongr. Anaesth., Prag, 1970.
112. Schwartz, D.A., and Horwitz, L.D.: Effects of ketamine on left ventricular performance. J. Pharmacol. Exp. Ther., 194:410, 1975.
113. Chamberlain, J.H., Seed, R.G.F.L., and Undre, N.: Myocardial depression by ketamine. Anaesthesia, 36:366, 1981.
114. Kaukinen, S.: The combined effects of antihypertensive drugs and anaesthetics (halothane and ketamine) on the isolated heart. Acta Anaesthesiol. Scand. 22:649, 1978.
115. Hill, E., Wong, K.C., Shaw, C.L., Sentker, C.R., and Blantnick, R.A.: Interactions of ketamine with vasoactive amines at normothermia and hypothermia in the isolated rabbit heart. Anesthesiology, 48:315, 1978.
116. Chang, P., Chan, K.E., and Ganendran, A.: Cardiovascular effects of 2-(chlorophenyl)-2-methylamino-cyclohexanone (CI-581). Br. J. Anaesth., 4a:391, 1969.
117. Johnston, M.: The cardiovascular effects of Ketamin in man. Anaesthesia, 31:873, 1976.
118. Corssen, G.: Unpublished data.
119. Ivankovich, A.D., El-Etr, A.A., Janeczko, G.F., and Maronic, J.P.: The effects of ketamine and of Innovar anesthesia on digitalis tolerance in dogs. Anesth. Analg., 54:106, 1975.
120. Hamilton, J.T., and Bryson, J.S.: The effects of ketamine on transmembrane potentials of Purkinje fibers of the pig heart. Br. J. Anaesth., 46:636, 1974.
121. Koehntop, D.E., Liao, J.-C., and VanBergen, F.H.: Effects of pharmacologic alterations of adrenergic mechanisms by cocaine, tropolone, aminophylline and ketamine on epinephrine-induced arrhythmias during halothane-nitrous oxide anesthesia. Anesthesiology, 46:83, 1977.
122. Smith, G., Thorburn, J., Vance, J.P., and Brown, D.M.: The effects of ketamine on the canine coronary circulation. Anaesthesia, 34:555, 1979.
123. Sonntag, H.: Koronare Haemodynamik unter Narkose-Einleitung mit Dehydrobenzperidol/Fentanyl und Ketamine, Langenbecks Arch. Chir., 332:301, 1972.
124. Merin, R.G.: The function of the heart: effects of anesthetics and adjuvant drugs. Refresher Courses in Anesthesiology, 6, 1978.
125. Folts, J.D., Afonso, S., and Rowe, G.G.: Systemic and coronary hemodynamic effects of ketamine in intact anaesthetized and unanesthetized dogs. Br. J. Anaesth., 47:686, 1975.
126. Kettler, D.: Hamodynamische Komponenten des myokardialen Energiebedarfs und Sauerstoffversorgung des Herzens bei verschiedenen Narkosen. Goettingen, Habilitationsschrift, 1971.
127. Sonntag, H., Heiss, H.W., Knowll, D., Fuchs, Ch., Regensburger, D., Schenk, H.D., and Bretschneider, H.J.: Der Einfluss von Ketamine auf den myokardialen Metabolismus. *In* Ketamin. Neue Ergebnisse in Forschung und Klinik. Edited by M. Gemperle, H. Kreuscher, and D. Langrehr. Berlin, Springer, 1973.
128. Diaz, F.A., Blanco, A.B., Beer, N., Velarde, H. Isquierdo, J.P., and Jaen, R.: Effects of ketamine on canine cardiovascular function. Br. J. Anaesth., 48:941, 1976.
129. Liao, J.C., Koehntop, D.E., and Buckley, J.J.: Dual effect of ketamine on the peripheral vasculature. Anesthesiology, 51:S116, 1979.
130. Gooding, J.M., Dimick, A.R., Tavokoli, M., and Corssen, G.: A physiologic analysis of cardiopulmonary responses to ketamine anesthesia in non-cardiac patients. Anesth. Analg., 56:813, 1977.
131. Idvall, J.: Ketamine infusions: pharmacokinetics and clinical effects. Br. J. Anaesth., 51:1167, 1979.
132. Tweed, W.A., Minuck, M., and Mymine, D.: Circulatory responses to ketamine anesthesia. Anesthesiology, 37:613, 1972

133. Takeshita, H., Okuda, Y., and Sari, A.: The effects of ketamine on cerebral circulation and metabolism in man. Anesthesiology, 36:69, 1972.

134. Dawson, B., Michenfelder, D., and Theye, A.: Effects of ketamine on canine cerebral blood flow and metabolism; modification by prior administration of thiopental. Anesth. Analg., 50:443, 1971.

135. Kreuscher, H., and Grote, J.: Effect of the phencyclidine derivative ketamine (CI-581) on brain circulation and oxygen utilization in dogs. Anaesthesist, 16:304, 1967.

136. Herrschaft, H., and Schmidt, H.: Der Einfluss von Ketamin auf die Hirndurchblutung beim Menschen. *In* Ketamin. Neue Ergebnisse in Forschung und Klinik. Edited by M. Gemperle, H. Kreuscher, and D. Langrehr. Berlin, Springer, 1973.

137. Herrschaft, H., and Schmidt, H.: Das Verhalten der globalen und regionalen Hirndurchblutung unter dem Einfluss von Propanidid, Ketamine und Thiopental-Natrium. Anaesthesist, 22:486, 1973.

138. Dhasmana, K.M., Saxena, P.R., Prakash, O., and Van der Zee, H.T.: A study on the influence of ketamine on systemic and regional hemodynamics in conscious rabbits. Arch. Int. Pharmacodyn. Therap., 269:323, 1984.

139. Lassen, N.A., and Christensen, M.S.: Physiology of cerebral blood flow. Br. J. Anaesth., 48:719, 1976.

140. Hagimori, M.: A study of cerebrospinal fluid pressure during anesthesia. Part I. Anesthesia with CI-581. Jpn. J. Anesth., 18:1475, 1969.

141. Hougaard, K., Hansen, A., and Brodersen, P.: The effect of ketamine on regional cerebral blood flow in man. Anesthesiology, 41:562, 1974.

142. List, W.F., Crumrine, R.S., Cascorbi, H.F., and Weiss, M.H.: Increased cerebrospinal fluid pressure with ketamine. Anesthesiology, 36:98, 1972.

143. Gardner, A.E., Olson, B.E., and Lichtiger, M.: Cerebrospinal-fluid pressure during dissociative anesthesia with ketamine. Anesthesiology, 35:226, 1971.

144. Evans, J., Rosen, M., Weeks, R.D., and Wise, C.: Ketamine in neurosurgical procedures. Lancet, i:40, 1971.

145. Gardner A.E., Dannemiller, F.J., and Dean, D.: Intracranial cerebrospinal fluid pressure in man during ketamine anesthesia. Anesth. Analg., 51:741, 1972.

146. Shapiro, H.M., Wyte, S.R., and Harris, A.B.: Ketamine anaesthesia in patients with intracranial pathology. Br. J. Anaesth., 44:1200, 1972.

147. Chbarrocas, E., Mercader, J.M., and Marques, R.: Effects of ketamine in cerebral angiography. Neuroradiology, 5:59, 1973.

148. List, W.F., and Cascorbi, H.F.: Druckanstieg im Liquor cerebrospinalis unter Ketamin. *In* Ketamin. Neue Ergebnisse in Forschung und Klinik. Edited by M. Gemperle, H. Kreuscher, and D. Langrehr. Berlin, Springer, 1973.

149. Taube, H.D., Gobiet, W., Liesegang, J., and Bock, W.J.: Intrakranielle Druckverhaeltnisse unter Ketamin. *In* Ketamin. Neue Ergebnisse in Forschung und Klinik. Edited by M. Gemperle, H. Kreuscher, and D. Langrehr. Berlin, Springer, 1973.

150. Tschakaloff, C.H.: Untersuchungen ueber das Verhalten des Hirnliquordrucks bei Ketamin Narkosen im Saeuglingsalter. *In* Ketamin. Neue Ergebnisse in Forschung und Klinik. Edited by M. Gemperle, H. Kreuscher, and D. Langrehr. Berlin, Springer, 1973.

151. Sari, A., Okuda, Y., and Takeshita, H.: The effect of ketamine on cerebrospinal fluid pressure. Anesth. Analg., 51:560, 1972.

152. Shapiro, H.M.: Intracranial hypertension: therapeutic and anesthetic considerations. Anesthesiology, 43:445, 1971.

153. Takahashi, K., Shima, T., Koga, Y., and Iwatsuki, K.: The effects of ketamine on the pulmonary hemodynamics in dogs. Jpn. J. Anaesth., 20:842, 1971.

154. Tarnow, J., Hess, W., Schmidt, D., and Eberlein, H.J.: Narkoseeinleitung bei Patienten mit koronarer Herzkrankheit: Flunitrazepam, Diazepam, Ketamin, Fentanyl. Anaesthesist, 28:9, 1979.

155. Spotoft, H., Korshin, J.D., Bredgaard-Sorensen, M., and Skovsted, P.: The cardiovascular effects of ketamine used for induction of anesthesia in patient with valvular heart disease. Can. Anaesth. Soc. J., 26:463, 1979.

156. Gassner, S., Cohen, M., Aygen, M., Levey, E., Ventura, E., and Shashdi, J.: The effect of ketamine on pulmonary artery pressure. An experimental and clinical study. Anaesthesia, 29:141, 1974.

157. Patschke, D., Brueckner, J.B., Reinecke, A., Schmicke, P., Tarnow, J., and Eberlein, H.J.: Der Einfluss der Ketamineanaesthesie auf die Nierendurchblutung. *In* Ketamin. Neue Ergebnisse in Forschung und Klinik. Edited by M. Gemperle, H. Kreuscher, and D. Langrehr. Berlin, Springer, 1973.

158. Waxman, K., Shoemaker, W.C., and Lippmann, M.: Cardiovascular effects of anesthetic induction with ketamine. Anesth. Analg., 59:355, 1980.

159. Langrehr, D., Alai, P., Andjelkovic, J., and Kluge, I.: Anesthesia with 2-(o-chlorophenyl)-2-

methylamino-cyclohexanone-HCL (CI-581): report of first findings in 500 cases. Anaesthesist, *16*:308, 1967.

160. Gjessing, J.: A clinical trial of ketamine. Presented at the International Symposium on "L'Anesthesie Vigile et SubVigile," Ostende, Belgium, April, 1969.

161. Dobson, M.B.: Anaesthesia with ketamine and thiopentone for short surgical procedures. Anaesthesia, *33*:268, 1978.

162. Matsuki, A., Kothary, S.P., and Zsigmond, E.K.: Lack of compensatory increase in plasma free norepinephrine during hypotension induced by intravenous thiamylal anesthesia. Anaesthesist, *22*:289, 1973.

163. Zsigmond, E.K., Kothary, S.P., Matsuki, A., Kelsch, R.C., and Martinez, O.: Diazepam for prevention of the rise in plasma catecholamines caused by ketamine. Clin. Pharmacol. Ther., *15*:223, 1974.

164. Jackson, A.P.F., Dhadphale, P.R., and Callaghan, M.L.: Haemodynamic studies during induction of anaesthesia for open heart surgery using diazepam and ketamine. Br. J. Anaesth., *50*:375, 1978.

165. Kumar, S.M., Kothary, S.P., and Zsigmond, E.K.: Plasma free norepinephrine and epinephrine concentrations following diazepam-ketamine induction in patients undergoing cardiac surgery. Acta Anaesthesiol. Scand., *22*:593, 1978.

166. Erdmann, W., Salt, P.J., Agoston, S., and Langrehr, D.: Antagonism of the circulatory effects of ketamine by diazepam in volunteers. Acta Anesth. Belg., *30*:239, 1979.

167. Zsigmond, E.K.: Reducing side effects in ketamine anesthesia. JAMA, *229*:392, 1974.

168. Sylvay, G., Weinreich, A.I., Lumb, P., Shiang, H.: Continuous infusion of ketamine for thoracic surgery using one-lung ventilation. *In* Trends in Intravenous Anesthesia. Edited by J.A. Aldrete and T.H. Stanley. Miami, Symposia Specialists Inc., 1980.

169. Wilson, R.D., Richey, J.V., Forestner, J.E., Hendrickson, M., Herrin, T.J., Norman, P.F., and Nigliazzo, A.: Cardiovascular effects of ketamine infusion. *In* Trends in Intravenous Anesthesia. Edited by J.A. Aldrete and T.H. Stanley. Miami, Symposia Specialists Inc., 1980.

170. Hatano, S., Nishiwada, M., and Matsumura, M.: Ketamine-diazepam anesthesia for abdominal surgery. A review of 1000 cases with continuous "Micro-Mini" drip administration technique. Anaesthesist, *27*:172, 1978.

171. Zsigmond, E.K., and Domino, E.F.: Ataract analgesia with diazepam-ketamine for induction of anesthesia. *In* Trends in intravenous anesthesia. Edited by J.A. Aldrete and T.H. Stanley. Miami, Symposia Specialists Inc., 1980.

172. Lilburn, J.K., Dundee, J.W., and Moore, J.: Ketamine infusions—observations on technique, dosage and cardiovascular effects. Anaesthesia, *22*:315, 1978.

173. Tarnow, J., and Hess, W.: Flunitrazepam-Vorbehandlung zur Vermeidung kardiovaskularer Nebenwirkungen von Ketamin. Anaesthesist, *28*:468, 1979.

174. Barclay, A., Houlton, P.C., and Downing, J.W.: Total intravenous anesthesia: a technique using Flunitrazepam, Ketamine, muscle relaxants, and controlled ventilation of the lung. Anaesthesia, *35*:287, 1980.

175. White, P.F.: Comparative evaluation of intravenous agents for rapid sequence induction-thiopental, ketamine, and midazolam. Anesthesiology, *57*:279, 1982.

176. Zsigmond, E.K., Kothary, S.P., Matsuki, and Martinez, O.A.: Ketamine-pancuronium induction on circulation and plasma catecholamines. Exerpta Medica International Congress Series No. 330, IV. Eur. Congr. Anesthesiol., 1974.

177. Matsuki, A., Zsigmond, E., Kelsch, R.C., and Kothary, S.P.: The effect of pancuronium bromide on plasma nor-epinephrine concentrations during ketamine induction. Can. Anaesth. Soc. J., *21*:315, 1974.

178. Bovill, J.G., and Dundee, J.W.: Attempts to control the cardiostimulatory effect of ketamine in man. Anaesthesia, *27*:309, 1972.

179. Longnecker, D.E., and Sturgill, B.C.: Influence of anaesthetic agents on survival following hemorrhage. Anesthesiology, *45*:516, 1972.

180. Wong, D.H.W., and Jenkins, L.C.: The cardiovascular effects of ketamine in hypotensive states. Can. Anaesth. Soc. J., *22*:339, 1975.

181. Weiskopf, R.B., Townsley, M.I., Riordan, K.K., Chadwick, K., Baysinger, M., and Mahoney, E.: Comparison of cardiopulmonary responses to graded hemorrhage during enflurane, halothane, isoflurane and ketamine anesthesia. Anesth. Analg., *60*:481, 1981.

182. Brueckner, J.B., Patschke, D., and Reineke, A.: Untersuchungen zur Wirkung von Ketamine im experimentellen haemorrhagischen Schock. *In* Ketamin. Neue Ergebnisse in Forschung und Klinik. Edited by M. Gemperle, H. Kreuscher, and D. Langrehr. Berlin, Springer, 1973.

183. Corssen, G., Reves, J.G., and Carter, J.R.: Neuroleptanesthesia, dissociative anesthesia and hemorrhage. Int. Anesthesiol. Clin., *12*:145, 1974.

184. Peter, K., Klose, R., and Lutz, H.: Ketanest zur Narkoseeinleitung beim Schock. Z. Prakt. Anaesth., *6*:396, 1970.

185. Virtue, R.W., Alanis, J.M., Mori, M., Lafarque, R.T., Vogel, H.K., and Metcalf, D.R.: An anes-

thetic agent: 2-orthochlorophenyl, 2-methylamino cyclohexanone CI-581. Anesthesiology, 28:823, 1967.

186. Stanley, V., Hunt, J., Willis, K.W., and Stephen, C.R.: Cardiovascular and respiratory function with CI-581. Anesth. Analg., 47:760, 1968.

187. Dillon, J.B.: Clinical experience with repeated ketamine administation for procedures requiring anesthesia. *In* Ketamin. Edited by H. Kreuscher. Berlin, Springer, 1969.

188. Iwatsuki, M., Aoba, Y., Sato, K., and Iwatsuki, N.: Clinical study of CI-581, a phencyclidine derivative. Tohoku J. Exp. Med., 93:39, 1967.

189. Zsigmond, E.K., Matsuki, A., Kothary, S.P., and Jallad, M.: Arterial hypoxemia caused by intravenous ketamine. Anesth. Analg., 55:692, 1968.

190. Rolly, G.: Use of ketamine as monoanesthetic in clinical anesthesia, acid-base status and oxygenation. *In* Ketamin. Edited by H. Kreuscher. Berlin, Springer, 1969.

191. Siepmann, H., and Podlesch, I.: Die Wirkung von verschieden hohen intramuskulaer verabreichten Ketamine Dosen im Saeuglings-und Kindesalter. *In* Ketamin. Neue Ergebnisse in Forschung und Klinik. Edited by M. Gemperle, H. Kreuscher, and D. Langrehr. Berlin, Springer, 1973.

192. Wilson, R.D., Traber, D.L., and McCoy, N.R.: Cardiopulmonary effects of CI-581—the new dissociative anesthetic. South. Med. J., 61:692, 1968

193. Lundey, P.M., Gowdy, C.W., and Colhouhn, E.H.: Tracheal smooth muscle relaxant effect of ketamine. Br. J. Anaesth., 46:333, 1974.

194. Wanna, H.T., and Gergis, S.D.: Procaine, Lidocaine, and ketamine inhibit histamine-induced contracture of guinea pig tracheal muscle in vitro. Anesth. Analg., 57:25, 1978.

195. Okumura, F., and Denborough, M.A.: Effects of anesthetics on guinea pig tracheal smooth muscle. Br. J. Anaesth., 52:199, 1980.

196. Hirshman, C.A.: Ketamine block of bronchospasm in experimental canine asthma. Br. J. Anaethesiol., 51:713, 1979.

197. Cabanas, A.: Effects of ketamine in normal and asthmatic airway smooth muscle of guinea pigs. Personal communication.

198. Waltemath, C.L., and Bergman, N.A.: Effects of ketamine and halothane on increased respiratory resistance provoked by ultrasonic aerosols. Anesthesiology, 41:473, 1974.

199. Huber, F.C., Reves, J.G., Gutierrez, J., and Corssen, G.: Ketamine: its effect on airway resistance in man. South. Med. J., 65:1176, 1972.

200. Corssen, G., Gutierrez, J., Reves, J.G., and Huber, F.C.: Ketamine in the anesthetic management of asthmatic patients. Anesth. Analg., 51:588, 1972.

201. Penrose, B.H.: Aspiration pneumonitis following ketamine induction for a general anesthetic. Anesth. Analg., 51:41, 1972.

202. Bosomworth, P.P.: Symposium on ketamine anesthesia. Anesth. Analg., 50:471, 1971.

203. Taylor, P.A., and Towey, R.M.: Depression of laryngeal reflexes during ketamine anesthesia. Br. Med. J., 2:688, 1971.

204. Editorial. Br. Med. J., 2:666, 1971.

205. Sage, M., and Laird, S.M.: Ketamine and the laryngeal reflexes. Br. Med. J., 2:670, 1972.

206. Yeung, M.L., and Lin, R.S.H.: Laryngeal reflexes in children under ketamine anesthesia. Br. J. Anaesth., 44:1089, 1972.

207. Alexander, J.P.: Ketamine anaesthesia. Br. Med. J., 3:46, 1971.

208. Coppel, D.L.: Ketamine anaesthesia (correspondence). Br. Med. J., 3:46, 1971.

209. Radney, P.A., and Badola, R.P.: Generalized extensor spasm in infants following Ketamine anesthesia. Anesthesiology, 39:459, 1973.

210. Vourc'h, G., Conseiller, C., and Lavante, A.: First clinical trials with ketamine. International Symposium Anesthesia: Vigile et Subvigile. Ostende, Belgium, April, 1969.

211. Maritano, M., Zaccagna, C.A., Vergano, F., and Musto, P.: Striated muscle fiber and CI-581. Minerva Anesthesiol., 35:86, 1969.

212. Martinez-Aguirre, E., and Wikinski, J.: Regional ketamine-induced depression of neuromuscular transmission in man. Acta Anaesthesiol. Belg., 30:183, 1979.

213. Bovill, J.G., Dundee, J.W., Coppel, D.L., and Moore, J.: Current status of ketamine anesthesia. Lancet, 1:1288, 1971.

214. Cronnelly, R., Dretchen, K.L., Sokoll, M.D., and Long, J.P.: Ketamine myoneural activity and interaction with neuromuscular blocking agents. Eur. J. Pharmacol., 22:17, 1973.

215. Johnston, R.R., Miller, R.D., and Way, W.L: The interaction of ketamine with d-tubocurarine, pancuronium, and succinylcholine in man. Anesth. Analg., 53:469, 1974.

216. List, W.F.: Serum potassium changes during induction of anesthesia. Br. J. Anaesth., 39:480, 1967.

217. Gal, T.J., and Malit, L.A.: The influence of ketamine induction of potassium changes and fasciculations following suxamethonium. Br. J. Anaesth., 44:1077, 1972.

218. Fuchs, S., and Kreuscher, H.: Untersuchungen ueber den Einfluss von Ketamine auf humorale Systeme des Menschen. *In* Ketamin. Edited by H. Kreuscher. Berlin, Springer, 1969.

219. Kreuscher, H., Baar, H.A., Boehm-Jurkovic, K., and Fischer, D.: Der Einfluss von Ketamine auf Herzzeitvolumen, Nierenzeitvolumen und Nierenfunktion. *In* Ketamin. Neue Ergebnisse in Forschung und Klinik. Edited by M. Gemperle, H. Kreuscher, and D. Langrehr. Berlin, Springer, 1973.

220. Bihler, K.: Nierenfunktion unter Ketamin beim alten Menschen. *In* Ketamin. Neue Ergebnisse in Forschung und Klinik. Edited by M. Gemperle, H. Kreuscher, and D. Langrehr. Berlin, Springer, 1973.

221. Pietras, J.R., Cromie, W.J., and Duckett, J.W.: Ketamine as a detumescent during hypospadia repair. J. Urol., *121*:654, 1979.

222. Gale, A.S.: Ketamine prevention of penile turgescence. JAMA, *219*:1629, 1972.

223. Langrehr, D., Stolp, W., Kluge, J., and Hans, A.: Ketamin-Anesthesia fuer geburtshilflich-gynaekologische Eingriffe. Z. Prakt. Anaesth., 3:145, 1970.

224. Dick, W., Johata, W.D., Milewski, P., and Traub, E.: Untersuchungen zum Verhalten des Uterustonus unter der Geburt waehrend der Ketamin Anaesthesie. *In* Ketamin. Neue Ergebnisse in Forschung und Klinik. Edited by M. Gemperle, H. Kreuscher, and D. Langrehr. Berlin, Springer, 1973.

225. Stolp, W., Langrehr, D., and Solkol, K.: Zur Anwendung von Ketamin in der geburtschilflichen Anaesthesie. Z. Geburtshilfe Perinatol., *169*:198, 1968.

226. Galloon, S., and Harley, P.: Ketamine and the pregnant uterus. Can. Anesth. Soc. J., 20:141, 1973.

227. Marx, G., Hwang, H.S., and Chandra, P.: Postpartum uterine pressure with different doses of ketamine. Anesthesiology, 50:163, 1979.

228. Matsuki, A., Shiga, T., Sanuki, K., Kudo, M., and Oyama, T.: Reduced triiodothyronine levels during and following ketamine-N_2O anesthesia in man. Jpn. J. Anaesth., 24:373, 1976..

229. Zsigmond, E.K., Kelsch, R.C., and Kothary, S.P.: Rise in plasma free-norepinephrine during anesthetic induction with ketamine. Phys. Drug Manual, 6:31, 1974.

230. Zsigmond, E.K., Kelsch, R.C., Kothary, S.P., and Vadnay, L.: Free nor-epinephrine concentrations during induction of anesthesia with ketamine. Rev. Bras. Anesth., 22:443, 1972.

231. Bovill, J.G., Clarke, R.S.J., Davis, E.A., and Dundee, J.W.: Some cardiovascular effects of ketamine in man. Br. J. Pharmacol. *41*:411, 1971.

232. Zsigmond, E.K.: Comment on plasma-free norepinephrine during ketamine anesthesia. Anesth. Analg. *51*:588, 1972.

233. Miller, E.D., Gianfagna, W., Ackerly, J.A., and Peach, M.J.: Converting-enzyme activity and pressor responses to angiotensin I and II in the rat awake and during anesthesia. Anesthesiology, 50:88, 1979.

234. Tanaka, K., and Pettinger, W.A.: Renin release and ketamine-induced cardiovascular stimulation in the rat. J. Pharmacol. Exp. Ther., *188*:229, 1974.

235. Fahringer, E.E., Foley, E.L., and Redgate, E.S.: Pituitary adrenal response to ketamine and the inhibition of the response by catecholaminergic blockade. Neuroendocrinology, *14*:151, 1974.

236. Nistico, G., Pisanti, N., Rotiroti, D., Preziosi, P., Cuocolo, R., DeMartino, G., and Nistico, G.M.: Effects of althesin and ketamine on resting and stress stimulated adrenocortical activity in rats. Br. J. Anaesth., 50:891, 1978.

237. Lin, M.T., Chen, C.F., and Pang, I.H.: Effects of ketamine on thermoregulation in rats. Can. J. Physiol. Pharmacol., 56:963, 1978.

238. Corssen, G., and Hoy, J.E.: A new parental anesthetic—CI-581: its effect on intraocular pressure. J. Pediatr. Ophthalmol. Strabismus, 4:20, 1967.

239. Schoeppner, H., Ulrich, W.D., Fries, E., and Schaedlich, M.: Zur Anwendung von CI-581 (Ketamin) in der Ophtalmologie. Wiss. Zeitschr. Humboldt Univ., *21*:87, 1972.

240. Yoshikawa, K., and Murai, Y.: The effect of ketamine on intraocular pressure in children. Anesth. Analg., 50:199, 1971.

241. Purschke, R.I., and Hassouna, I.: Der Einfluss von Ketamin auf den intraokularen Druck. Z. Prakt. Anaesth., 8:227, 1973.

242. Rubli, E.: Uber den Einfluss von Halothan, Cyclopropan und Ketamin auf den normalen intraokularen Druck bei Kindern. Anaesthesist, 20:337, 1971.

243. Mevhann, W.: Ketamin Narkose in der Augenheilkunde. Klin. Monatsbl. Augenheilkd., *161*:109, 1972.

244. Rudolph, P.: Der intraoculaere Druck waehrend Ketaminanesthesie und Halothannarkose. Anaesthesist, 23:245, 1974.

245. Adams, A.: Ketamine in paediatric ophthalmic practice. Anaesthesia, 28:212, 1973.

246. Harris, J.E., Letson, R.D., and Buckley, J.: The use of CI-581, a new parental anesthetic, in ophthalmic practice. Trans. Am. Ophthalmol. Soc., 66:206, 1968.

247. Peuler, M., Glass, D.D., and Arens, J.F.: Ketamine and intraocular pressure. Anesthesiology, 43:575, 1975.

248. Ausinsch, B., Rayburn, R.L., Munson, E.S., and Levy, N.S: Ketamine and intraocular pressure in children. Anesth. Analg., *55*:773, 1976.
249. Kitamura, S., Ogli, K., Kozaki, M., and Yamazaki, Y.: Lacrimation under ketamine anesthesia. Jpn. J. Anesth., *20*:749, 1971.
250. Bruce, D.L., and Wingard, D.W.: Anesthesia and the immune response. Anesthesiology, *34*:271, 1977.
251. Wilson, R.D., Priano, L.L., Traber, D.L., Sakai, H., Daniels, J.C., and Ritzman, S.E.: Investigation of possible immunosuppression from ketamine and 100% oxygen in normal children. Anesth. Analg., *50*:464, 1971.
252. Cullen, B.F., and Cretien, P.B.: Ketamine and in-vitro lymphocyte transformation. Anesth. Analg., *52*:518, 1973.
253. Fine, J., Weissman, J., and Finestone, S.C.: Side-effects after ketamine anesthesia: transient blindness. Anesth. Analg., *53*:72, 1974.
254. Lassner, J.: Erfahrungen mit Ketamin im Selbstversuch. *In* Ketamin. Edited by H. Kreuscher. Berlin, Springer, 1969.
255. Albin, M.S., and Janeta, P.J.: Reducing side-effects in ketamine anesthesia. JAMA, *226*:414, 1973.
256. Garfield, J.M.: A comparison of psychologic responses to ketamine and thiopental-nitrous oxide-halothane anesthesia. Anesthesiology, *36*:329, 1972.
257. Fine, J., and Finestone, S.C.: Sensory disturbances following ketamine anesthesia: recurrent hallucination. Anesth. Analg., *52*:428, 1973.
258. Collier, B.B.: Ketamine and the conscious mind. Anaesthesia, *27*:120, 1972.
259. Wilson, R.D., Traber, D.L., and Evans, B.L.: Correlation of psychologic and physiologic observations from children undergoing repeated ketamine anesthesia. Anesth. Analg., *48*:995, 1969.
260. Wulfsohn, N.L.: Ketamine dosage for induction based on lean body mass. Anesth. Analg., *51*:299, 1972.
261. Harris, J.A., Biersner, R.J., Edwards, D., and Bailey, L.W.: Attention, learning and personality during ketamine emergence. Anesth. Analg., *54*:169, 1975.
262. Sussman, D.R.: A comparative evaluation of ketamine anesthesia in children and adults. Anesthesiology, *40*:459, 1974.
263. Ginsberg, H., and Gerber, J.A.: Ketamine hydrochloride: a clinical investigation in 60 children. S. Afr. Med. J., *43*:627, 1969.
264. Hollister, G.R., and Burn, J.M.B.: Side effects of ketamine in pediatric anesthesia. Anesth. Analg., *53*:264, 1974.
265. Spoerel, W.E., and Kandel, P.F.: CI-581 in anaesthesia for tonsillectomies in children. Can. Anaesth. Soc. J., *17*:172, 1970.
266. Cronin, M.M., Bousfield, J.D., Hewitt, G.B., McEllan, I., and Boulton, T.B.: Ketamine anesthesia for radiotherapy in small children. Anaesthesia, *27*:135, 1972.
267. Dundee, J.W., Bovill, J.G., Clarke, R.S.J., and Pandit, S.K.: Problems with ketamine in adults. Anaesthesia, *26*:86, 1971.
268. Coppell, D.L., Bovill, J.G., and Dundee, J.W.: The taming of ketamine. Anaesthesia, *28*:293, 1973.
269. Bovill, J.G., Clarke, R.S., Davis, E.A., Dundee, J.W., Pandit, S.K., and Moore, J.: Clinical studies of induction agents. XXXVIII. Effects of premedication and supplements on ketamine anaesthesia. Br. J. Anaesth., *43*:600, 1971.
270. Khorramzadeh, E., and Lotfy, A.O.: Personality predisposition and emergence phenomena with ketamine. Psychosomatics, *17*:94, 1976.
271. Hejja, P., and Galloon, S.: A consideration of ketamine dreams. Can. Anaesth. Soc. J., *22*:100, 1975.
272. Morgan, M., Loh, L., Singer, L., and Moore, P.H.: Ketamine as the sole anaesthetic agent for minor surgical procedures. Anaesthesia, *26*:158, 1971.
273. Sadove, M.S., Hatano, S., Zahed, B., Redlin, T., Arastounejad, P., and Roman, V.: Clinical study of droperidol in the prevention of the side effects of ketamine anesthesia: preliminary report. Anesth. Analg., *50*:388, 1971.
274. Foldes, F.F.: The prevention of the psychotomimetic effects of ketamine. *In* Ketamin. Neue Ergebnisse in Forschung und Klinik. Edited by M. Gemperle, H. Kreuscher, and D. Langrehr, Berlin, Springer, 1973.
275. Figallo, E.M., Casall, H., Tantisira, B., Wadhwa, R.K., and Taylor, F.H.: Ketamine as the sole anaesthetic agent for laparoscopic sterilization. Br. J. Anaesth., *49*:1159, 1977.
276. Dunn, S.R., Walker, J.S., Aston, D.L., and Cripps, D.: Effects of anesthetic technique on blood loss in termination of pregnancy. Br. J. Anaesth., *45*:633, 1973.
277. Krantz, M.L.: Ketamine in obstetrics: comparison with methoxyflurane. Anesth. Analg., *53*:890, 1974.
278. Dundee, J.W., Bovill, J., Knox, J.W.D., Clarke, R.S.J., Black, G.W., Love, S.H.S., Moore, J.,

Elliott, J., Pandit, S.K., and Coppel, D.L.: Ketamine as an induction agent in anaesthetics. Lancet, *1*:1370, 1970.

279. Kothary, S.P., and Zsigmond, E.K.: A double-blind study of the effective antihallucinatory doses of diazepam prior to ketamine anesthesia. Clin. Pharmacol. Ther., *21*:108, 1977.

280. Korttila, K., and Levanen, J.: Untoward effects of ketamine combined with diazepam for supplementing conduction anaesthesia in young and middle-aged adults. Acta Anasthesiol. Scand., *22*:640, 1978.

281. Ayim, E.N., and Makatia, F.X.: The effects of diazepam on ketamine anaesthesia. East Afr. Med. J., *53*:377, 1976.

282. Erbguth, P.H., Reiman, B., and Klein, R.L.: The influence of chlorpromazine, diazepam and droperidol on emergence from ketamine. Anesth. Analg., *51*:693, 1972.

283. Loh, L., Singer, L., Morgan, M., and Moore, P.H.: Influence of diazepam on the emergence reactions following ketamine anaesthesia. Can. Anaesth. Soc. J., *18*:421, 1972.

284. Kapferer, J.M.: Kombination von Ketamin mit Valium und Dehydrobenzberidol. *In* Ketamin. Neue Ergebnisse in Forschung und Klinik. Edited by M. Gemperle, H. Kreuscher, and D. Langrehr. Berlin, Springer, 1973.

285. Dundee, J.W., and Lilburn, J.K.: Ketamine-lorazepam: attenuation of the psychic sequelae of ketamine by lorazepam. Anaesthesia, *37*:312, 1977.

286. Kothary, S.P., and Pandit, S.K.: Orally administered diazepam and lorazepam-sedative and amnesic effects. Anesthesiology, *53*:518, 1980.

287. Freuchen I., Ostergaard, J., Kuehl, J.B., and Mikkelsen, B.O.: Reduction of psychomimetic side-effects of Ketalar (ketamine) by Rohypnol (flunitrazepam). A randomized double-blind trial. Acta Anaesthesiol. Scand., *20*:97, 1976.

288. Houlton, P.J.C., and Downing, J.W.: General anaesthesia with intravenous flunitrazepam, continuous ketamine infusion and muscle relaxant. S. Afr. Med. J., *54*:1048, 1978.

289. Reves, J.G.: Benzodiazepines. *In* Pharmacokinetics of Anaesthesia. Edited by C. Prys-Roberts and C.C. Hug. Blackwell, Oxford, 1984.

290. El-Naggar, M., Kintanar, D., Rodenas, J., and Collins, V.: Ketamine as an induction agent and an adjunct to nitrous oxide-oxygen, curare anesthesia sequence. Anesthesiol. Rev., *1*:11, 1975.

291. Ginsberg, H., and Gerber, J.A.: CI-581: a clinical report on 100 patients. S. Afr. Med. J., *42*:1177, 1968.

292. Magbagbeola, J.A.O., and Thomas, N.A.: Effect of thiopentone on emergence reactions to ketamine anaesthesia. Can. Anaesth. Soc. J., *21*:321, 1974.

293. O'Neil, A.A., Winnie, A.P., Zadigian, M.E., and Collins, V.J.: Premedication for ketamine anesthesia: phase I: the "classic" drugs. Anesth. Analg., *51*:475, 1972.

294. Pender, J.W.: Dissociative anesthesia. JAMA, *215*:1126, 1971.

295. Sun, S.: Postanesthetic action of ketamine on the central nervous system. *In* Ketamin. Neue Ergebnisse in Forschung und Klinik. Edited by M. Gemperle, H. Dreuscher, and D. Langrehr. Berlin, Springer, 1973.

296. Albin, M.S.: Evaluation in patients subjected to ketamine anesthesia and other anesthesia agents. Abstract presented at the meeting of the American Society of Anesthesiologists. New York, October, 1970.

297. Corssen, G., Oget, S., and Reed, P.C.: Computerized evaluation of psychic effects of ketamine. Anesth. Analg., *50*:397, 1971.

298. Thompson, G.E.: Ketamine-induced convulsions. Anesthesiology, *37*:662, 1972.

299. Bennett, D.R.: Ketamine anesthesia in brain-damaged epileptics. Neurology, *23*:449, 1973.

300. Fisher, M.: Use of ketamine hydrochloride in the treatment of convulsions. Anaesth. Intensive Care, *2*:266, 1974.

301. Corssen, G., Little, S.G., and Tavakoli, M.: Ketamine and epilepsy. Anesth. Analg., *53*:319, 1974.

302. Celesia, G.G., Chen, R.C., and Bamforth, B.J.: Effects of ketamine in epilepsy. Neurology. *25*:169, 1975.

303. Rainey, J.M.. and Crowder, M.K.: Prevalence of phencyclidine in street drug preparations. N. Engl. J. Med., *290*:466, 1974.

304. Shaffer, L.L.: Ketamine. JAMA, *229*:763, 1974.

305. Rainey, J.M., and Crowder, M.K.: Ketamine or phencyclidine. JAMA, *230*:824, 1974

306. Eastman, J.W., and Cohen, S.N.: Hypertensive crisis and death associated with phencyclidine poisoning. JAMA, *231*:1270, 1975.

307. Rita, L., Cox, J.M., Seleny, F.L., and Tolentino, R.L.: Ketamine hydrochloride for pediatric premedication. I. Comparison with pentazocine. Anesth. Analg., *53*:375, 1974.

308. Nicoletti, R.I.: Pediatric premedication with intramuscular ketamine. Rev. Bras. Anest., *20*:337, 1970.

309. Sehatti, G., Erdmann, W., Frey, R., and Partheniadis, E.: Ketamine: Ein Praemedikationsmittel in der Kinderanaesthesie. *In* Ketamin. Neue Ergebnisse in Forschung und Klinik. Edited by M. Gemperle, H. Kreuscher, and D. Langrehr. Berlin, Springer, 1973.

310. Liang, H.S., and Liang, H.G.: Minimizing emergence phenomena: sub-dissociative dosage of ketamine in balanced surgical anaesthesia. Anesth. Analg., *54*:312, 1975.
311. Reves, J.G., Vinik, H.R., and Wright, D.: Midazolam efficacy for intramuscular premedication: a double-blind placebo, hydroxyzine, controlled study. Presented at the Annual Meeting of the American Society of Anesthesiologists. Las Vegas, October, 1982.
312. Corssen, G., and Reves, J.G.: Monitoring depth of ketamine anesthesia. *In* Clinical Anesthesia. Edited by J.F. Artusio and W.H.L. Dornette. Philadelphia, F.A. Davis Co., 1973.
313. Pandit, S.K., Kothary, S.P., and Kumar, S.M.: Low-dose intravenous infusion technique with ketamine. Anaesthesia, *35*:669, 1980.
314. Aldrete, J.A., and McDonald, J.S.: Low-dose ketamine-diazepam prevents adverse reactions. *In* Trends in Intravenous Anaesthesia. Edited by J.A. Aldrete and T.H. Stanley, Miami, Symposia Specialist, 1980.
315. Saint-Maurice, C., Laguente, G., Courturier, C., and Goutail-Flaud, F.: Rectal ketamine in pediatric anesthesia. Br. J. Anaesth., *51*:573, 1979.
316. Wessels, J.V., Allen, G.W., and Slogoff, S.: The effects of nitrous oxide on ketamine anesthesia. Anesthesiology, *39*:382, 1973.
317. White, P.F., Johnston, R.R., and Pudwill, C.R.: Interaction of ketamine and halothane in rats. Anesthesiology, *42*:179, 1975.
318. Corssen, G.: Recent developments in the anesthetic management of burned patients. J. Trauma, *7*:152, 1967.
319. Corssen, G., and Oget, S.: Dissociative anesthesia for the severely burned child. Anesth. Analg., *50*:95, 1971.
320. Wilson, R.D., Nichols, R.J., and McCoy, N.R.: Dissociative anesthesia with CI-581 in burned children. Anesth. Analg., *46*:719, 1967.
321. Roberts, F.W.: A new intramuscular anaesthetic for small children: a report of clinical trials of CI-581. Anaesthesia, *22*:23, 1967.
322. Wilson, R.D., Traber, D.L., and Evans, B.L.: Correlation of psychologic and physiologic observations from children undergoing repeated ketamine anesthesia. Anesth. Analg., *49*:995, 1969.
323. Larson, D.L.: Shriners Burn Institute —early care of the acutely burned child. Nebr. Med. J., *54*:733, 1969.
324. Abston, S.: A surgeon's appraisal of ketamine. South. Med. J., *63*:1085, 1970.
325. Wilson, R.D., Knapp, C., Traber, D.L., and Evans, B.L.: A new method for safe management of the child with a contracted neck. South. Med. J., *63*:1420, 1970.
326. Klose, R., and Peter, L.: Clinical studies concerning ketamine as the sole agent for burned patients. Anaesthesist, *22*:121, 1973.
327. Ensel, J., Zanello, E., and Winkler, C.: Anesthesia in burn patients under 5 years of age. Anaesth. Analg., *30*:1093, 1973.
328. Horatz, K., and Speh, B.: Ketamin in der operativen Frakturenbehandlung bei alten und Risikopatienten. *In* Ketamin. Neue Ergebnisse in Forschung und Klinik. Edited by M. Gemperle, H. Kreuscher, and D. Langrehr. Berlin, Springer, 1973.
329. Oduntan, S.A., and Gool, R.Y.: Clinical trial of ketamine (CI-581). Can. Anaesth. Soc. J., *17*:411, 1970.
330. Szappanyos, G., Gemperle, M., and Rifat, K.: Selective indications for ketamine anaesthesia. Proc. R. Soc. Lond. [Biol.], *64*:1156, 1971.
331. Lorhan, P.H., and Lippmann, M.: A clinical appraisal of the use of ketamine hydrochloride in the aged. Anesth. Analg., *50*:448, 1971.
332. Nettles, D.C., Herrin, T.J., and Mulen, J.G.: Ketamine induction in poor-risk patients. Anesth. Analg., *52*:59, 1973.
333. Zegfeld, C.: Allgemeine Erfahrungen mit Ketamin als Einleitungsnarkotikum. *In* Ketamin. Edited by H. Kreuscher. Berlin, Springer, 1969.
334. Langrehr, D., and Neuhaus, R.: Ketamin-indikation zur Anwendung bei Risikopatienten. *In* Ketamin. Neue Ergebnisse in Forschung und Klinik. Edited by M. Gemperle, H. Kreuscher, and D. Langrehr. Berlin, Springer, 1973.
335. Kapferer, J.M.: Ketamin bei geriatrischen Patienten. *In* Ketamin. Neue Ergebnisse in Forschung und Klinik. Edited by M. Gemperle, H. Kreuscher, and D. Langrehr. Berlin, Springer, 1973.
336. Barson, P., and Arens, J.F.: Ketamine as an induction anesthetic for poor-risk patients. South. Med. J., *67*:1398, 1974.
337. Vaughan, R.W., and Stephen, C.R.: Abdominal and thoracic surgery in adults with ketamine, nitrous oxide, and d-tubocurarine. Anesth. Analg., *53*:271, 1974.
338. Stephen, C.R., Johnston, E., and Burleson, J.: Induction of anesthesia with ketamine in adults. Proceedings of the Annual Meeting of the American Society of Anesthesiology. New York, 1970.
339. Stephen, C.R.: Induction of anesthesia with ketamine. AANA J., *41*:37, 1973.
340. Peter, K., Van Ackern, K. and Frey, B.: Die Wirkung verschiedener Narkotika auf Herz und Kreislauf bei der Narkoseeinleitung im fruehen haemorrhagischen Schock. Z. Prakt. Anaesth., *7*:263, 1972.

341. Chasapakis, G., Kekis, N., Sakkalis, C., and Kolios, D.: Use of ketamine and pancuronium for anaesthesia for patients in hemorrhagic shock. Anesth. Analg., 52:282, 1973.

342. Bond, A.C., and Davies, C.K.: Ketamine and pancuronium for the shocked patient. Anaesthesia, 29:59, 1974.

343. Spieckermann, P.G., Braun, U., Hellberg, K., Lohar, B., Kettler, R.D., Nordeck, E., and Brettschneider, H.J.: Uberlebens-und Wiederbelebungszeit des Herzens waehrend Ketamin-Barbiturat- und Halothan-Narkose. Z. Prakt. Anaesth., 5:365, 1970.

344. Kassel, H.: Allgemeine Erfahrungen mit Ketamin bei Risikopatienten. *In* Ketamin. Edited by H. Kreuscher. Berlin, Springer, 1969.

345. Muncibi, S., and Santorini, R.: Utilizzazione della Ketamina in ortopedia e traumatologia. Minerva Anesthesiol., 39:370, 1973.

346. Cavalli, P.L., and Morsica, C.: Il Ketalar nella anestesia ortopedica, traumatologica ed oculistica. Minerva Anesthesiol., 40:328, 1974.

347. Carbone, M., Scotto, M.L., and Pelelli: L'uso della Ketamina come anestetico traumatologia incruenta. Minerva Anesthesiol., 40:408, 1974

348. Caro, D.: Trial of ketamine in an accident and emergency. Anaesthesist, 29:227, 1974.

349. Guertner, Th., Erdelyi, M., and Sommerlad, W.: Erfahrungen mit Ketamin in der Traumatologie. *In* Ketamin. Neue Ergebnisse in Forschung und Klinik. Edited by M. Gemperle, H. Kreuscher, and D. Langrehr. Berlin, Springer, 1973.

350. Fischer, K.: Ketamine in der Traumatologie. *In* Ketamin. Neue Ergebnisse in Forschung und Klinik. Edited by M. Gemperle, H. Kreuscher, and D. Langrehr. Berlin, Springer, 1973.

351. Schlag, G.: Die Bedeutung des Ketamins in der Traumatologie. *In* Ketamin. Neue Ergebnisse in Forschung und Klinik. Edited by M. Gemperle, H. Kreuscher, and D. Langrehr. Berlin, Springer, 1973.

352. Fischer, K.: Ketamine in der Herzchirurgie. *In* Ketamin. Neue Ergebnisse in Forschung und Klinik. Edited by M. Gemperle, H. Kreuscher, and D. Langrehr. Berlin, Springer, 1973.

353. Corssen, G., Allarde, R., Brosch, F., and Arbenz, G.: Ketamine as the sole anesthetic in open-heart surgery. A preliminary report. Anesth. Analg., 49:1025, 1970.

354. Sanchez, R., Canseco, J.L.T., Acuna, L., and Mireles, M.: The use of ketamine in patients undergoing cardiac surgery. Anaesthesist, 20:152, 1971.

355. Lillehasen, P., Aune, H., and Stovner, J.: Ketamine-pancuronium induction in patients with aortic stenosis. Acta Anesthesiol. Scand., 19:193, 1975.

356. Petrajitis, B., Szappanyos, G., Etienne, A., Gemperle, M., and Rifat, K.: Ketamine in open heart surgery. *In* Ketamin. Neue Ergebnisse in Forschung und Klinik. Edited by M. Gemperle, H. Kreuscher, and D. Langrehr. Berlin, Springer, 1973.

357. Sefer, St.: Erfahrungen mit Ketamin bei kardiochirurgischen Eingriffen. *In* Ketamin. Neue Ergebnisse in Forschung und Klinik. Edited by M. Gemperle, H. Kreuscher, and D. Langrehr. Berlin, Springer, 1973.

358. Corssen, G.: Ketamine for high-risk cardiac patients. Anesthesiology, 36:413, 1972.

359. Lippman, M.: Emergency closed mitral commissurotomy using ketamine anesthesia: report of a case. Anesthesiology, 35:543, 1971.

360. Chari, P., and Pandit, S.K.: Ketamine as an induction agent in anaesthesia for closed mitral valvotomy. Surv. Anesthesiol., 18:56, 1974.

361. Bland, J.W., Dunbar, R.W., Kaplan, J.A., and Guffin, A.: Anesthetic technic using profound hypothermia for correction of congenital heart defects in infants and small children. South. Med. J., 69:831, 1976.

362. Ochsner, J.L., Lawson, N.W., Mills, N.L., King, T.D., and Williams, L.C.: Technic of deep hypothermia and circulatory arrest in the neonate and infants. South. Med. J., 69:607, 1976.

363. Levin, R.M., Seleny, F.L., and Streczyn, M.V.: Ketamine-pancuronium-narcotic technic for cardiovascular surgery in infants—a comparative study. Anesth. Analg., 54:800, 1973.

364. Radnay, P.A., Arai, T., and Nagashima, H.: Ketamine-gallamine anesthesia for great-vessel operations in infants. Anesth. Analg., 53:365, 1974.

365. Savege, T.M., Colvin, M.P., Weaver, E.J.M., Bond, C., Drake, J., and Inniss, R.: A comparison of some cardiorespiratory effects of althesin and ketamine when used for induction of anaesthesia in patients with cardiac disease. Br. J. Anaesth., 48:1071, 1976.

366. Pinaud, M., Souron, R., and Nicholas, F.: Ketamine anesthesia for implantation of a permanent pacemaker: hemodynamic study. Anesth. Analg., 36:531, 1976.

367. Eisenkraft, J.B., Dimich, I., and Miller, R.: Ketamine-diazepam anaesthesia in a patient with carcinoid syndrome. Anaesthesia, 36:881, 1981.

368. Jackson, A.P.F., Dhadphale, P.R., and Callaghan, M.L.: Haemodynamic studies during induction of anaesthesia for open-heart surgery using diazepam and ketamine. Br. J. Anaesth., 50:375, 1978.

369. Dhadphale, P.R., Jackson, A.P.F., and Alseri, S.: Comparison of anesthesia with diazepam and ketamine vs. morphine in patients undergoing heart-valve replacement. Anesthesiology, 51:200, 1979.

370. Hatano, S., Keane, D.M., Boggs, R.E., El-Kaggar, M.A., and Sadove, M.S.: Diazepam-ketamine anaesthesia for open heart surgery—a micro-mini-drip administration technique. Can. Anaesth. Soc. J., 23:648, 1976.
371. Reves, J.G., Lell, W.A., McCracken, L.E., Kravetz, R.A., and Prough, D.S.: Comparison of morphine and ketamine. Anesthetic techniques for coronary surgery: a randomized study. South. Med. J., 71:33, 1978.
372. Kaplan, J.A., Bland, J.W., and Dunbar, R.W.: The perioperative management of pericardial tamponade. South. Med. J., 69:417, 1976.
373. Lumb, P.D., Silvay, G., Weinreich, A.I., and Shiang, H.: A comparison of the effects of continuous ketamine infusion and halothane on oxygenation during one-lung anesthesia in dogs. Can. Anaesth. Soc. J., 26:394, 1979.
374. Stanley, V., Hunt, J., Willis, K.W., and Stephen, C.R.: Cardiovascular and respiratory function with CI-581. Anesth. Analg., 47:760, 1968.
375. Szappanyos, G.G.: The use and advantage of "ketalar" (CI-581) as anaesthetic agent in pediatric cardiac catheterisation and angiography. Anaesthesist, 18:365, 1969.
376. Faithfull, N.S., and Haider, R.: Ketamine for cardiac catheterization. An evaluation of its use in children. Anaesthesia, 26:318, 1971.
377. Dillon, J.B.: Rational use of ketamine as an anaesthetic. Proc. R. Soc. Lond. [Biol.], 64:1153, 1971.
378. Coppel, D.L., and Dundee, J.W.: Ketamine anesthesia for cardiac catheterization. Anaesthesia, 27:25, 1972.
379. Neemeatallah, F.A.: Ketamine anaesthesia versus basal narcosis for cardiac catheterization in children. Middle East J. Anaesth., 3:433, 1972.
380. Samuelson, P.N.: Anesthesia for pediatric cardiac catheterisation. Symposium of Pediatric Cardiac Anesthesia, American Academy of Pediatrics. Maui, Hawaii, March, 1982.
381. Manners, J.M.: Anaesthesia for diagnostic procedures in cardiac disease. Br. J. Anaesth., 43:276, 1971.
382. Serra, G.C., Cardona, S., Giudice, C., LiRosi, G., and Musci, D.: Impiego della ketamina nel paziente asmatico e nelle condizioni broncospatiche. Acta Anaesth. Ital., XXIV:519, 1973.
383. Fischer, M.M.: Ketaine hydrochloride in severe bronchospasm. Anaesthesia, 32:771, 1977.
384. Betts, G.K., and Parkin, C.E.: Use of ketamine in an asthmatic child: a case report. Anesth. Analg., 50:420, 1971.
385. Marx, G.: Obstetric anesthesia in the presence of medical complications. Clin. Obstet. Gynecol., 17:165, 1974.
386. Akamatsu, T.J., Bonica, J.J., Rehmet, R., and Eng. M.: Experiences with the use of ketamine for parturition: I. Primary anesthetic for vaginal delivery. Anesth. Analg., 53:284, 1974.
387. Janeczko, J.G., El-Etr, A.A., and Younes, S.: Low-dose ketamine anesthesia for obstetrical delivery. Anesth. Analg., 53:828, 1974.
388. Hyman, M.D.: The use of small doses of ketamine in obstetrics. Anesthesiol. Rev., Feb., 1974.
389. Craft, J.B., Levinson, G., and Shnider, S.M.: Inhalation analgesia versus low-dose ketamine for labor and delivery. Weekly Anesth. Update. Lesson 30, Vol. 1, 1978.
390. Bassel, G.M.: The present role of ketamine in obstetric-anesthesia. West. J. Med., 135:393, 1981.
391. Galbert, M.W., and Gardner, A.E.: Ketamine for obstetrical anesthesia. Anesth. Analg., 52:926, 1973.
392. Sellick, B.A.: Cricoid pressure to control regurgitation of stomach contents during induction of anesthesia. Lancet, 2:404, 1961.
393. Meer, F.M., Downing, J.W., and Coleman, A.J.: An intravenous method of anaesthesia for caesarean section. Part II: Ketamine. Br. J. Anaesth., 45:191, 1973.
394. Crawford, J.: Awareness during operative obstetrics under general anesthesia. Br. J. Anaesth., 43:179, 1971.
395. Peltz, B., and Sinclair, M.D.: Induction agents for caesarian section: a comparison of thiopentone and ketamine. Anaesthesia, 28:34, 1973.
396. Maduska, A.L.: Ketamine in obstetrics: where are we? Some personal reflections. Anesthesiol. Rev., Jan., 1978, p. 38.
397. Marx, G.F., Cabe, C.M., Kim, Y.I., and Eidelman, A.I.: Neonatal blood pressures. Anaesthesist, 25:318, 1976.
398. Bunodiere, M., Green, M., Bunodiere, N., Deligne, P., and Guilmet, C.: Le chlorhydrate de ketamine pour l'anesthesie en obstetrique. Anesth. Analg., 32:187, 1975.
399. Marx, G.F.: Obstetric anesthesia in the presence of medical complications. Clin. Obstet. Gynecol., 17:165, 1974.
400. Corssen, G.: Ketamine in obstetric anesthesia. Clin. Obstet. Gynecol., 17:249, 1974.
401. McDonald, J.S., Mateo, C.V., and Reed, E.C.: Modified nitrous oxide or ketamine hydrochloride for caesarean section. Anesth. Analg., 51:975, 1972.

402. Roopnarinesingh, S., and Kalipersadnech, S.: Manual removal of the placenta under ketamine. Anaesthesia, 29:486, 1974.

403. Rucci, F.S., and Caroli, G.: Ketamine and eclampsia. Br. J. Anaesth., 46:546, 1974.

404. Austin, T.R.: Ketamine hydrochloride: a potent analgesic. Br. Med. J., 2:943, 1976.

405. Hodgkinson, R., Marx, G.F., Kim, S.S., and Miclat, N.M.: Neonatal neurobehavioral tests following vaginal delivery under ketamine, thiopental and extradural anesthesia. Anesth. Analg., 56:548, 1977.

406. Hodgkinson, R., Bhatt, M., Kim, S.S., Grewal, G., and Marx, G.F.: Neonatal behavioral tests following cesarean section under general and spinal anesthesia. Am. J. Obstet. Gynecol., 132:670, 1978.

407. Jastak, J.T., and Goretta, C.: Ketamine as a continuous-drip anesthetic for outpatients. Anesth. Analg., 52:341, 1973.

408. Westhues, G.: Klinische Erfahrungen mit der intramuskulaeren Anwendung von Ketamin bei Kindern. *In* Ketamin. Edited by H. Kreuscher. Berlin, Springer, 1969.

409. Podlesch, I.: Erfahrungen mit Ketamin bei ophtalmologischen Eingriffen im Kindesalter. *In* Ketamin. Edited by H. Kreuscher. Berlin, Springer, 1969.

410. Dangel, P.: Ketamin in der paediatrischen Chirurgie. *In* Ketamin. Edited by H. Kreuscher. Berlin Heidelberg New York, Springer, 1969.

411. Gemperle, G.N., Gemperle, M., and Szappanyos, G.: Unsere Klinischen Erfahrungen mit Ketamine in der Kinderchirurgie (100 Faelle). *In* Ketamin. Edited by H. Kreuscher. Berlin, Springer, 1969.

412. Brunkhorst, B., Horatz K., and Koenig, G.: Die Anwendung von Ketamin vorwiegend in der Kinder- und Neurochirurgie. *In* Ketamin. Edited by H. Kreuscher. Berlin, Springer, 1969.

413. Eckart, I.: Erfahrungen mit Ketamin bei Kindern. *In* Ketamin. Edited by H. Kreuscher. Berlin, Springer, 1969.

414. Zook, E.G., Roesch, R.P., Thompson, L.W., and Bennett, J.E.: Ketamine anesthesia in pediatric plastic surgery. Plast. Reconstr. Surg., 48:241, 1971.

415. Keilty, S.R., and Bridges, J.M.: Ketamine for minor procedures in children. Lancet, 1:631, 1972.

416. Meadows, A.T., Mayer, B.W., and Naiman, J.L.: Ketamine for minor procedures in children. Lancet, 1:632, 1972.

417. Lotfy, A.O., Esmaili, M.H., and Amir-Jahed, A.K.: Ketamine anesthesia for ano-rectal surgery. Am. J. Proctol., 31:26, 1980.

418. Ensel, J., Durand, J.P., and Delegue, L.: Notre experience de la Ketamine en anesthesiologie infantile. Anesth. Analg., 28:903, 1971.

419. Page, P., Morgan, M., and Loh, L.: Ketamine anaesthesia in paediatric procedures. Acta Anaesthesiol. Scand., 16:155, 1972.

420. Holten-Jensen, A.M., Egebo, K., Hansen, A., and Sturup, A.G.: Ketalar (CI-581). Experience from 200 anesthesias. Nord. Med., 84:1231, 1970.

421. Zohairy, A.F.M., and Siddiqi, S.M.W.: The use of ketamine HCL in minor surgery. Middle East J. Anaesth., 31:123, 1971.

422. Casale, F.F., and Sil, B.: Ketalar in minor surgery. Med. J. Zambia, 5:165, 1971.

423. Falls, H.F., Hoy, J.E., and Corssen, G.: CI-581: an intravenous or intramuscular anesthetic for office ophthalmic surgery. Am. J. Ophthalmol., 61:1093, 1966.

424. Harrison, G.G.: Some recent advances in anaesthesia of interest to ophthalmic surgeons. S. Afr. Med. J., 40:400, 1971.

425. Schoeppner, H., Ulrich, W.D., Friis, E., and Schaedlich, M.: Zur Anwendung von CI-581 (Ketamin) in der Ophthalmologie. Math. Nat. R., XXI, 1972.

426. Edlinger, E.: Die Anwendung von Ketamin in Augneheilkunde bei extrabulbaeren Eingriffen. *In* Ketamin. Neue Ergebnisse in Forschung und Klinik. Edited by M. Gemperle, H. Kreuscher, and D. Langrehr. Berlin, Springer, 1973.

427. Aplvor, D.: Ketamine in paediatric ophthalmological surgery. An evaluation of its efficacy and postoperative effects. Anaesthesia, 28:501, 1973.

428. Newell, F.W.: Current trends in ophthalmic anesthesia. Ophthalmic Surg., 6:15, 1975.

429. Stoecker, L.: Klinische Erfahrungen mit Ketamin bei Eingriffen im Zahn-Mund-und Kieferbereich. *In* Ketamin. Edited by H. Kreuscher. Berlin, Springer, 1969.

430. O'Brien, D.N.: An evaluation of ketamine, droperidol and nitrous oxide in pedodontic outpatients. J. Dent. Child., Jan.-Feb., 42:31, 1975.

431. Allen, G.D.: Minor anesthesia. J. Oral Surg., 31:330, 1973.

432. Sobczak, O.M.: Use of ketamine in pediatric dentistry. Anesth. Analg., 54:248, 1975.

433. Young, R.A., and Epker, B.N.: Ketamine hydrochloride in outpatient oral surgery in children. J. Oral Maxillofac. Surg., 29:703, 1971.

434. Carrel, R.: Ketamine: a general anesthetic for unmanageable ambulatory patients. J. Dent. Child., 40:288, 1973.

435. Cohenour, K., Gamble, J.W., Metzgar, M.T., and Ward, R.L.: A composite general anesthesia for pediatric outpatients. J. Oral Maxillofac. Surg., 36:594, 1978.

436. Alling, C.C.: Outpatient sedation and general anesthesia. Ala. J. Med. Sci., *13*:40, 1978.
437. Greenfield, W.: Neuroleptanalgesia and dissociative drugs. Dent. Clin. North. Am., *17*:263, 1973.
438. Bamber, D.B., and McEvan, T.E.: Ketamine for outpatient dental conservation in children. Anaesthesia, 28:446, 1973.
439. Kaplan, D., and Hirchowitz, A.S.: The dental treatment of problem children under ketamine analgesia. S. Afr. Med. J., *49*:313, 1975.
440. Brockmueller, V.K.D.: Ketamine for oral and maxillofacial surgery. Dtsch. Zahnaerztl. Z., *26*:974, 1971.
441. Roper, A.L., and Kramer, R.J.: Ketamine anesthesia in minor otologic procedures. Laryngoscope, *81*:1423, 1971.
442. Chuden, H.G.: Klinische Erfahrungen mit Ketamine bei der Adenotonsillektomie. Anaesthesist, *20*:155, 1971.
443. Guenzler, W., and Strehlau, D.: Erfahrungen mit Ketamin bei 400 Tonsillektomien nach Sluder. Anaesthesist, *21*:213, 1972.
444. Stanca, A., Frederici, L., Giomarelli, G.P., and De Bernardinis, G.B.: L'uso del ketalar nelle adenotonsillectomie. Minerva Anesthesiol., *39*:228, 1973.
445. Saarnivaara, L.: Comparison of thiopentone, althesin and ketamine in anaesthesia for otolaryngological surgery in children. Br. J. Anaesth., *49*:363, 1977.
446. Bryant, W.M.: Ketamine anesthesia and intranasal or intraoral operations. Plast. Reconstr. Surg., *51*:562, 1973.
447. Blanc, V.F., Weber, M.L., Leduc, C., LaBerge, R., Desjardins, R., and Perreault, G.: Acute epiglottitis in children: management of 27 consecutive cases with nasotracheal intubation with special emphasis on anesthetic considerations. Can. Anaesth. Soc. J., 24:1, 1977.
448. Barson, P.K., Scott, M.L., Lawson, N.W., and Ochsner, J.L.: Ketamine for bronchoscopy of children. South. Med. J., *67*:1403, 1974.
449. Wilson, G.H., Fotias, N.A., and Dillon, J.B.: Ketamine: a new anesthetic for use in pediatric neuroroentgenologic procedures. AJR, *106*:434, 1969.
450. Bennett, J.A., and Bullimore, J.A.: The use of ketamine hydrochloride anaesthesia for radiotherapy in young children. Br. J. Anaesth., *45*:197, 1973.
451. Sanford, F.G., and Jones, C.W.: Immobilization for radiotherapy by ketamine. Anesthesiol. Rev., *3*:16, 1976.
452. Mayhew, J.F., and Rachel, J.: Ketamine: its use in the pediatric patient for radiotherapy. J. AANA, *45*:178, 1977.
453. Catton, D.V.: Intramuscular ketamine-repeated injections. Can. Anaesth. Soc. J., *20*:227, 1973.
454. Piwoz, S., and Goldstein, B.: The use of ketamine anesthesia in radiation therapy. Radiology, *109*:725, 1973.
455. Bozorgi, N., Stepto, R.C., Havdala, H., Prenzla, M., and Salvo, B.: The use of ketamine anesthesia for laparoscopy. Obstet. Gynecol., *39*:636, 1972.
456. Azar, I., and Ozomey, E.: The use of ketamine for abdominal tubal ligation. Anesth. Analg., *52*:39, 1973.
457. Ruibe-Ramirez, L.C., Camerena, R., Hernandez, F., and Diaz, M.: Outpatient laparoscopic sterilization: a review of complications in 2,000 cases. J. Reprod. Med., *18*:103, 1977.
458. McKenzie, R., and Tantisira, B.: Culdoscopy: a new use for ketamine. Anesth. Analg., 52:353, 1973.
459. Galloon, D.: Ketamine for dilation and curettage. Can. Anaesth. Soc. J., 18:600, 1971.
460. Hervey, W.H., and Hustead, R.F.: Ketamine-patient acceptance. Anesth. Analg., *51*:647, 1972.
461. Corssen, G., Groves, E.H., Gomez, S., and Allen, R.J.: Ketamine: its place in anesthesia for neurological diagnostic procedures. Anesth. Analg., *48*:181, 1969.
462. Faure, C., Fihey, A., and Lupold, M.: Notes De technique, L'encephalographie gazeuse sous anesthesie generale au chlorhydrate de ketamine chez l'enfant. J. Radiol., *56*:717, 1975.
463. Dundee, J.W., and Wyant, G.M.: Dissociative anesthesia. *In* Intravenous Anaesthesia. Edited by J.W. Dundee and G.M. Wyant. Edinburgh, Churchill Livingston, 1974.
464. Muhlmann-Weil, M.: Unsere Erfahrungen mit Ketamine in der Neuroradiologie (Carotisangiography). Anaesthesist, *19*:313, 1970.
465. Wyte, S.R., Shapiro, H.M., Turner, P., and Harris, A.B.: Ketamine-induced intracranial hypertension. Anesthesiology, *36*:174, 1972.
466. Szappanyos, G., Gemperle, M., and Gemperle, G.: The utilization of ketamine as an adjunct with spinal and epidural analgesia. *In* Ketamine. Edited by Kreuscher. Berlin, Springer, 1969.
467. Boegl, P., and Hutschenreuter, K.: Die Kombination der Ketamin-narkose mit einer Leitungsanaesthesie. *In* Ketamin. Neue Ergebnisse in Forschung und Klinik. Edited by M. Gemperle, H. Kreuscher, and D. Langrehr. Berlin, Springer, 1973.
468. Erdemir, H.A., Huber, F.C. and Corssen, G.: Dissociative anesthesia with ketamine: a suitable adjunct to epidural anesthesia. Anesth. Analg., *49*:623, 1970.

469. Thompson, G.E., and Moore, D.C.: Ketamine, diazepam, and Innovar: a computerized comparative study. Anesth. Analg., 50:548, 1971.
470. Beekhuis, G.J., and Kahn, D.L.: Anesthesia for facial cosmetic surgery. Low dosage ketamine-diazepam anesthesia. Larynogoscope, 88:1709, 1978.
471. Sears, B.E.: Experience with ketamine anesthesia. J. Natl. Med. Assoc., Jan., 1975.
472. Kamm, G.: Ketamine anesthesia in a developing country. Anaesthesist, 22:415, 1973.
473. Abbey, N.D.: Letter to the editor: ketamine. Can. Med. Assoc. J., 106:749, 1972.
474. Corssen, G.: The use of ketamine hydrochloride for relief of pain and suffering in disaster situations. In Disaster Medicine. Edited by R. Frey and P. Safar. Berlin, Springer, 1980.
475. Ahnefeld, F.W., Haug, H., and Israng, H.H.: Ketamin im Katastrophenfall. In Ketamin. Edited by H. Kreuscher. Berlin, Springer, 1969.
476. Ahnefeld, F.W., Haug, H., and Israng, H.H.: Ketamin—ein Anaesthetikum fuer Katastrophen—und Notfallsituationen. Wehrmed. Mschr., 4:108, 1974.
477. Wilson, R.D.: Personal communication.
478. Erdmann, W.: Ketamine-benzodiazepines-alloferin-air anesthesia in disaster situations. Proceeding of the 3rd International Meeting of Disaster Medicine, Monaco, 1979.
479. Rust, M., Landauer, B., and Kolb, E.: The value of ketamine in emergency situations. Anaesthesist, 27:205, 1978.
480. Cromartie, R.: Rapid anesthesia induction in combat casualties with full stomachs. Anesth. Analg., 55:74, 1976.
481. Beeking, C.: Anwendung der Kombination von Ketamin und Diazepam als Dauertropf-Infusions-Narkose in Katastrophen situationen. Anestheziol. Reanimatol., 5:21, 1980.
482. D'Arcy, E.J., Fell, R.H., Ansell, B.M., and Arden, G.P.: Ketamine and juvenile chronic polyarthritis (Still's disease). Anaesthesia, 31:624, 1976.
483. Schoening, B., Banniza, U., and Koch, H.: Ketamin und Diazepam zur Anaesthesie bei infantiler Cerebralparese. Anaesthesist, 23:14, 1974.
484. Kamvyssi-Dea, S., Kritikou, P., Exarhos, N., and Skalkeas, G.: Anaesthetic management of reconstruction of the lower portion of the trachea. Br. J. Anaesth., 47:82, 1975.
485. Ellis, R.H., Hinds, C.J., and Gadd, L.T.: Management of anaesthesia during tracheal resection. Anaesthesia, 31:1076, 1976.
486. Bernhardi, L.A.: Ketamine: a dissociative anesthetic agent. J.A.O.A., 73:458, 1974.
487. Hamann, R.A., and Cohen, P.J.: Anesthetic management of a patient with epidermolysis bullosa dystrophica. Anesthesiology, 34:389, 1971.
488. Lee, C., and Nagel, E.L.: Anesthetic management of a patient with recessive epidermolysis bullosa dystrophica. Anesthesiology, 43:122, 1975.
489. Patrikh, R.K., and Moore, M.R.: Anaesthetics in porphyria: intravenous induction agents. Br. J. Anaesth., 47:907, 1975.
490. Rizk, S.F., Jacobson, J.H., and Silvay, G.: Ketamine as an induction agent for acute intermittent porphyria. Anesthesiology, 46:305, 1977.
491. Parikh, R.K., and Moore, M.R.: Effect of certain anesthetic agents on the activity of rat hepatic delta-aminolaevulinate synthase. Br. J. Anaesth., 50:1099, 1978.
492. Kostrzewski, E., and Gregor, A.: Ketamine in acute intermittent porphyria—dangerous or safe? Anesthesiology, 49:376, 1978.
493. Rizk, S.F.: Ketamine is safe in acute intermittent porphyria. Anesthesiology, 51:184, 1979.
494. Nieder, R.M.: Ketamine treatment of priapism. JAMA, 221:195, 1972.
495. Sklar, G.S., Reiss, R.F., and Fox, J.W.C.: Preferential use of ketamine in von Willebrand's disease. Anesthesiol. Rev., Sept., 1977.
496. Brewer, C.L., Davidson, J.R.T., and Hereward, S.: Ketamine (ketalar): a safer anaesthetic for ECT. Br. J. Psychiatry, 120:679, 1972.
497. Orecchia, C., Marullo-Reedtz, G., and Bram, S.: CI-581 e terapia elettroconvulsivante. Minerva Anesthesiol., 66:711, 1969.
498. Empt, J., and Kugler, J.: Analgesie bei Trigeminus Neuralgie. In Ketamin. Neue Ergebnisse in Forschung und Klinik. Edited by M. Gemperle, H. Kreuscher, and D. Langrehr. Berlin, Springer, 1973.
499. Kassel, H.: Ketanest-Anaesthesie bei Uraemie. In Ketamin. Neue Ergebnisse in Forschung und Klinik. Edited by M. Gemperle, H. Kreuscher, and D. Langrehr. Berlin, Springer, 1973.
500. Flynn, R.W.: Ketamine in the management of a case of lymphosarcoma cutis. Br. J. Anaesth., 46:699, 1974.
501. Defalque, R.J.: Ketamine for blind nasal intubation. Anesth. Analg., 50:984, 1971.
502. Clausen, L., Sinclair, D.M., and Van Hasselt, C.H.: Intravenous ketamine for postoperative analgesia. South. Afr. Med. J., 49:1437, 1975.
503. Ito, Y., and Ichiyanagi, K.: Post-operative pain relief with ketamine infusion. Anaesthesia, 29:222, 1974.
504. Shantha, T.R.: Ketamine for the treatment of hiccups during and following anesthesia: a preliminary report. Anesth. Analg., 52:822, 1973.

505. Tavakoli, M., and Corssen, G.: Control of hiccups by ketamine: a preliminary report. Ala. J. Med. Sci., *11*:3, 1974.
506. Salem, R.: An effective method for the treatment of hiccups during anesthesia. Anesthesiology, 28:463, 1967.
507. Condi, M.: Utilisation de la ketamine dans le traitement du delirium tremens et des delires medicaux. Anesth. Analg., 29:377, 1972.
508. Editorial. Ketamine—a new anesthetic. Can. Med. Assoc. J., *105*:1278, 1971.
509. Steward, D.J.: Letter to the editor. Can. Med. Assoc. J., *106*:750, 1972.
510. Sappington, A.A., Corssen, G., Becker, A.T., and Tavakoli, M.: Effects of ketamine on patient responsiveness during the various phases of a single induced anxiety session. Ala. J. Med. Sci., *14*:121, 1977.
511. Lockhart, C.H., and Jenkins, J.: Ketamine-induced apnea in patients with increased intracranial pressure. Anesthesiology, *37*:92, 1972.
512. Elliot, E., Hanid, T.K., Arthur, L.J.H., and Kay, B.: Ketamine anaesthesia for medical procedures in children. Arch. Dis. Child., *51*:56, 1976.
513. Brewer, C.: Psychosis and ketamine. Br. Med. J., 2:349, 1972.
514. Reames, E., and Rosenblatt, R.: Ketamine anesthesia of a catotonic-schizophrenic patient. Anesthesiology, *51*:577, 1979.
515. Guerra, F.: Ketamine may exacerbate psychiatric illness. Anesthesiology, 53:177, 1980.
516. Sefrin, P.: Klinische Erfahrung mit ketamine. Anaesthesiologie, 43:525, 1972.
517. Wadhwa, R.K., and Tantisira, B.: Parotidectomy in a patient with a family history of hyper-thermia. Anesthesiology, *40*:191, 1974.
518. Meltzer, H.Y., Hassan, S.F., Moretti, R., Hengefeld, C., and Brueckner, D.: Effect of ketamine on creatine phosphokinase levels. Lancet, *1*:1195, 1975.
519. Latarjet, J., Brunet, E., Banssillon, V.G., and Petit, P.: La Ketamine en Chirurgie Viscerale. Anesth. Analg., *30*:721, 1973.
520. Szappanyos, G., Gemperle, M., and Rifat, K.: Ketamine anaesthesia in visceral surgery. *In* Ketamin. Neue Ergebnisse in Forschung und Klinik. Edited by M. Gemperle, H. Kreuscher, and D. Langrehr. Berlin, Springer, 1973.
521. Panacciulli, E., Sordi, L., and Trazz, R.: The hallucinogen CI-581 in its use in anesthesiology. G. Ital. Mal., *20*:61, 1966.
522. Gruhl, D.W.: Kombinations-Narkose mit kleinen Ketaminedosen fuer kurze Eingriffe. Anaesthe-sist, *21*:62, 1972.
523. Ngai, S.H., and Wirklund, R.A.: Levodopa and surgical anesthesia. Neurology, 22:38, 1972.
524. Kaplan, J.A., and Cooperman, L.H.: Alarming reactions to ketamine in patients taking thyroid medication-treatment with propanolol. Anesthesiology, 35:229, 1971.

Chapter 8

NEUROLEPTANALGESIA AND NEUROLEPTANESTHESIA

Neuroleptanalgesia (NLA) is a curious syndrome characterized by apathy, immobility, and analgesia that is produced by the administration of a combination of a narcotic analgesic, e.g., fentanyl (Sublimaze), and a major tranquilizer, e.g., droperidol (Inapsine). With the addition of other agents, e.g., inhalation anesthetics (usually nitrous oxide) and muscle relaxants, NLA converts to neuroleptanesthesia (NLAN).

HISTORY

In the 1950s, Laborit and Huguenard re-examined the conventional approach to general anesthesia, i.e., profound depression of central nervous system (CNS) activity, with potentially dangerous effects on vital functions.[1,2] Seeking selective neurovegetative blockade ("multifocal inhibition") of cellular, autonomic, and endocrine mechanisms normally activated in response to stress, they developed a "lytic cocktail" containing an analgesic (meperidine), two tranquilizers (chlorpromazine and promethazine), and atropine. Unfortunately, the resultant state of "artificial hibernation" was often associated with circulatory depression and delayed awakening. Hence, the new technique did not achieve widespread popularity.

Hayward-Butt concurrently devised "ataralgesia," a similar approach to tranquility and freedom from pain that involved the use of an analgesic (meperidine), a tranquilizer (mepazine), and an analeptic (aminophenazole).[3] This method, too, was not widely accepted. Interestingly, several years later, Dardalhon labeled a diazepam-phenoperidine-droperidol combination "narco-ataralgesia."[4] Still another combination of diazepam and pentazocine, which produced "somnoanalgesia," was introduced by Aldrete.[5]

Further research then came to "neurolepsis," a syndrome first observed by Delay in animals and then in humans receiving haloperidol; the first member of the butyrophenones, a new group of tranquilizers, this drug was synthesized by Janssen.[6,7] The syndrome includes inhibition of various psychic, vegetative, and motor functions, tending toward catalepsy and suppressing apomorphine-induced vomiting. DeCastro and Mundeleer then combined the new narcotic analgesic, phenoperidine (a meperidine derivative also synthesized by Janssen, et al.) with the haloperidol in the first demonstration of NLA as a detached, pain-free state of consciousness without severe circulatory depression.[8] NLA achieved by using haloperidol and phenoperidine rapidly gained popularity in Europe as an alternative to general anesthesia.[9]

Further pharmacologic research by Janssen and colleagues produced even more potent drugs, namely the butyrophenone tranquilizer, droperidol, as well as the narcotic analgesic, fentanyl.[10-12] DeCastro and Mundeleer found the new fentanyl-droperidol combination superior to the earlier pair of phenoperidine and haloperidol, with more rapid onset of analgesia, less respiratory depression, and fewer extrapyramidal side-effects.[13]

While use of NLA and NLAN with fentanyl and droperidol became widespread throughout Europe, numerous variations in technique were tried, causing confusion about choice of drug, methods of administration, and indications for, and contraindications to, NLA, and consequently increasing lack of confidence in its efficacy.

Henschel, one of the earliest enthusiasts in Europe of the use of NLA, was influential in bringing this situation under control. He arranged an international symposium in Bremen in 1963 to discuss methodologic problems relating to NLA. The "standard" method of inducing and maintaining NLA that evolved from this meeting still provides a useful frame of reference for anesthesiologists today.[14]

Clinical anesthesiologists still disagree as to the use of fentanyl and droperidol as separate drugs rather than as a combination in a fixed mixture. In the United States, the administration of droperidol and fentanyl in a fixed mixture (Innovar; Thalamonal in Europe) is widely accepted as an effective and safe method for achieving the neuroleptanalgesic state. The reason behind this acceptance may be that droperidol was not available as a separate drug until 1971, when the United States Food and Drug Administration approved its use as a separate component of the neuroleptanalgesic mixture. The individual use of these two drugs will probably gain popularity in the United States as anesthesiologists accumulate more experience with their administration.

The use of other tranquilizer-narcotic combinations has been proposed by various investigators. The tranquilizers substituted for droperidol include benzperidol, trifluperidol, and diazepam. Some clinicians administer morphine instead of fentanyl simply because morphine is less expensive. Although phenoperidine, until recently, was the analgesic drug of choice in some Scandinavian countries, various clinical investigators believe that dextromoramide may be best for stereotactic procedures or for use in pediatric patients. More recently, DeCastro proposed a combination of an analgesic and a narcotic antagonist to produce "sequential anesthesia" as another alternative to NLA.[15] Currently, the use of the neuroleptic, droperidol, and the narcotic analgesic, fentanyl, seems the best means to achieve NLA, either as separate drugs or combined as Innovar.

NEUROLEPTANALGESIA (NLA)

Neuroleptic Drugs: Phenothiazines and Butyrophenones

Neuroleptic drugs can be divided into two categories, phenothiazines, with propylamino side chains (Fig. 8–1A), and butyrophenones, which are butylamino derivatives (Fig. 8–2A). The butylamines appear to be "stronger" neuroleptic agents than are the propylamines.[16]

Among the phenothiazines, chlorpromazine is used most often (Fig. 8–1B). Substitution of a piperazine ring at the amine group increases neuroleptic potency, as with prochlorperazine (Fig. 8–1C). Methylation of the carbon atom

A.

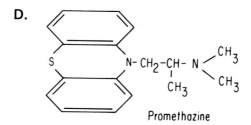

Anilino Propylamines

B.

Chlorpromazine

C.

Prochlorperazine

D.

Promethazine

Fig. 8–1.   Phenothiazines.

chain, as in promethazine (Fig. 8–1*D*), enhances antihistaminic, but lessens neuroleptic, activity.

The butyrophenone neuroleptic agents are fluorinated derivatives. Insertion of a substituted piperidine ring onto the basic butyrophenone structure (Fig. 8–2*A*) enhances potency, as is noted in haloperidol (Fig. 8–2*B*). Anilino-piperidino sub-stitution at the amine group increases both specificity and potency, as in dro-peridol (dehydrobenzperidol) (Fig. 8–2*C*) and spiroperidol (Fig. 8–2*D*), the most potent of the available neuroleptics.[17,18] The phenothiazines and related com-pounds, with weak neuroleptic properties (e.g., rauwolfia alkaloids), have been totally supplanted for use in NLA by the butyrophenones.

The predominant characteristic of butyrophenones in humans is a peculiar

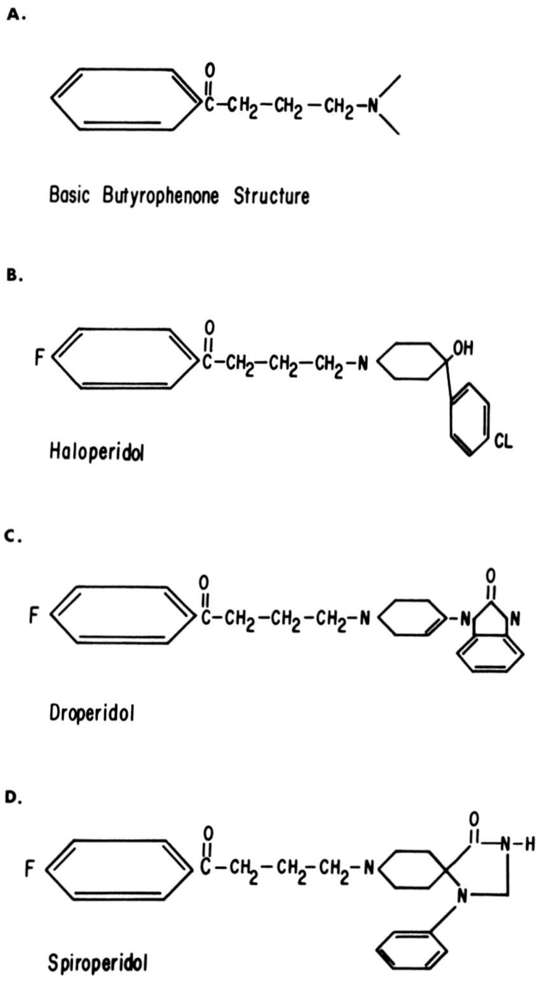

A.

Basic Butyrophenone Structure

B.

Haloperidol

C.

Droperidol

D.

Spiroperidol

Fig. 8–2. Butyrophenones.

type of CNS depression resulting in modest sedation but marked tranquility, cataleptic immobility, and antiemetic effects.[6,8,16] Side-effects, especially after large doses, may include extrapyramidal dyskinesia, restlessness, hyperactivity, chills and shivering, agitation ("inner anxiety"), hallucinations, and bizarre sensations of weightlessness and loss of body image.[16,19] Function of the reticular activating system is well maintained, and electroencephalographic (EEG) alpha rhythm is not appreciably altered.[20] The sedative and tranquilizing effects last 2 to 8 hours, but altered consciousness may persist for as much as 12 hours.

Neuroleptic drugs of high potency, e.g., droperidol, when used at low doses, are behaviorally active with few nonspecific effects. The weak neuroleptic agents, e.g., phenothiazines and rauwolfia alkaloids, in the large doses required to be effective, are more likely to be associated with side-effects, such as orthostatic hypotension, hypothermia, and soporific, antihistaminic, and adrenolytic activity.[16]

CELLULAR MODE OF ACTION

The neuroleptic potency of butyrophenones is closely related to their ability to form a monolayer on biologic membranes, reducing the surface tension of the membrane and decreasing its permeability.[7,21] This action seems to be specific for cell membranes in the CNS excited by dopamine, norepinephrine, and serotonin, the permeability of which is regulated by the competitive inhibition of glutamic acid by γ-aminobutyric acid (GABA).[18] Because the chemical structure of the butylamino portion of the butyrophenones closely resembles that of GABA, presumably these neuroleptic agents can occupy GABA receptors on the postsynaptic membrane, thereby reducing synaptic transmission and resulting in a build-up of dopamine in the intersynaptic cleft.[7] Neuroleptic drugs also inhibit the re-uptake of dopamine and norepinephrine into the storage granules of the presynaptic terminals.[7,22] These combined effects result in a build-up of dopamine in the intersynaptic cleft;[18] the balance of dopamine and acetylcholine in certain key sites in the brain is then upset, e.g., the extrapyramidal nigro-striatum system, and leads to the inhibition of "operant" behavior induced by the neuroleptic agents.[23]

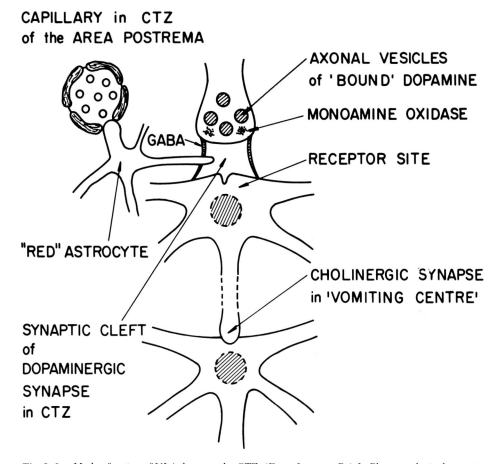

Fig. 8–3. Mode of action of NLA drugs at the CTZ. (From Janssen, P.A.J.: Pharmacological aspects. *In* Neuropsychopharmacology. Edited by D. Bente and P. Bradley. Amsterdam, Elsevier, 1965.)

The chemoreceptor trigger zone (CTZ) is the site of emetic action of apomorphine (Fig. 8–3).[24] "Red" astrocytes transport neurolept molecules from the capillary to dopaminergic synapses in the CTZ, where they occupy GABA receptors. Apomorphine depolarizes the red astrocytes, causing the release of dopamine in the synaptic cleft. Because the GABA receptors are occupied, however, transmission is blocked and the vomiting center remains inactive. Hence, neuroleptic drugs are potent antiemetics, as shown in Table 8–1, which illustrates the comparison of CTZ blocking activity of these drugs in dogs and their clinical potency in humans, with that of chlorpromazine.[18]

HALOPERIDOL (HALDOL)

Pharmacokinetics. In humans, haloperidol delivered intravenously acts within 5 to 10 minutes; its effects may last 24 to 48 hours. Tritium-labeled haloperidol is excreted mostly in the urine and feces within 24 hours of administration (urinary excretion is maximal in the first 4 hours), but radioactivity is detectable for as many as 96 hours after administration.[25,26]

Pharmacology. Haloperidol is a potent, long-acting neuroleptic drug. Its effects are characteristic for the butyrophenones, including cataleptic immobility with inhibition of spontaneous motor activity and suppression of amphetamine-induced stereotyped movements in animals.

The drug is an effective antiemetic.[27] Its cardiovascular effects are negligible, except for a moderate alpha-adrenergic blocking action that may cause orthostatic hypotension. Respiratory function is unimpaired, but renal vasodilatation is attenuated.[28] Side-effects include agitation, dyskinesia, and extrapyramidal reactions.

Clinical Applications. Haloperidol has largely been replaced in NLA by droperidol (except in some Scandinavian countries), because extrapyramidal muscle activity and postoperative psychic disturbances are less frequent with the latter agent. At present, haloperidol is used principally to treat various psychotic states.[29,30] It is an effective antagonist of hallucinatory and delirious reactions caused by LSD, mescaline, and alcohol.[31] Used with meperidine in obstetrics, haloperidol provides maternal tranquility without interfering with the normal course of labor or causing fetal depression.[32]

Table 8–1. Antiemetic Action of NLA Drugs

	CTZ Blocking Activity	Comparative Clinical Dosage
Phenothiazines		
Chlorpromazine	1	1
Prochlorperazine	2	2–10
Perphenazine	50	10
Butyrophenones		
Haloperidol	50	90
Droperidol	700	200
Spiroperidol	4000	700
Rauwolfia		
Reserpine	weak	90

(From Janssen, P.A.J.: Pharmacological aspects. *In* Neuropsychopharmacology. Edited by D. Bente and P. Bradley. Amsterdam, Elsevier, 1965.)

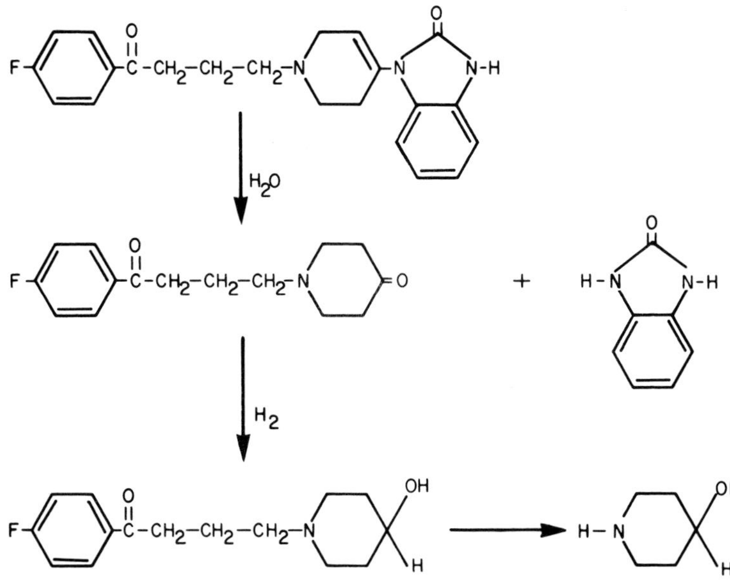

Fig. 8–4. Metabolism of droperidol. (From Janssen, P.A.J.: Zur Frage des Abbaus und der Ausscheidung der beider Neuroleptanalgesie zur Anwendung Kommenden Pharmaka. *In* Die Neuroleptanalgesie. Edited by W.F. Henschel. Berlin, Springer, 1966.)

DROPERIDOL (DEHYDROBENZPERIDOL, INAPSINE, AND DROLEPTAN)

Pharmacokinetics. Droperidol is rapidly distributed throughout the body. Its action begins within 3 to 10 minutes of delivery and lasts 2 to 4 hours; alteration of consciousness may persist for as many as 12 hours. The metabolism of droperidol is illustrated in Figure 8–4.[33] The benzimidazolone group in the 4 (para) position of the parent droperidol (I) is hydrolyzed, leaving the parafluorobutyrophenone-4-piperidone derivative (II), which is then reduced to tertiary alcohol (III); this alcohol in turn is dealkylated to a simple 4-piperidinol, leaving a fluorinated benzyl residue. Because these reactions occur fairly rapidly, the maximum period of activity of droperidol is limited to 2 to 4 hours. After an initial steep alpha (distribution) slope, plasma decay curves of droperidol in humans show a moderately rapid decline during the beta (metabolism/excretion) phase, reaching fairly low levels 4 hours after administration (Fig. 8–5).[34] The drug is extensively (85 to 90%) bound to plasma proteins. There is a remarkable discrepancy between the concentration of radiolabeled droperidol in the brain and in the blood; after 4 hours, 20% of the total radioactive dose persists in the brain, whereas the blood level has decreased to 4% after 4 hours. Droperidol and its metabolites are excreted in urine and feces.[25] About 10% of the drug appears unchanged in the urine.[35]

Pharmacology

Central Nervous System. Droperidol mimics the actions of the phenothiazines but is considerably more potent and more specific.[10,36,37] In humans, droperidol produces the neuroleptic syndrome, characterized by psychomotor slowing, emotional quieting, and affective indifference. The subject appears placid, drowsy, and indifferent to the surroundings; the patient tends to fall asleep but is readily arousable. Somnolence is less marked than with phenothiazines. Although during the semiconscious state (termed mineralization by European investigators) the

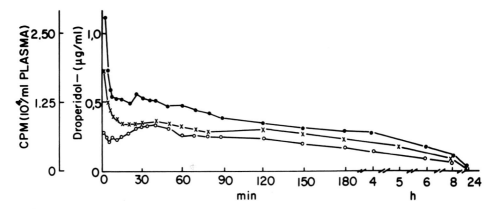

Fig. 8–5.   Droperidol in plasma. _____. = plasma 0.31 mg/kg dose curve; x___x = plasma 0.27 mg/kg dose curve; o___o = serum 0.03 mg/kg dose curve.

face of the patient is expressionless, with eyes closed as if asleep, he or she remains in contact; the patient is still able to respond to questions clearly but slowly, in a monotonous voice, and to obey commands promptly.

Analgesia. Droperidol alone has no analgesic effect; it also does not potentiate the action of narcotic analgesics, although it may prolong their duration of activity.[38,39] An antianalgesic action has been reported, however.[40]

Cardiovascular System. Only in excessive doses does droperidol cause significant depression of myocardial contractility.[41–43] Its usual cardiovascular effects are mainly those of moderate alpha-adrenergic blockade with decreased peripheral and pulmonary vascular resistance and transient mild to moderate hypotension;[10,33,44,45] this latter finding is suggestive of its potential use as an "afterload" reducer.[45] It appears that droperidol-induced alpha-adrenergic blockade is not specific; there is documentation of isolated pulmonary arteries and saphenous veins in which the amplitude of spontaneous contraction is significantly depressed by the drug.[46] It was recently suggested that the effect of droperidol on the vascular system may be the result of a less specific antivasoconstrictor action.[47]

Because of the adrenolytic effect of the drug, postural hypotension frequently occurs.[48] Although the vascular effect is ordinarily not profound, dangerous hypotensive reactions, including death, have been reported in patients already receiving other vasodilator therapy.[49] Conversely, the use of droperidol can be beneficial during vascular surgery to modify undesirable hypertension associated with cross-clamping the abdominal aorta.[50] Droperidol, with or without fentanyl, reportedly causes vasoconstriction of the cerebral vasculature, reducing cerebral blood flow (without altering O_2 consumption) in dogs and man.[51–53] This fact has been disputed, however, such as when hypocapnia occurs.[54] A dopamine-induced increase in renal blood flow is not significantly impaired by the administration of droperidol during normovolemia.[55]

Droperidol does not have positive inotropic effects when included in preparations designed to contract isolated rabbit papillary muscle isometrically, but it does produce a dose-dependent decrease in the level of stress developed by the patient.[56] Droperidol, administered at a dose of 1 mg/kg, to neurally intact dogs in preparation for right-heart bypass, caused a significant increase in left ventricular end-diastolic pressure, indicating that large doses of droperidol may depress left ventricular performance.[57] Except in large doses, droperidol does not exert any significant effects on myocardial contractility, and is therefore not associated with prolonged circulatory depression in humans.[41–43]

Droperidol is also effective in protecting against epinephrine-induced arrhythmias, a result probably related to a quinidine-like reduction in pacemaker activity and lengthening of the refractory period.[42,58–62] The drug also exerts significant antiarrhythmic effects during anesthesia with halothane or cyclopropane (and presumably other general anesthetics).[58,63–65] Fewer ventricular cardiac arrhythmias occurred during anesthesia with droperidol-phenoperidine than with halothane during dental extractions.[66]

Respiratory System. Droperidol does not significantly alter respiratory function.[67] Indeed, it may even lessen fentanyl-induced respiratory depression.[68]

Hepatic System. Droperidol does not affect liver function.[69]

Endocrine System. Droperidol has little influence on adrenocortical function, but does increase growth hormone and blood glucose levels.[70,71]

Metabolism. Droperidol reduces total body oxygen consumption by 20 to 30%.[72] Blood viscosity and hematocrit determinations also show a decrease.[73]

Complications. Droperidol-induced peripheral vasodilatation may cause increased intraoperative bleeding, although this result seems a small price to pay for protection against the deleterious effects of massive vasoconstriction.[74]

Occasionally, patients feel jittery and ill-at-ease ("inner anxiety"), especially after receiving large doses of droperidol; moderate to marked restlessness and apprehension may also occur with small (2.5 mg) doses.[75] These effects may occur more frequently in patients under stress, and in those who are apprehensive and anxious.

Extrapyramidal side-effects may manifest as varying degrees of dyskinesia, especially of the face, neck and pharyngeal muscles, with speech and swallowing difficulties, grimacing, trismus, oculogyric spasms, or torticollis.[76–78] The frequency and severity of these effects are less than occurs with the phenothiazines, and they usually are dose related, although dyskinesia may result from ordinary, small doses.[79,80] Such extrapyramidal activity responds promptly to the intravenous use of diphenhydramine, benztropine (Cogentin), or other antiparkinsonian agents.[78]

Hallucinations and bizarre sensations of weightlessness and loss of body image may occur, usually after large doses of droperidol.[81] The incidence of undesirable reactions to droperidol can be significantly reduced by the concurrent administration of diazepam.[82]

Clinical Applications

Preanesthetic Medication. Droperidol is a useful preanesthetic medication because of its sedative, tranquilizing, and antiemetic effects.[83] With an average dose of 5 mg delivered intramuscularly 1 to 2 hours preoperatively, the patient soon becomes sedated, tranquil, detached, indifferent, calm, quiet, and remains cooperative and responsive to instruction. For patients undergoing outpatient surgical procedures, droperidol in combination with atropine may be a superior preanesthetic medication than those preparations that include the use of other tranquilizers or narcotics, because it significantly reduces the incidence of postoperative nausea and vomiting, thereby permitting earlier discharge.[84] Whether use of this drug combination reduces the need for postoperative analgesics is debatable.

A droperidol syrup administered orally in doses of 0.3 to 0.6 mg/kg, combined with atropine, is useful for application in children 2 to 9 years of age before otolaryngologic, orthopedic, and general surgical procedures.[85] The drug is palatable, well absorbed, and produces good sedative and antisalivary actions, with a low incidence of postoperative vomiting. The additional use of diazepam in syrup form offers no advantage over droperidol alone.

Droperidol is a potent antipsychotic agent. Administered with atropine as preanesthetic medication for ketamine anesthesia, droperidol eliminates emergence delirium reactions, markedly improving both patient and physician acceptance of ketamine anesthesia.[86]

Nausea and Vomiting. The antiemetic effects of droperidol are well established.[87–89] Although the drug is especially effective against narcotic-induced and post-anesthetic emesis, its efficacy in preventing or controlling motion sickness is questionable.[90]

Obstetrics. Droperidol is a useful adjunct to general anesthesia for obstetric procedures.[91,92] Doses of 5 to 10 mg delivered intramuscularly or intravenously usually provide maternal tranquility and detachment; the amount of general anesthetic required for cesarean section may also be markedly reduced.

"Awake" Intubation of the Trachea. This procedure can be facilitated by the use of droperidol (2.5 to 5 mg intravenously) in conjunction with diazepam.[93]

Shock. Droperidol (7.5 to 20 mg intravenously) may contribute importantly to the therapy of incipient shock.[94] In patients suffering from myocardial infarction, acute cardiorespiratory insufficiency, or a combination of the two conditions, droperidol delivered intravenously (7.5 to 20 mg) may help to reverse incipient shock by inhibiting the sympathetic aspects of prioprioceptive reflex processes. In addition, its alpha-adrenergic blocking effect may serve as a valuable guide to blood volume status in shock or shocklike states.[74] If blood or fluid replacement therapy is adequate, alpha-adrenergic blockade should improve tissue perfusion without significantly altering arterial blood pressure. Conversely, a drop in blood pressure level after injection of droperidol indicates inadequacy of circulating blood volume, requiring further transfusion, fluid therapy, or both. Placing the patient in a position with the head down to facilitate venous return may also be beneficial.

Psychiatric Emergencies. The antipsychotic action of droperidol is useful in psychiatric emergencies.[95] Acutely agitated patients can be controlled quickly by administering 10 mg of droperidol intravenously without the use of other antipsychotic drugs.

Analgesic Drugs

GENERAL PHARMACOLOGIC CHARACTERISTICS

Narcotic analgesic components of NLA must meet certain requirements, including rapid onset and short duration of action, with minimal depression of circulatory and cerebral cortical function. The last criterion is especially important for patients who must be alert and cooperative throughout the operation. Profound respiratory depression is an unavoidable concomitant of narcotic analgesics once modest dosage is exceeded, despite the continuing intensive search for an exception to this dictum. Therefore, ventilatory support is usually required.

For the past 20 years, four analgesics have been used in NLA: fentanyl, phenoperidine, dextromoramide, and pentazocine. In appropriate dosage, all four drugs induce a level of analgesia that is adequate for minor surgical procedures. Except for pentazocine, which has both opiate and antagonist properties, larger doses can provide complete surgical analgesia with minimal alteration of cortical function, so the patient remains awake and cooperative.

Two new synthetic derivatives of fentanyl, sufentanyl and alfentanyl, appear to offer some advantages over currently available drugs. Sufentanyl, approximately 10 times as potent as fentanyl, lacks significant cardiovascular effects. Alfentanyl is less potent than fentanyl and is shorter-acting. For further discussion of fentanyl and its congeners, see Chapter 3.

PHENOPERIDINE

Chemistry. Phenoperidine (DL-ethyl 1-(3-hydroxy-3-phenylpropyl)-4-phenyl-4-piperidinecarboxylate) is a synthetic narcotic that is chemically related to meperidine (Fig. 8–6).

Metabolism and Excretion. Fifty percent of a given dose of phenoperidine is excreted unchanged in the urine. The remainder of the drug undergoes metabolic breakdown, first to meperidine and then to meperidinic acid, of which 75% is recovered in the urine.[81]

Pharmacology

Central Nervous System (CNS). Phenoperidine produces intense analgesia without significant sedation. In analgesic potency, the drug is intermediate between morphine and fentanyl: phenoperidine (2 mg intramuscularly) is equianalgesic with morphine (10 mg intramuscularly) in humans.[79] After intravenous administration, analgesia ensues within 2 to 3 minutes and lasts 60 to 90 minutes.

Phenoperidine stimulates the CTZ and also increases muscle tone. Other excitatory effects are species specific: low doses cause morphine-like excitement in mice and cats, but sedation and lead-pipe muscular rigidity are noted in rats.[9]

Cardiovascular System. Cardiovascular function is minimally affected. Bradycardia that may occur is attributed to central vagal stimulation.[96]

Respiratory System. Phenoperidine is a potent respiratory depressant, causing apnea in doses greater than 0.05 mg/kg. A peculiar dissociative action on the CNS may result in respiratory arrest before analgesia is complete. The drug obtunds pharyngeal and laryngeal reflexes, enabling tracheal intubation without the use of muscle relaxant and without coughing or "bucking" in response to the tracheal stimulus. Prolonged postoperative intubation, if required, is well tolerated by the conscious patient.

Clinical Applications. Phenoperidine in combination with haloperidol or droperidol provides effective NLA.[4,97–99]

DEXTROMORAMIDE (PALFIUM)

Chemistry. Dextromoramide ((S)-(+)-1-[3-methyl-4-(4-morpholinyl-1-oxo-2,2-diphenylbutyl] pyrrolidine) is a methadone derivative (Fig. 8–6) synthesized by Janssen, et al., in 1957.[9]

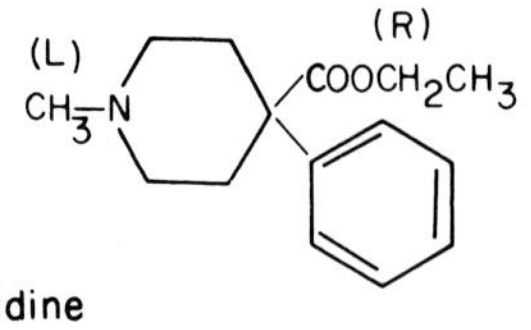

A. Meperidine

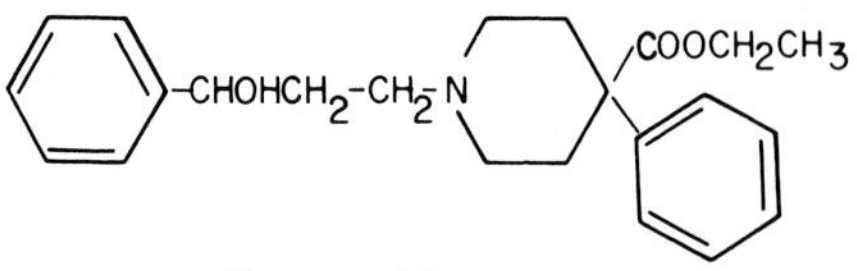

B. Phenoperidine

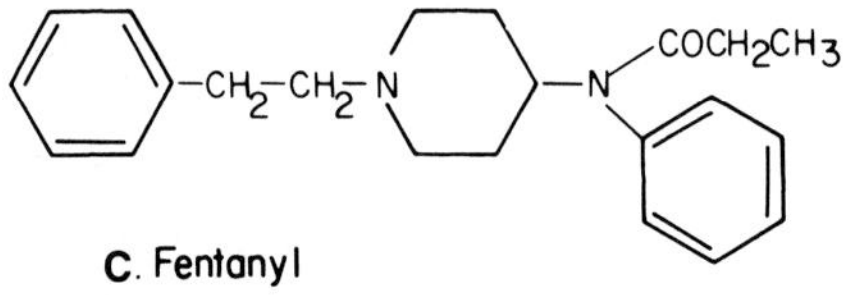

C. Fentanyl

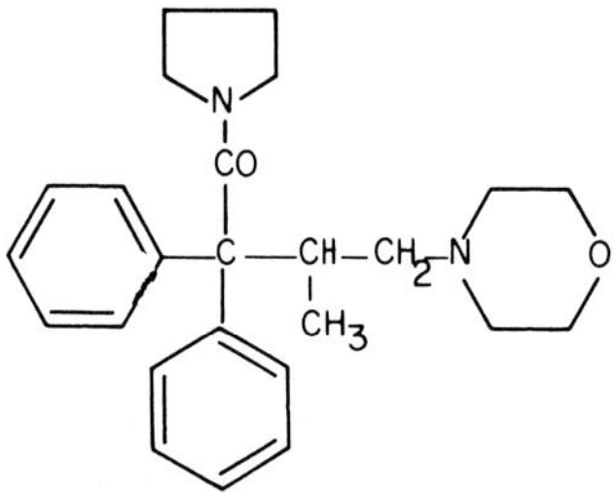

D. Dextromoramide

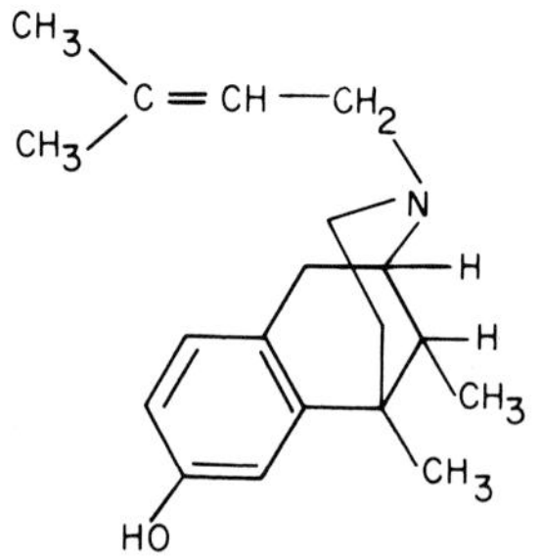

E. Pentazocine

Fig. 8–6. Structural formulae of meperidine and its derivatives.

Pharmacology

Central Nervous System. Dextromoramide, used as an analgesic, is somewhat more potent than morphine given intravenously—5 mg are equivalent to about 10 mg of morphine.[100] The onset of its analgesic effect is more rapid, but the duration of its effect is somewhat shorter than that of morphine or meperidine.[101,102] Dextromoramide differs from other commonly used narcotic analgesics in two respects: it is nearly as effective orally as parenterally, and it causes less sedation.[100] The addictive liability of the drug is similar to that of other narcotics.[103]

Clinical Applications. Dextromoramide can be used alone or with other neuroleptic agents for surgical patients in whom periods of wakefulness are required during the course of anesthesia, as in the surgical treatment of epileptic disorders. The drug can also be used in the control of obstetric after-pain.[100] Side-effects, such as dizziness, nausea, and vomiting, do occur with single doses of dextromoramide in excess of 5 mg.[101]

PENTAZOCINE (TALWIN AND FORTRAL)

Chemistry. Pentazocine (2-dimethylallyl-5,9-dimethyl-2-hydroxybenzomorphan) (Fig. 8–6) is an opiate agonist-antagonist.

Pharmacology

Central Nervous System. Pentazocine has analgesic and very weak opiate antagonist effects. Although its precise mechanism of action is not known, pentazocine is believed to be a competitive antagonist at mu opiate receptors and an agonist at kappa and sigma opiate receptors.[31] Pentazocine does not antagonize morphine-induced respiratory depression, but it may precipitate opiate withdrawal symptoms in patients who regularly receive opiates.[31]

When used as an analgesic, pentazocine is approximately one half as potent as morphine given intravenously—20 mg are equivalent to 10 mg of morphine.[104,105] With the intramuscular delivery of pentazocine, analgesia is established within 20 minutes and lasts 2 to 3 hours.

Cardiovascular and Respiratory System. In the absence of significant heart disease, pentazocine given in recommended dosage does not significantly affect cardiovascular function. The period of respiratory depression noted with pentazocine use is shorter than that associated with equipotent doses of morphine.

Complication and Side-Effects. It was anticipated that, as an opiate antagonist, pentazocine would be free of addictive liability and significant psychotomimetic action. After its release for clinical use, however, numerous instances of emotional and physical dependence were reported, usually in patients with a history of drug abuse.[65] In addition, abrupt discontinuance of pentazocine after extended use may result in withdrawal symptoms, such as abdominal cramps, rhinorrhea, anxiety, and fever.

Clinical Applications. A 20- to 30-mg dose of pentazocine, intramuscularly, may be used for pain relief in obstetrics.[106] When used with droperidol, it provides effective NLA for neurodiagnostic procedures, with maintenance of excellent cardiovascular stability.[107] Pentazocine used in conjunction with diazepam ("pentazepam") produces an NLA-like state termed somnoanalgesia; in this state, the patient appears to be asleep but is cooperative and is able to respond to spoken commands (see Chapter 9).[5]

Alphaprodine (Nisentil)

When alphaprodine was used to produce NLA, cardiovascular stability was less secure than when either fentanyl or meperidine was used in combination with droperidol and nitrous oxide.[108]

Innovar (Thalamonal, Leptanal, Leptophen)

Innovar is a fixed-ratio combination of droperidol (2.5 mg/ml) and fentanyl (50 μg/ml). Its pharmacologic profile is essentially that of its separate components, with some minor differences.[109,110]

Central Nervous System (CNS)

Site of Action. Innovar acts at subcortical sites in the brain. Thalamic and hypothalamic injections of Innovar in cats cause deep sedation and tranquilization; during Innovar-induced surgical analgesia, neither EEG nor single-cell unit activity in the feline auditory cortex is depressed.[111,112]

EEG and Behavioral Changes. Neither droperidol nor fentanyl significantly affects the human EEG findings (Fig. 8–7). With the exception of a transient increase in amplitude and a decrease in frequency after the intravenous delivery of fentanyl (0.3 mg) as well as an apparent activation of alpha rhythm during early recovery from the drug effect, the EEG findings remained unchanged.[113]

In human volunteers, 10 ml of Innovar (i.e., 25 mg droperidol, 0.5 mg fentanyl) given intravenously produced no significant EEG changes during injection or the subsequent 20 minutes. The subjects remained reactive and rousable but analgesic and indifferent.[113] Deep breathing was frequently encouraged to avoid

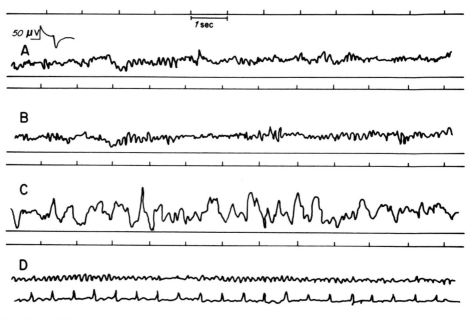

Fig. 8–7. EEG effects of NLA. Recordings from left fronto-occipital region in an 87-year-old man. *A,* control: *B,* 5 minutes after 20 mg droperidol given intravenously. *C,* 27 seconds after 0.3 mg fentanyl given intravenously. Note increase in amplitude and decrease in frequency. *D,* 15 minutes later. Alpha rhythm has returned and appears to be activated and stabilized. (From Doenicke, A., Kugler, J., Schellenberger, A., and Guertner, T.: The use of electroencephalography to measure recovery time after intravenous anesthesia. Br. J. Anaesth., 38:580, 1966.)

sleep and hypoxia during these first 20 minutes. Unstimulated, they then slept several hours, still readily rousable, with accompanying EEG sleep patterns. Usually for about 10 hours subjects experienced alternating periods of sleep and waking.[113]

Effect on Oxygen Consumption. NLA reduces whole body O_2 consumption by 40 to 45%.[72]

Effect on CBF and ICP. Innovar decreases CBF in dogs without altering cerebral O_2 consumption, suggesting that the effect is due to cerebral vasoconstriction.[52,53] The degree of change in CBF is insignificant in normal man, provided hypercapnia is avoided.[114] Normal or elevated ICP, however, can be moderately reduced with the use of even small (2 ml) doses of Innovar in patients with normal or raised ICP maintained in a state of hypocapnia with controlled ventilation.[51,54,115]

Cardiovascular System. Innovar in usual doses produces minimal depression of myocardial function in animals and in humans, including geriatric patients.[110,116–122] Heart rate tends to slow as a result of fentanyl-induced vagal stimulation.[123] Myocardial oxygen consumption is reduced in dose-related fashion, with a corresponding decrease in coronary artery flow.[124] Total peripheral resistance decreases, as a result of alpha-adrenergic blockade by droperidol, and the capacitance vessels dilate (Fig. 8–8); pre-load and arterial blood pressure levels are reduced.[118,120,125,126] Central venous pressure may rise in the presence of increased thoraco-abdominal muscle tone as well as rigidity.[110,118]

In hemorrhagic shock, homeostatic reflex mechanisms remain relatively unimpaired by Innovar.[127] Renal blood flow is increased through the cortex but is not appreciably altered in the medulla.[128] Innovar also exerts an antiarrhythmic action, again attributable to droperidol.[129]

Respiratory System. The depressant effects of Innovar on respiratory rate and tidal volume are essentially those related to fentanyl.[37,118,130–132] Droperidol does not enhance, and indeed may even partially attenuate, this depression.[68,133] Innovar may cause a significant decrease in functional residual capacity, even in the absence of chest wall rigidity.[134]

Innovar-induced respiratory depression must be countered by assisted or controlled ventilation.[118] The depression may be enhanced by concomitant use of pentobarbital or diazepam.[135,136] On the other hand, arterial Po_2 values tend to be higher during recovery from NLAN than from anesthesia with halothane and nitrous oxide, probably because NLAN patients, being almost immediately alert, responsive, and pain-free, are able to breathe deeply and cough on command.[137]

Musculoskeletal System. The rigidity of abdominal and chest wall muscles occasionally noted with Innovar use is caused by the fentanyl component of the drug. It may be precipitated by nitrous oxide and can be prevented or treated with muscle relaxant drugs.[138–140]

Hepatic System. Liver function is not significantly altered by Innovar or its components.[69,140–143] The tone of the sphincter of Oddi in guinea pigs seems unaffected by Innovar, but fentanyl administered alone may be spasmogenic.[144]

Genitourinary System. Renal function is not significantly altered by Innovar.[145] Glomerular filtration rate is increased and active tubular transport of sodium is enhanced.[146] Full doses of fentanyl may increase urine osmolarity and reduce urinary output because of release of antidiuretic hormone (ADH).[147] Rapid infusion of lactated Ringer's solution produces a greater diuretic response during NLA than during light levels of conventional anesthesia.[147]

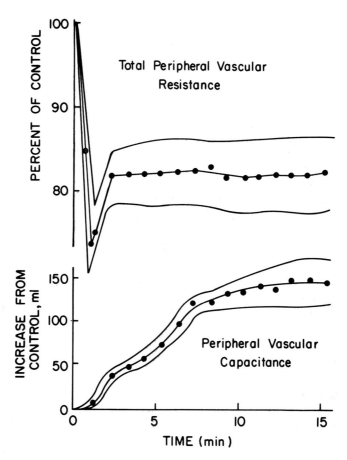

Fig. 8–8. Changes in peripheral vascular resistance and capacitance in dogs after droperidol (0.5 mg/kg) and fentanyl (0.01 mg/kg) given intravenously. *Solid lines,* mean values; *shaded area,* standard errors of the mean. Capacitance changes lagged behind resistance changes. (Dixon, S.H., Nolan, S.P., Stewart, S., and Morrow, A.G.: Neuroleptanalgesia: effects of Innovar on myocardial contractility, total peripheral vascular resistance and capacitance. Anesth. Analg., *49*:331, 1970.)

Miscellaneous Effects. Blood glucose levels do not rise significantly during NLA before the surgical incision is made.[148] Thereafter, the rise varies with the degree of surgical stress, being greatest during intra-abdominal surgery.[148] Innovar is nonirritating to veins and muscle tissue; hence, the drug may be injected intravenously or intramuscularly with impunity.

Innovar depresses vestibular function.[149] It suppresses the nystagmus produced by caloric stimulation of the external auditory canal (Fig. 8–9), but not that related to galvanic stimulation of the same area; this disparity suggests that the site of this depression lies within the labyrinthine part of the vestibular system.[150] The effect occurs within 10 minutes of the intravenous injection of 2 ml of Innovar IV and lasts for more than 3 hours.[150] Whether the fentanyl or the droperidol component of Innovar is responsible has not been established.[151,152]

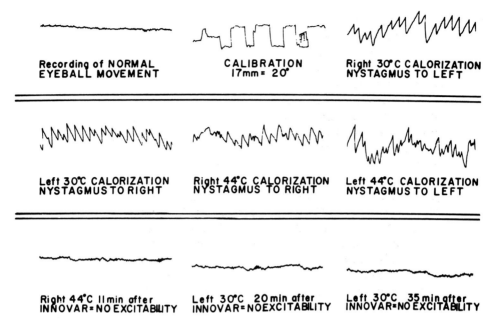

Fig. 8–9. Effect of Innovar on vestibular function. Electronystagmographic record after 2 ml of Innovar given intravenously. (From Dowdy, E.G., and Moore, W.T.: Droperidol and fentanyl combination: effect on the human labyrinth. Anesthesiology, *30*:604, 1969.)

Complications and Side-Effects

RESPIRATORY DEPRESSION

Induction of NLA or NLAN is invariably accompanied by respiratory depression that is caused by fentanyl, whether the drug is administered separately or in combination as Innovar. Before the onset of full anesthesia or muscle paralysis, the patient can breathe deeply on command. If they are unable to do so, assistance to or control of respiratory exchange to avoid hypoxia must be instituted promptly and maintained throughout the operation and into the recovery period until spontaneous ventilation is deemed adequate.[140]

MUSCULAR RIGIDITY

Rigidity of trunk muscles, attributable to large doses or rapid administration of fentanyl during induction, may markedly impede respiratory exchange, even with high positive-pressure ventilation (face mask and breathing bag). Frightening subjective stiffness of the chest wall, lasting several minutes, has been observed after the administration of Innovar (2 ml intramuscularly) for anesthetic premedication. In both instances, the patients, quietly reassured, were able to breathe deeply upon request until the sensations subsided spontaneously.[153]

During induction of NLAN, rigidity may be precipitated by nitrous oxide.[138,139] Succinylcholine promptly corrects the situation, which may be prevented by prior administration of any desired muscle relaxant. (Obviously, should awareness remain, respiratory assistance with bag and mask will counter unpleasant sensations of suffocation accompanying neuromuscular blockade.)

EXTRAPYRAMIDAL EFFECTS

The onset of these effects may be immediate during recovery from NLA or NLAN or may be delayed by 24 to 48 hours. They are attributable to the butyrophenone component of Innovar and occurred more frequently during its initial use when doses were two to three times higher than those currently administered.[14] A realistic estimate of the incidence of these effects is 0.2%.[154] The most common extrapyramidal symptoms noted after administration of droperidol or Innovar are dystonic contractions of facial, neck, and pharyngeal muscles, with perioral and periorbital spasms, grimacing, torticollis, trismus, and speech and swallowing difficulties. More rarely, parkinsonian symptoms may be observed, e.g., cog-wheel rigidity, mask-like faces, and resting tremors of the extremities; pre-existing parkinsonism may be temporarily worsened. These manifestations, usually transient (although persistence for days has been reported), have been ascribed to antagonism of dopaminergic effects in the basal ganglia, probably by droperidol blockade of post-synaptic receptors.[78,155,156] Mild akathisia (motor restlessness) has also been reported after the use of Innovar.[156] These variations in extrapyramidal activity are usually self-limited, but may infrequently require therapy with antiparkinson drugs, e.g., benztropine (Cogentin), diphenhydramine (Benadryl), and atropine.

HYPERTENSION

Sustained severe hypertension may occur during NLAN.[157] This change in pressure may be due to the release of catecholamines caused by insufficient analgesia; to inadequate correction of the hypoxia or hypercarbia of fentanyl-induced respiratory depression; or to the direct action of fentanyl in stimulating or facilitating the release of catecholamines, predominantly epinephrine.[158,159] Avoidance of potentially disastrous consequences, e.g., in the presence of cerebrovascular anomalies, may require the administration of hypotensive agents, such as sodium nitroprusside or trimethaphan (Arfonad).[157]

HYPOTENSION

Hypotension that occurs during induction of NLA or NLAN, suggestive of hypovolemia, usually responds to parenteral fluid therapy, but may also require the use of vasopressors. Orthostatic hypotension may follow inappropriate positioning or moving of the patient receiving Innovar.

BRADYCARDIA

Fentanyl-induced bradycardia rarely occurs after premedication with antisialogogues, e.g., atropine or glycopyrrolate. Should bradycardia result, it is readily reversible with vagolytic doses of atropine.

AWARENESS DURING NLAN

This potential concomitant of light anesthesia, especially in the drug-paralyzed patient who is unable to communicate, may also occur with Innovar administration, but the incidence of awareness is less with Innovar.[160]

OTHER COMPLICATIONS

Neurologic, psychic, and autonomic disturbances during the first few hours of recovery from NLAN include claustrophobia, nausea and vomiting associated with postural changes, diaphoresis, and elevation of body temperature.[161] Dizziness, blurred vision, and hallucinatory episodes, sometimes associated with periods of mental depression, may also occur. Chills and shivering during recovery from NLAN, as with other anesthetic regimens, reflects a disturbance of thermoregulation; with Innovar use, the droperidol component is probably responsible. Reduced ability to concentrate may be apparent the next day, gradually subsiding thereafter. Such postoperative disturbances may be more evident if they are not masked by the effect of sedatives and other drugs.[113]

COMPLICATIONS ASSOCIATED WITH INNOVAR FOR PREANESTHETIC MEDICATION

Use of Innovar in this setting may result in unpleasant subjective symptoms, including restlessness, apprehension, and dyskinesia. Some patients may even refuse to undergo the procedure, despite previous consent;[162,163] this refusal is especially common in patients planning to undergo sterilization, possibly because of the greater emotional impact of this procedure.[163]

Clinical Use

During NLA, the patient is sedated but awake throughout the operation, with no need for other depressant or anesthetic agents. Autonomic overreaction to surgical trauma, especially excessive vasoconstriction, is reduced, promoting good tissue perfusion. NLA is suitable for operations, the success of which is facilitated by cooperation of a conscious patient, e.g., certain otologic or neurosurgical procedures. If, as is more usual, consciousness is not essential for the procedure, the use of NLAN, a unique variety of balanced anesthesia produced by the addition of nitrous oxide to NLA, may be preferable. Although NLAN is suitable for minor and brief operations, its use is more appropriate for major, traumatic, and lengthy procedures, including open-heart, thoracic, abdominal, orthopedic, genitourinary, and neurologic surgical procedures, especially in elderly and high-risk patients.[154,164–167]

The potent analgesic and tranquilizing effects of the drugs used for NLAN enable avoidance of deep anesthesia. The technique offers important advantages, including smooth induction, cardiovascular stability during anesthesia, minimal adverse effects on other organ systems, and smooth rapid recovery, with minimal nausea and vomiting.[140,154,167–174] Peristalsis and renal function rapidly return to normal function because of minimal intraoperative inhibition.

Administration of NLA Agents

Droperidol and fentanyl can be used separately or in combination (Innovar) intramuscularly, in intermittent intravenous increments, or by continuous intravenous infusion, e.g., 250 ml balanced salt solution containing 10 ml Innovar or 20 ml (1 mg) fentanyl, with or without droperidol (12.5 to 25 mg). Note that the analgesic effects of a single intravenous dose of fentanyl lasts 30 to 60 minutes, whereas the tranquilizing effects of droperidol last at least 2 to 4 hours, with some alteration of consciousness for as many as 12 hours.

Preanesthetic Medication

It is useful to administer droperidol (2.5 to 5.0 mg intramuscularly or slowly by intravenous route) 45 to 60 minutes before surgery either alone or with 0.05 to 0.1 mg of fentanyl (both separately or combined as 2.0 ml of Innovar together with an antisialogogue). This early introduction enables an initial appraisal of patient response to the NLA drugs before their use in the operating room. Within 10 to 15 minutes, the patient is usually tranquil, sedated, apathetic, and indifferent, with minimal impairment of cardiorespiratory functions. A later bonus is a markedly reduced incidence of postoperative nausea and vomiting.[175]

Supplementation with other CNS depressants, e.g., barbiturates, narcotics, or tranquilizers, is rarely necessary. If such drugs are added, one must recall that their action may be potentiated by the NLA drugs, and thus all drug doses should be adjusted accordingly. Infants and children seem particularly susceptible to the sedative actions of droperidol; hence, preanesthetic medication of pediatric patients with Innovar is still controversial.[176]

Induction

While vital signs are monitored closely, Innovar (2 to 4 ml) is administered intravenously at a slow rate (if delivery is by infusion, the rate may be fairly rapid, e.g., 100 drops/minute) for about 5 minutes or until the respiratory rate begins to slow. If droperidol and fentanyl are used separately, 5 to 10 mg of droperidol are intravenously administered first, with subsequent slow intravenous delivery of fentanyl (0.1 to 0.2 mg). When the rate of respiration has slowed to 10 to 12 breaths/minute and a decline in systolic blood pressure (10 to 25 mm Hg) is noted, the operation may begin.

Maintenance

Throughout the surgical procedure, arterial pressure, pulse, and respiratory rate determinations should be monitored frequently and verbal contact with the patient should be maintained. If lightening of NLA occurs, signaled by increases in blood pressure, heart and respiratory rate, or both, with or without slight movements of the extremities, intravenous injections of Innovar (0.5 to 1.0 ml) or fentanyl (0.05 to 0.1 mg) are given. Alternatively, the intravenous infusion of these drugs used for induction is resumed until the vital signs return to their initial NLA values. Drug infusions are stopped when the respiratory rate decreases to 10 breaths/minute. Although the depressed patient will usually breathe deeply on command, occasionally verbal contact is lost and apnea ensues. Obviously, artificial respiration must then be promptly instituted with a face mask or an endotracheal tube. Fortunately, narcotic antagonists are rarely needed; hence, analgesia is unimpaired. Nevertheless, equipment and drugs for resuscitation should be readily available.

Recovery

The patient recovering from NLA is usually calm and cooperative, but indifferent, and occasionally in need of support because of respiratory depression. Surveillance is essential to guard against this possible depression. Although still controversial, use of doxapram as a "chemical ventilator" may be considered. Continuing analgesia commonly obviates the postoperative use of analgesics. Should narcotics be administered, one fourth to one third of the usual dose is ample.

NLA with Haloperidol and Phenoperidine

This drug combination is still used in some Scandinavian countries.[9] After an initial intravenous dose of 2 mg of phenoperidine, a mixture of 20 mg phenoperidine, 2 mg haloperidol, and 2.3 mg Hydergine in 500 ml of 5% glucose in water is administered by intravenous infusion (Hydergine, a vasodilator, is added to prevent peripheral cyanosis). Initially, the drip rate is at maximum while verbal contact with the patient is maintained. Respiratory depression that usually precedes the establishment of full analgesia is countered by instructing the patient to breathe deeply (this is feasible because of unimpaired cortical function). Tracheal intubation is accomplished with the aid of succinylcholine delivered intravenously. Further muscular relaxation, if needed, is provided by intermittent intravenous doses of d-tubocurare. The NLA infusion is stopped 15 to 20 minutes before the end of the procedure and a narcotic antagonist is administered intravenously if spontaneous respiration is not quickly resumed.

Awakening is usually prompt. Should continued endotracheal intubation be required postoperatively for any reason, the presence of the tube is ordinarily well tolerated. Analgesia commonly persists for 6 to 8 hours postoperatively; then, pain medication may become necessary. Analgesic drug dosage should then be only 50% of that needed after ordinary anesthesia.

Phenoperidine may also be administered by intermittent intravenous injection in increments smaller than 2 mg if spontaneous breathing is to be maintained; the increments may be as large as 5 mg if ventilation is manually or mechanically controlled. The effect of each dose lasts approximately 60 minutes.

NEUROLEPTANESTHESIA (NLAN)

Preanesthetic Medication

Premedication for NLAN is as described for NLA. Because the skilled anesthesiologist is guided by the clinical effects of the drugs used, rather than by formulas based on body weight, the effects of the premedication must be assessed about 30 minutes after its delivery, adjusting drug dosage accordingly.

Induction

Most patients, with no oral intake of liquids or solids after midnight of the preceding day, are relatively dehydrated on arrival in the anesthesia room. Intravenous infusion of 200 to 300 ml of balanced salt solution before induction of NLAN (unless contraindicated by the cardiopulmonary status) helps to minimize drug-induced circulatory depression.

The next step involves the administration of a test dose of Innovar (1 to 2 ml intravenously). If the blood pressure level is relatively unaltered, drug administration may continue. If, however, the test dose is followed by a decline in systolic blood pressure of 25% or greater, hypovolemia has ensued. Further injection of Innovar is then halted until an additional 250 to 500 ml of balanced salt solution can be rapidly infused; the patient should maintain a moderate head-down position to improve venous return. (In the presence of compromised cardiac reserve, such fluid therapy should be instituted cautiously to avoid sudden circulatory overload.) Once circulatory volume and arterial pressure have been restored, induction of NLAN may proceed.

Minimal tranquilization, sedation, and apathy after premedication and the test dose of Innovar or its components validate the safety of the administration of full doses of Innovar (0.1 to 0.15 ml/kg intravenously) to a maximum of 10 ml to induce NLAN; profound NLA effects or hypotension call for sharp reduction in dosage.[177] Elderly, toxic, cachectic, and other high-risk patients may require only 0.05 ml/kg or less, to a total dose of 3 to 5 ml of Innovar, in contrast to a dose of 6 to 8 ml for the average patient. Comparable doses of droperidol (15 to 20 mg) and fentanyl (0.3 to 0.4 mg) may be administered separately if preferred; infusions of solutions of Innovar or its components may be substituted (see the previous section entitled *Administration of NLA Agents* for some suggested dilutions).[178–180]

The doses selected may be administered as single or fractional intravenous bolus injections or by rapid intravenous infusion, while vital signs are closely monitored. With the onset of somnolence and apathy, further injections of NLA drugs are suspended or infusions are slowed. An endotracheal tube is then inserted, after the delivery of a muscle relaxant drug, and the administration of nitrous oxide and oxygen in proportions of 2:1 (or 1:1 for patients at risk) is begun, by either manual or mechanical ventilation.

An alternate proposal for induction of NLAN begins with a barbiturate-muscle relaxant sequence for tracheal intubation, followed by the introduction of nitrous oxide and *then* infusion of a mixture of droperidol and fentanyl in balanced salt solution.[180]

Maintenance

Signs of lightening of NLAN include increases in heart rate, systolic or diastolic blood pressures, lacrimation, sweating, mydriasis, and purposeful body movements (if the surgical procedure does not require complete neuromuscular blockade). Such signs signal the need for the administration of additional increments or infusion of fentanyl. Additional doses of muscle relaxants are administered as required. The suggestion to administer fentanyl (0.05 to 0.1 mg intravenously) at regular 45- to 50-minute intervals to minimize seesaw ("Schaukel") effects in cardiovascular parameters inevitably implies full to excessive drug dosage, and therefore is not recommended.[181]

Because of its prolonged duration of action, droperidol, either alone or as a component of Innovar, should not be administered after the induction period unless an intravenous infusion of Innovar is used. Such an infusion should be terminated when a satisfactory NLAN state has been established, with the use of slightly more than one half of the total dose. Another exception is for procedures that are longer than 7 to 8 hours, in which case the reinforcing doses of Innovar should not exceed one third to one half of the initial dose. Maintenance of NLAN with Innovar rather than fentanyl alone may otherwise result in overtranquilization of the patient, with undue prolongation of post-anesthetic recovery. In high-risk and geriatric patients, a 50:50 mixture of nitrous oxide and oxygen will frequently suffice to maintain the NLAN state.

Further injections of fentanyl should be avoided during the last 30 minutes of an operation to minimize the subsequent need for narcotic antagonists. Similar avoidance of muscle relaxants, if possible, during the last 60 minutes will facilitate reversal with appropriate drugs as needed.

Recovery

Recovery from NLAN is usually smooth and rapid, with the patient becoming responsive within 3 to 5 minutes after discontinuing the administration of nitrous oxide. In the recovery room, patients tend to be drowsy, detached, and free of pain, nausea, and vomiting. Less analgesic medication is required than after other general anesthetics.[182] Adequate spontaneous ventilation returns gradually, and patients may need ventilatory assistance as long as adequate respiratory exchange is not fully restored.

Physostigmine (Antilirium) is an effective antagonist of disorientation or somnolence that may follow the use of large doses of droperidol or Innovar.[183,184] A 2-mg dose of physostigmine given intravenously (1 mg/minute) usually awakens the patient within 2 to 4 minutes, without bradycardia or salivation. When the effects of the drug wear off, in 30 to 45 minutes, the patient may become mildly drowsy, readily rousable, and no longer disoriented.[184] Use of this preparation is particularly helpful in neurosurgical patients, in whom early assessment of neurologic deficits sustained during the procedure is required.[185]

If naloxone is used to counteract fentanyl-induced respiratory depression during emergence from NLAN, fractional doses, e.g., 0.1 mg intravenously, are preferable to a single bolus dose of 0.4 mg, to avoid "overshoot" response of hypertension, tachycardia, and increased cardiac output.[186]

A modification in the technique of the separate use of droperidol and fentanyl to induce and maintain NLAN has been proposed by Foldes, et al.[187] These authors recommend beginning with a bolus of droperidol (0.15 mg/kg intravenously), waiting several minutes for neurolepsis to ensue, then administering fentanyl (0.02 to 0.06 mg intravenously) at 2-minute intervals until the rate of respiration reaches 12 breaths/minute or lower. The administration of nitrous oxide-oxygen is begun after the first or second increment of fentanyl; spontaneous respiration is assisted throughout the period that the patient is anesthetized. Muscle relaxation for short procedures is provided by using succinylcholine; d-tubocurare is recommended for patients requiring endotracheal intubation for prolonged surgery. Analgesia is maintained with the administration of fentanyl (0.01 to 0.04 intravenously).

One advantage of the method proposed by Foldes and colleagues is that of keeping blood levels of fentanyl low by gradually administering the drug until its analgesic effect is optimal. Disadvantages include prolonged induction time and the occasional development of hypercarbia in the spontaneously breathing patient; the potentially serious metabolic sequelae of this state are less likely to occur with controlled respiration.

Pediatric Use of NLAN

NLAN has long been considered unsuitable for use in infants and children under the age of 2 years because of the higher susceptibility to the CNS depressant and extrapyramidal effects of droperidol in this patient group.[188,189] In addition, minute-to-minute control of the depth of anesthesia is less precise than is noted with the use of a barbiturate and a muscle relaxant drug, a combination that promotes speedier induction of and reduces the dosage of droperidol and fentanyl required for subsequent NLAN.[181] The barbiturate-muscle relaxant technique is suitable for very short surgical procedures, i.e., under 45 minutes, with the use of inhalational anesthetics. Finally, NLAN has limited usefulness for brief procedures; the long-acting droperidol may cause unduly sustained listlessness, although cardiorespiratory functions are unimpaired.[188,189]

To avoid denying the benefits of NLAN to this age group, the droperidol dosage should be increased.[180,181] The droperidol to fentanyl ratio of 50:1 as in Innovar may be reduced to 12.5:1 for children older than 1 year of age and to 10:1 for infants younger than 1 year of age.[180] Suggested infusion drip rates are as follows: infants younger than age 1 year receive a mixture of 10 mg droperidol and 1 mg fentanyl in 500 ml balanced salt solution administered at a drop per minute rate of 0.8 × kg/body weight; the same volume of solution for patients older than age 1 year contains 12.5 mg droperidol and 1 mg fentanyl and is administered at a drop per minute rate of 0.5 × kg/body weight. For example, an infant under age 1 year weighing 5 kg would receive 4 drops/minute of the 10:1 mixture and a child weighing 20 kg would receive 10 drops/minute of the 12.5:1 mixture, decreasing (or increasing) the drip rate about 15 minutes after induction according to the response of the patient. Clearly, these suggested starting rates are merely averages to be adjusted according to individual variations in physical state and response. In a rare instance, when even doubling of the drip rate fails to achieve satisfactory NLAN, injection of Innovar (1 to 2 ml intravenously) may remedy the defect; the recommended average drip rate may then be resumed. Note that, during the initial NLAN induction phase, the infusion rate is relatively high to avoid a gap between the rapidly waning hypnotic action of the barbiturate and the gradually increasing NLAN effects.

For longer operations performed on patients in this age group, an illustrative technique, slightly modified from the original, is as follows:[190]

1. Omit premedication.
2. Before induction of anesthesia, infuse lactated Ringer's solution rapidly to compensate for dehydration in the starved child and the alpha-adrenergic blocking action of droperidol.
3. Inject 0.3 mg/kg droperidol, 0.01 mg/kg fentanyl, and 0.06 to 0.2 mg atropine intravenously according to physical state, weight, and age. When the drugs take effect, in approximately 30 seconds, administer oxygen through a face mask. Assist respiration for approximately 2 minutes while the induction drugs achieve their full effect, as judged by maximal pupillary constriction. Give 0.07 mg/kg pancuronium intravenously, wait 2 minutes, and then insert an endotracheal tube.
4. Maintain controlled respiration with a 60:40 mixture of nitrous oxide and oxygen by using appropriate ventilatory settings. For repair of tracheo-esophageal fistula, reduce inspiratory pressures to the minimum effective level until the alimentary connection has been severed. Give additional supplements of fentanyl (0.001 mg/kg intravenously) as indicated by increases in pulse rate, blood pressure, sweating, lacrimation, or mydriasis. Avoid further delivery of fentanyl during the last 30 minutes of the operation. Administer more pancuronium as needed; follow with appropriate drugs for reversal of muscle relaxation at the end of surgery (except in certain infants with tracheo-esophageal fistula, as mentioned in the section entitled, *Pediatric Surgery*).
5. Return of consciousness, ability to suck, and adequate spontaneous respiration are prompt, usually within a few minutes after discontinuing nitrous oxide. Use of opiate antagonists is rarely required.

CLINICAL APPLICATIONS OF NLA AND NLAN

The special attributes of droperidol, fentanyl, and Innovar, including pre-, intra-, and postoperative cardiovascular stability, analgesia, and antiemetic action, as well as calmness and indifference to discomfort while awake, can be exploited in a variety of clinical areas.

Ophthalmologic Surgery

The antiemetic effect of the droperidol fraction of Innovar is particularly valuable in preanesthetic medication and NLA for intraocular operations, especially cataract extraction, after which retching or vomiting could jeopardize the results of the procedure.[171,191–197] During NLA, a retrobulbar block is well tolerated; the patient remains calm, but is able to respond to questions or to maintain awkward positions with ease. Intraocular pressure is not affected or is slightly decreased by NLA, and the relative lack of cardiovascular toxicity is beneficial to the high proportion of elderly, hypertensive patients requiring ophthalmologic procedures.[198,199] Should patient wakefulness or cooperation not be required, NLAN is equally suitable and offers the added benefit of more direct control of ventilation if depressed by fentanyl. Anesthesia can be kept superficial, with the exception of the phase during which the endotracheal tube is placed. The postoperative course is usually smooth, with no need for the administration of adjunctive sedative, analgesic, or antiemetic preparations.

Otorhinolaryngologic Surgery

NLA is useful for many of these procedures, especially with the patient sitting or semirecumbent and participating actively during hearing or other tests. NLA also provides the otologist with good operating conditions for lengthy and delicate operations on the middle ear without significant discomfort to the patient.[200] In stapes operations, untoward bleeding in the graft area can be overcome by infiltrating the area with a local anesthetic containing epinephrine for vasoconstriction. NLA and preanesthetic medication with droperidol or Innovar substantially lessen the otherwise prolonged and intense nausea and vomiting commonly observed during recovery from these procedures.[201–203] NLAN is similarly advantageous for the patient who need not be awake during the procedure. In addition, the ensuing early ambulation reduces the possibility of arterial embolism.[202]

NLAN is useful for tonsillectomy and adenoidectomy in children, because airway reflexes are obtunded and the endotracheal tube is well tolerated, facilitating swift surgical manipulations. Awakening is prompt, with analgesia lasting for at least 3 hours.[204]

Oral Surgery

Innovar, 1 to 2 ml given intravenously immediately before instituting local or regional anesthesia, is usually sufficient to render the patient quiet, detached, and cooperative.[205] More extensive dental extractions and other intraoral operations involving the gingiva and tongue can be performed with NLA similarly complementing local anesthesia.[206] Note that if these procedures are performed in an outpatient setting, the patient must not be discharged before the sedative and tranquilizing effects of Innovar have essentially subsided and the patient is alert. It is especially important to assess the blood pressure level while the patient is in the upright position to ensure that no residual adrenergic blocking effects, which may compromise circulatory homeostasis and cause orthostatic hypotension, are present.

Meniere's Disease and Related Labyrinthine Disorders

Innovar, 1 to 2 ml intravenouly, can terminate an acute attack of Meniere's disease within 10 minutes.[149] Spontaneous nystagmus of central or peripheral origin and positional alcohol-induced nystagmus can similarly be suppressed by Innovar.[207,208]

"Awake" Intubation of the Trachea

NLA facilitates patient cooperation during tracheal intubation while the patient is awake.[209,210] The antiemetic action of the droperidol component minimizes the danger of vomiting and subsequent regurgitation during induction of NLA in the patient with a "full" stomach.[211]

Endoscopy and Bronchoscopy

NLA evokes psychic indifference while retaining responsiveness and cooperation of the patient undergoing endoscopy.[212,213] Continuous infusion and fractional dose NLA techniques are both useful.[179,214] Note that successful endoscopy requires good topical anesthesia, readily performed during NLA.[215,216]

If the NLA drugs are used separately, droperidol is administered prior to surface anesthetization, followed by fractional doses of fentanyl. NLA is especially advantageous in patients undergoing bronchoscopy in that spontaneous respiration keeps airway dynamics intact.[171] In upper alimentary endoscopy, retching and vomiting are avoided and the performance of a detailed examination is then facilitated.[213,217]

Cardiac Catheterization

Cardiac catheterization is often performed in high-risk patients of all ages, in whom maintenance of cardiovascular stability during prolonged immobilization in abnormal positions is vital. NLA, with the use of Innovar or droperidol and fentanyl separately, by the fractional or infusion method, minimizes the discomfort experienced during catheterization without significant alteration in hemodynamics; the exception is that of fentanyl-induced lowering of the pulmonary artery pressure, which should be taken into account for proper interpretation of hemodynamic measurements.[218]

Ketamine may be preferred for use in infants and children undergoing cardiac catheterization (see Chapter 7), but NLA is also effective in this age group.[219] By employing 0.025 ml/kg of Innovar intramuscularly, to a maximum of 1 ml, 30 minutes before the start of the procedure, rapid, safe, and effective sedation is provided without significant respiratory or cardiovascular depression. The patient is readily rousable but is quiet if undisturbed, usually remaining sedated 2 to 4 hours.[219]

"Awake" Pronation

When the patient must be prone for various plastic, orthopedic, neurologic, and other surgical procedures, it may be desirable for the patient to remain awake and breathing spontaneously through an endotracheal tube. He or she may then assist in turning, moving cephalad or caudad, and raising for placement of bolsters to assess subjective comfort of the final position before the beginning of surgery. This awakened state is feasible with the use of NLA.[220] Respiration can be paced by verbal command whenever necessary. If loss of consciousness is desired, NLAN may be induced by the addition of nitrous oxide.

Supplementation to Local and Regional Anesthesia

NLA can facilitate the establishment and maintenance of regional anesthesia blocks, providing a cooperative patient who is comfortable, sedated, indifferent to the surroundings, and able to tolerate unusual positions, and even endotracheal intubation, if required.[221–224]

Neurodiagnostic Procedures

NLA is appropriate for patients scheduled for angiography, pneumoencephalography, ventriculography, and myelography, in whom general anesthesia is less desirable.[225–230] Side-effects of headaches and vomiting are substantially lessened with NLA, and the hypertensive response to the injection of air into the ventricular system is rarely observed in patients who received NLA.[226] Postural hypotension, which may occur when the patient is placed upright, responds promptly to positional change, the use of vasopressors, or both measures. If retrograde amnesia for the procedure is desired, a mixture of nitrous oxide and oxygen may be administered briefly (30 to 60 seconds) at the end of the examination.[153]

Focal Neurosurgical Procedures

Excision of epileptogenic foci in the cerebral cortex to treat seizure disorders refractory to drug therapy is guided by EEG recordings from electrodes placed directly upon the cerebral cortex for precise localization of the offending focal lesion(s) and its (their) extirpation. The combination of local anesthesia and heavy sedation commonly used for these protracted manipulations (as many as 12 hours or more) is unsatisfactory because the patient ultimately becomes restless and begins to move. With NLA, the procedure is expedited and the side-effects are eliminated.[153] In addition, because NLA does not significantly alter the EEG, efforts to locate the epileptogenic focus are not hindered.

NLA is also useful for stereotactic procedures, such as cryothalamotomy. In the treatment of carbamazepine (Tegretol)-resistant tic douloureux by alcohol injection, NLA provides good working conditions for eliciting the paresthesias required for accurate placement of the needle.[231]

Neurosurgery

In contrast to the increases in CBF and ICP observed with halothane and other inhalational anesthetics in patients with space-occupying intracranial lesions, both parameters show small but significant reductions with droperidol and fentanyl use, especially with concomitant hyperventilation. The risk of craniotomy is thereby minimized in these patients.[51,54,232,233] NLAN offers specific advantages for neurosurgical procedures.[234–236] Induction of anesthesia is expeditious, cardiovascular stability is ensured, and the brain gradually decreases in volume in response to moderate hyperventilation and a reduction in $Paco_2$.[237] Some operations, e.g., resection of epileptogenic foci, require occasional intraoperative communication with the patient.[140,174,238,239] Discontinuing the administration of nitrous oxide results in prompt awakening and response to commands, e.g., to move an extremity, open the eyes, show the tongue, and nod or turn the head. The patient is meanwhile free of pain and has no later recollection of the event.

Intracranial manipulations are usually not painful and require only small, infrequent intravenous doses of fentanyl. Nevertheless, adequate respiratory support is essential to counteract the respiratory depressant effects of the drug.[240] Similarly, in the presence of space-occupying lesions, fentanyl and other narcotics should be excluded from the preanesthetic medication to avoid respiratory depression with resultant hypercarbia and elevation of ICP.[241]

Hypotension, associated with inadequate circulating blood volume, should be corrected immediately with appropriate intravenous fluid therapy, positional change, and the administration of vasopressors if necessary, to avoid a potentially hazardous decrease in intracranial perfusion pressure.[54]

When hypothermia is combined with NLAN for intracranial procedures, the time periods required for cooling and rewarming are significantly shorter than those associated with halothane or methoxyflurane anesthesia.[235] In addition, hypertonic solutions used to reduce ICP and brain volume are less frequently required.

Another advantage of NLAN for neurosurgical procedures is the rapid return of consciousness, usually within 3 to 5 minutes after nitrous oxide is discontinued. Early assessment of sensorium and quick detection of any neurologic deficit are then possible.

Cardiac Surgery

Two major problems in cardiac anesthesia are (1) the limited physiologic reserve of most cardiac patients, and (2) the excessive vasoconstriction that results from the release of vasoactive amines, despite high flow rates, during cardiopulmonary bypass (low perfusion shock is one example of such vasoconstriction).[242] NLAN offers these patients the desiderata of myocardial stability, intra- and postoperatively, including a lack of myocardial depression, unimpaired response of the myocardium to the inotropic and chronotropic effects of catecholamines, and moderate alpha-adrenergic blockade, improving tissue perfusion during bypass and during recovery. Additional desirable features of NLAN for use in cardiac surgery patients are prolonged analgesia and tolerance of the endotracheal tube in situ, facilitating ventilatory support and tracheal toilet as required.[188,243–255] These advantages of NLAN were confirmed in a series of 101 patients (47 male and 54 female subjects, ranging in age from 3 weeks to 60 years), the cardiac defects and corrective operative procedures of whom are listed in Table 8–2.[188] When comparing 50 consecutive patients in the series with another group of 50 patients who had open-heart surgery during halothane-nitrous oxide anesthesia, arterial pressures were significantly higher in those individuals who received NLAN (Table 8–3).[188] Characteristically, the diastolic pressures remained unchanged, but the systolic pressures were significantly lower in those patients who received halothane, confirming the benign effect of NLAN on cardiovascular function.

Figure 8–10 shows the polygraph record obtained during replacement of the tricuspid valve and closure of the atrial septal defect in a 36-year-old man with Ebstein's anomaly.[188] Three months before the time of this operation, the patient sustained a cardiac arrest during induction of halothane anesthesia; he was successfully resuscitated. When the surgical procedure was rescheduled, induction of NLAN with 6 ml Innovar (15 mg droperidol, 0.3 mg fentanyl) given intravenously was uneventful; the operation was completed during 2½ hours on bypass. The first arterial blood pressure reading upon restoration of effective heart action, after termination of bypass, was 136/80 mm Hg. Recovery was unremarkable.

Note that NLAN drugs should be administered slowly to avoid the possibility of even transient overdosage, which is an ever present hazard of rapid injection of undiluted potent drugs. The use of dilute solutions of NLAN drugs may be preferred for this reason.[244]

NLAN-induced decreases in perfusion pressure and oxygen demand may result

Table 8–2. Cardiac Surgery During NLAN in 101 Patients

Type of Cardiac Defect	No. of Patients	Type of Surgery
Ventricular septal defect	41	Closure of defect (2 repeat)
Atrial septal defect	13	Closure of defect (1 repeat)
Pulmonic stenosis (valvular and/or infundibular)	9	Repair of stenosis
Acquired mitral valve disease (mitral valve stenosis and/or insufficiency)	19	Mitral valvuloplasty (12 patients) Mitral valve replacement (7 patients)
Congenital or acquired aortic valve disease (aortic valve stenosis and/or insufficiency)	11	Aortic valvuloplasty (6 patients) Aortic valve replacement (5 patients)
Tetralogy of Fallot	4	Total correction
Ostium Primum	2	Closure of defect
Transposition of great vessels	1	Creation of atrial septum defect
Atrioventricularis communis	1	Repair of atrioventricularis communis
Total	101	

(From Corssen, G., Chodoff, P., Domino, E.F., and Kahn, D.R.: Neuroleptanalgesia and anesthesia for open heart surgery. Pharmacologic rationale and clinical experience. J. Thorac. Cardiovasc. Surg., 49:901, 1965.)

Table 8–3. Arterial Blood Pressure Determinations Made During Open-Heart Surgery in 50 Consecutive Patients During NLAN and 50 During Halothane-Nitrous Oxide Anesthesia

		Mean Preperfusion Pressure	Mean Postperfusion Pressure	Significance*
Neurolept	Systolic B.P.	113.3	121.0	$p < 0.05$
	Diastolic B.P.	69.6	73.2	N.S.
Halothane	Systolic B.P.	100.2	93.2	$p < 0.05$
	Diastolic B.P.	61.1	61.2	N.S.
		Neurolept	Halothane	Significance**
Perfusion Pressure		98.5	82.0	$p < 0.001$
Age		18.2	23.25	N.S.

*Paired comparison
**Group comparison
(From Corssen, G., Chodoff, P., Domino, E.F., and Kahn, D.R.: Neuroleptanalgesia and anesthesia for open heart surgery. Pharmacologic rationale and clinical experience. J. Thorac. Cardiovasc. Surg., 49:901, 1965.)

in compensatory increases in heart rate and myocardial O_2 consumption. Another potential drawback of NLAN is the droperidol-induced hypotension that can occur in relatively hypovolemic patients during open-heart surgery.[256] The need for cautious induction of anesthesia with droperidol, fentanyl, and oxygen is obvious.

NLAN is suitable for use in patients requiring pacemaker implantation.[257] In vascular surgery, including aortofemoral bypass, aneurysmectomy, and throm-

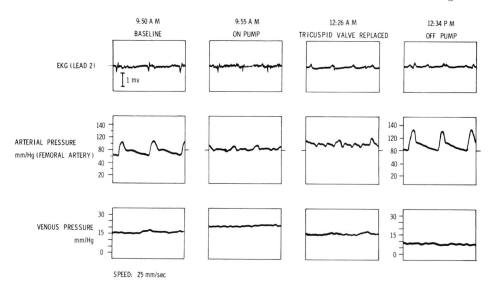

Fig. 8–10. Polygraph record of 36-year-old man during NLAN for correction of Ebstein's anomaly. (From Corssen, G., Chodoff, P., Domino, E.F., and Kahn, D.R.: Neuroleptanalgesia and anesthesia for open heart surgery. Pharmacologic rationale and clinical experience. J. Thorac. Cardiovasc. Surg., 49:901, 1965.)

boendarterectomy, NLAN seems superior to halothane-nitrous oxide for maintaining cardiovascular homeostasis and acid-base equilibrium.[258]

Hemorrhagic Shock

The decreased peripheral vascular resistance that results from droperidol-induced alpha-adrenergic blockade aids the patient in shock by reducing cardiac work and myocardial O_2 consumption. Decreased resistance in combination with rapid intravenous fluid therapy restores effective cardiovascular function, usually without the need of vasopressor agents. This property of droperidol can be lifesaving as illustrated in Figure 8–11.[259]

A 46-year-old woman underwent emergency splenectomy after an automobile accident. Several hours later, she was returned to the operating room with signs of impending shock and abdominal distention, indicative of renewed abdominal bleeding. She was conscious, with dusky, moist, cold skin; peripheral pulses and arterial blood pressure were undetectable, but her carotid pulse was faintly palpable.

Droperidol (15 mg intravenously) was administered, followed in 3 minutes by orotracheal intubation with the patient awake and cooperative. Her forehead became warm and dry and her skin color improved with oxygen administration under positive pressure. Fentanyl (0.15 mg intravenously) was then delivered over a 1-minute period, with subsequent inhalation of a 50% mixture of nitrous oxide and oxygen. Consciousness was lost within 30 seconds and the operation began. A liter of blood was found in the abdominal cavity, and a bleeding artery was promptly identified and ligated. Blood pressure was then determined to be 105/65 mm Hg, and the pulse rate was 100 beats per minute. She awakened pain-free shortly after extubation. Blood loss was estimated at 2200 ml, and was replaced with 2100 ml of whole blood. Her postoperative recovery was uneventful.

In short, NLAN is clearly suitable for the patient in hypovolemic shock who requires immediate surgery.

Catastrophes

NLA and NLAN are suitable for the care of mass casualty victims requiring immediate surgical intervention.[260] Prerequisites for the safe use of droperidol

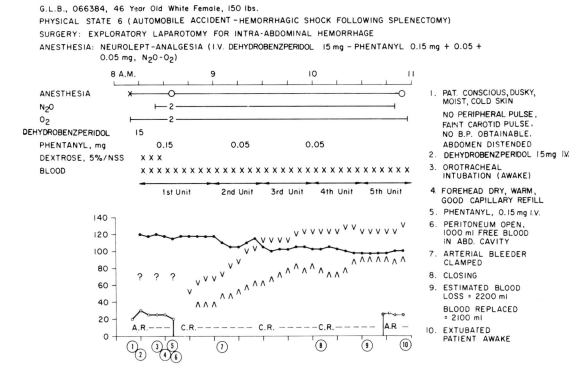

Fig. 8–11. NLAN in a patient in hemorrhagic shock. (From Corssen, G., and Chodoff, P.: Clinical management of the patient in shock: Neuroleptanalgesia. Clin. Anesth., 2:137, 1965.)

and fentanyl are the presence of an anesthesiologist and a minimum of resuscitative equipment, such as Ambu-type bags, face masks, endotracheal tubes, and oxygen. Without this equipment, the administration of NLA or NLAN might be too hazardous for such high-risk patients, but other agents (e.g., ketamine) could be more appropriate (see Chapter 7).

Removal of Pheochromocytoma

In theory, NLAN appears ideal for the patient undergoing removal of pheochromocytoma. Droperidol reduces the pressor response to epinephrine and protects against epinephrine-induced arrhythmias, and the combined effects of droperidol and fentanyl should be expected to maintain cardiovascular stability without excessive blood pressure fluctuations of ventricular arrhythmias in response to manipulation of the tumor.[58–60,261–263] Indeed, numerous investigators attest to the efficacy of droperidol, NLA, or NLAN for use in this setting.[264–267] Marked hypertension associated with the use of droperidol was reported.[268] In our own series of seven patients in whom a pheochromocytoma was surgically removed during NLAN, hypertension from tumor manipulation in one young man could not be controlled with increasing doses of droperidol, but it responded promptly to intravenous doses of chlorpromazine (12.5 mg to a total of 50 mg).[153] Whether in some patients with pheochromocytoma droperidol causes central stimulation of the sympathoadrenal system, directly stimulates the tumor cells to release catecholamines, or inhibits catecholamine uptake into the nerve terminals is not clear.[268]

In any case, NLAN is still recommended for use during removal of pheochromocytoma, because the unusual hypertensive response to droperidol is well controlled with alpha-adrenergic receptor blockade with phentolamine.[268] NLAN, through its droperidol component, protects the heart against epinephrine-induced arrhythmias and also exerts minimal depressant action on cardiac and renal function.

Urologic Surgery

NLAN is advantageous for use in patients with renal malfunction because it increases the glomerular filtration rate and augments active tubular transport of sodium.[146,269] In addition, in the presence of oliguria secondary to acute circulatory failure, droperidol increases urinary volume, apparently through inhibition of the sympathetic reflexes.[94] NLAN is also a useful anesthetic technique for use in patients in chronic kidney failure who must undergo renal transplantation.[270] Smaller than usual (one third to one half less) doses of NLA drugs are required for both induction and maintenance of NLAN; nitrous oxide concentrations need not exceed 50%, thereby assuring even greater cardiovascular stability without impairing analgesia during the procedure.

Biliary Surgery

NLAN is suitable for these operations because it has no adverse effects on liver function or liver parenchyma.[271] The criticism that the tonus of the sphincter of Oddi is increased by fentanyl (as with morphine), with resultant elevation of biliary duct pressure,[272,273] has been countered by clinical observations that, although fentanyl alone can achieve this end, the effect is attenuated by the accompanying droperidol.[272]

Hand Surgery

NLA can be a valuable adjunct in hand surgery, e.g., for determination of the precise length of tendon graft required. Extensive dissection of muscles and tendons is feasible with a fully cooperative patient helping the surgeon to analyze and treat complex impairments of the hands.[274]

Pediatric Surgery

NLAN is suitable for all age groups, although the dosage of droperidol should be reduced in children under the age of 2 years (see previous discussion of techniques of administration). Prerequisites for the safe use of NLAN in neonates are a well-functioning intravenous line, strict individual dosage plan, avoidance of fluid overload, and maintenance of minute-by-minute control of depth of anesthesia. The technique is especially recommended for use during lengthy and traumatic operations associated with considerable blood loss, such as in the correction of congenital anomalies of intestinal and respiratory organs. Note that infants with tracheo-esophageal fistula, who require ventilatory support preoperatively or demonstrate excessive spillage of gastric contents into the lungs, should continue to receive automatic ventilation during immediate postoperative recovery.

Obstetrics

NLA alone offers optimal conditions for a smooth, uncomplicated vaginal delivery, with the mother awake and cooperative.[275,276] The administration of Innovar, 2 ml intramuscularly, can also provide satisfactory sedation and analgesia in conjunction with local or regional blocks and the subanesthetic concentrations of nitrous oxide in oxygen.[277]

In one technique, 3 to 5 ml of Innovar are administered intramuscularly according to the weight and emotional state of the mother, when uterine contractions become strong and regular and the cervix is dilated to about 4 cm.[278] Subsequent increments of Innovar (0.5 to 1.0 ml intramuscularly) may be given at 30-minute intervals until the cervix is fully dilated. Delivery is usually uneventful, with no need for general or regional anesthesia.

In an alternative technique 5 ml Innovar (i.e., 12.5 mg droperidol and 0.25 mg fentanyl) in 500 ml of 5% glucose in water is delivered by continuous intravenous infusion at the same point in labor, when contractions are strong and regular and the cervix has dilated to about 3 to 5 cm.[279] The initial 50 to 100 ml are infused rapidly within 10 to 20 minutes, after which the rate is slowed and regulated by patient response until the cervix is fully dilated. The infusion is then stopped, although occasionally a further slow drip is needed until the fetal head has crowned.[279]

For cesarean section, NLA may be combined with local analgesia; the administration of droperidol in fractional intravenous doses of 2.5 mg, to a total of 10 to 15 mg, is followed by thorough infiltration of the region between the pubis and umbilicus with a local anesthetic solution. Once the cord is clamped, fentanyl may be added intravenously in doses of 0.05 mg for further analgesia.[280]

Whereas NLA is suitable for uncomplicated vaginal delivery with the mother awake, NLAN may be preferred for cesarean section and other complicated obstetric manipulations during which the patient should be asleep.[275] Preanesthetic medication with droperidol (0.5 mg intramuscularly) together with an antisialagogue is followed by intermittent injections or continuous intravenous infusion of Innovar, the total induction dose of which is strictly limited to 3 to 5 ml. The trachea is intubated with the aid of a muscle relaxant, and nitrous oxide (50% in oxygen) is administered until delivery. Fentanyl supplementation is not instituted until the cord is clamped.

The advantages of NLA and NLAN in obstetrics include minimal interference with uterine motility, i.e., no significant prolongation of labor, provided that recommended dosage of Innovar (especially its fentanyl component) is not exceeded; cardiovascular stability; amnesia; and prolonged postoperative analgesia with minimal nausea and vomiting. Note that for uncomplicated delivery, NLA is preferable to NLAN: the technique is simpler, obviating tracheal intubation; avoidance of the use of general anesthetics minimizes the risk of adverse effects on the fetus; and the awake mother is able to participate actively in the delivery.

Porphyria and Thiopental Anaphylaxis

NLAN may be a safe alternative to general anesthesia in patients with hereditary hepatic porphyria or with known idiosyncratic reaction to barbiturates, in whom these drugs can cause life-threatening complications.

Tetanus

NLA is effective in the treatment of tetanus requiring prolonged respiratory assistance. Innovar may be administered either in increments of 2 ml intravenously every 30 minutes to 2 hours, depending on the severity of the disease, or by intravenous infusion of 60 ml in 500 ml of a balanced salt solution to a total of 300 ml per day.[281,282] Diazepam may be added if more sedation is required.[283] NLA offers patients with tetanus pain control as well as tolerance of the endotracheal tube, thereby facilitating prolonged mechanical ventilation. Cardiovascular stability is maintained. Organ toxicity is absent, as are adverse effects on gastrointestinal motility, even when the therapy lasts to and exceeds 30 days. Extrapyramidal symptoms are rare and are promptly suppressed by antiparkinsonian drugs.

CONTRAINDICATIONS

Treatment with monoamine oxidase inhibitors (MAOi) can cause severe potentiation of the hypotensive effects of fentanyl or other narcotic analgesics. Therefore, patients should not receive NLA or NLAN unless MAOi therapy has been discontinued for at least 14 days.

NLA is not recommended for use in patients with addictions to alcohol or narcotic agents who often require excessively large doses of Innovar. The unsuspected, unadmitted addict is always at risk.[284] Patients with Parkinson's disease are also not good candidates for NLA because droperidol and other butyrophenones can initiate extrapyramidal side-effects and may even exacerbate symptoms of parkinsonism in patients receiving levodopa.[155] (Note, however, that Innovar is especially suitable for stereotactic operations for the surgical treatment of Parkinson's disease, when patient cooperation is required for success of the procedure.[285])

PRECAUTIONS

Innovar should be used with great caution in patients with head injuries or those undergoing resection of brain tumors to avoid hypercarbia and the accompanying increase in ICP that may follow untreated drug-induced respiratory depression. The possibility of postural impairment of respiratory exchange, e.g., in the prone position, requires constant monitoring, with prompt institution of respiratory support if necessary. Similarly, in patients with impaired pulmonary function resulting from chronic obstructive lung disease or other causes, Innovar may further decrease pulmonary function by suppressing respiratory drive. Respiration should then be assisted or controlled before hypoxia and hypercarbia develop. Should narcotic antagonists be required later to reverse the respiratory depression, the patient must be closely monitored to ensure that respiratory depression does not recur should the effects of the Innovar outlast those of the antagonist. Innovar-induced decreases in pulmonary arterial pressure can affect diagnostic and surgical procedures in which interpretation of such measurements determines the clinical management.

Liver and Kidney Dysfunction. NLA drugs should be administered cautiously to patients with liver or kidney dysfunction, because both of these organs participate in their metabolism and excretion.

Central Nervous System Depressants and Innovar. Because the effects of CNS depressants, e.g., barbiturates, tranquilizers, narcotics, and general anesthetics, are enhanced by Innovar when these drugs are used together, their dosage should be mutually reduced.

GENERAL REMINDERS

Preanesthetic medication with Innovar and the intravenous test dose at the start of NLA or NLAN enables assessment of the susceptibility of the patients to the drugs, thus preventing overdosage. An initial hypotensive response suggests hypovolemia and the need for fluid replacement. Because fentanyl is a potent respiratory depressant, early manual or mechanical ventilatory support is essential to avoid asphyxia. Fentanyl-induced chest wall rigidity can be prevented by the use of muscle relaxants; pancuronium may be the drug of choice because it tends to increase the heart rate, partially countering the vagotonic effects of fentanyl. Profound bradycardia may otherwise be corrected with the intravenous application of atropine.

After induction of NLA or NLAN, analgesia should be maintained with supplemental doses of fentanyl, not Innovar, to avoid overtranquilization and prolonged recovery. During the immediate post-anesthetic recovery period, close monitoring of respiratory and circulatory function is essential, with frequent arousal of the patient to encourage deep breathing. Adequate reversal of the effects of narcotic and muscle relaxant drugs should be ensured. Equipment for cardiopulmonary resuscitation that is in good working order should be at hand.

REFERENCES

1. Laborit, H., and Huguenard, P.: Practique de l'hibernotherapie en chirurgie et en médicine. Paris, Masson, 1954.
2. Laborit, H.: Stress and cellular function. Philadelphia, Lippincott, 1959.
3. Hayward-Butt, J.T.: Ataralgesia: operations without anesthesia. Lancet, 2:972, 1957.
4. Dardalhon, P.: Narco-ataralgesie avec le melange phenoperidine + dehydrobenzperidol. Ann. Anesth. Franc., 7:233, 1966.
5. Aldrete, J.A.: Somnoanalgesia with Pentazepam. *In* Trends in Intravenous Anesthesia. Edited by J.A. Aldrete and T.H. Stanley. Miami, Symposia Specialists, 1980.
6. Delay, J.: Psychopharmacology Frontiers. Boston, Little Brown, 1959.
7. Janssen, P.A.J.: The pharmacology of haloperidol. Int. J. Neuropsychiatr., 3(Suppl. 1):10,, 1967.
8. DeCastro, J., and Mundeleer, P.: Anesthesie sans barbituriques; la neurolept analgesie (R 1406, R 1625, hydergine, procain). Anesth. Analg., 16:1022, 1959.
9. Nilsson, E., and Janssen, P.: Neuroleptanalgesia, an alternative to general anesthesia. Acta Anaesthesiol. Scand., 5:73, 1961.
10. Janssen, P.A.J., Niemegeers, C.J.E., Schellekens, K.H.L., Verbruggen, F.J., and VanHueten, J.M.: The pharmacology of dehydrobenzperidol, (R 4749), a new potent and short-acting neuroleptic agent chemically related to haloperidol. Arzneimittelforschung, 13:205, 1963.
11. Janssen, P.A.J.: A review of the chemical features associated with strong morphine-like activity. Br. J. Anaesth., 34:260, 1962.
12. Janssen, P.A.J., and Eddy, N.: Compounds related to pethidine. IV. New general chemical methods of increasing the analgesic activity of pethidine. J. Med. Chem., 2:32, 1960.
13. DeCastro, J., and Mundeleer, P.: Dehydrobenzperidol and phentanyl. Two new anesthetics which open new possibilities in neuroleptanalgesia. Proceeding of the Symposium of Neuroleptanalgesia, First European Congress of Anesthesiology, Vienna, 1962.
14. Henschel, W.F.: Die Entwicklung der Neuroleptanalgesie bis zu ihrer heutigen Stellung in der Anaesthesie. *In* Die Neuroleptanalgesie. Edited by W.F. Henschel. Berlin, Springer, 1966.
15. DeCastro, J.: Twenty-five years of neuroleptanalgesia—concepts, evolution, actual trends. Proceedings of the First International Symposium of History of Modern Anesthesia. Rotterdam, 1982.
16. Edmonds-Seal, J., and Prys-Roberts, C.: Pharmacology of drugs in neuroleptanalgesia. Br. J. Anaesth., 42:207, 1970.
17. Janssen, P.A.J.: Chemical and pharmacological classification of neurolept drugs. Proceedings of the Interdisciplinary Week on Neuroleptics, Liege, 1969.
18. Janssen, P.A.J.: Pharmacological aspects. *In* Neuropsychopharmacology. Edited by D. Bente and P. Bradley. Amsterdam, Elsevier, 1965.
19. Saarne, A.: Experience with haloperidol as a premedicant. Acta Anaesthesiol. Scand., 7:21, 1962.

20. Marshall, B.M., and Gordon, R.A.: Electroencephalographic monitoring in anesthesia with droperidol and fentanyl. Can. Anaesth. Soc. J., 15:357, 1968.
21. Seeman, P.M., and Bialy, H.S.: The surface activity of tranquillizers.. Biochem. Pharmacol., 12:1181, 1963.
22. Roos, B.E.: Effects of certain tranquillisers on the level of homovanillic acid in the corpus striatum. J. Pharm. Pharmacol., 17:820, 1965.
23. Hillarp, N.A., Guxe, K., and Dahlstrom, A.: Demonstration and mapping of central neurones containing dopamine, noradrenaline, and 5-hydro-oxytryptamine and their reactions to psychopharmaca. Pharmacol. Rev., 18:727, 1966.
24. Borison, H.L., and Wang, S.C.: Physiology and pharmacology of vomiting. Pharmacol. Rev., 5:193, 1953.
25. Soudijn, W., Van Wijngaarden, I., and Allewijn, F.: Distribution, excretion, and metabolism of neuroleptics of the butyrophenone type. Eur. J. Pharmacol., 1:47, 1967.
26. Johnson, P.D., Charalampos, K.D., and Braun, G.A.: Absorption and excretion of tritiated haloperidol in man. Int. J. Neuropsychiat., 3:(Suppl. 1)24, 1967.
27. Drybert, V.: Haloperidol (Serenase) in the prevention of postoperative nausea and vomiting. Acta Anaesthesiol. Scand., 6:37, 1964.
28. Yeh, B.K., and Goldberg, L.I.: Attenuation of dopamine renal and mesenteric vasodilation by haloperidol: evidence for a specific dopamine receptor. J. Pharmacol. Exp. Ther., 168:303, 1969.
29. Goldstein, B.J.: Haloperidol in controlling the symptoms of acute psychoses. Curr. Psychiatr. Ther., 8:232, 1966.
30. Jones, B., Lehman, H.E., Saxena, M.A., and Ban, T.A.: Treatment of chronic schizophrenic patients with haloperidol and chlorpromazine combined. Curr. Psychiatr. Ther., 10:276, 1966.
31. Brown, A.S.: Neuroleptanalgesia. Int. Anesthesiol. Clin., 7:159, 1969.
32. Lawson, J.I.M., and McGowan, S.W.: Haloperidol in obstetrics. Lancet, 1:1205, 1962.
33. Janssen, P.A.J.: Zur Frage des Abbaus und der Ausscheidung der bei Neuroleptanalgesie zur Anwendung kommenden Pharmaka. In Die Neuroleptanalgesie. Edited by W.F. Henschel. Berlin, Springer, 1966.
34. Schaer, H., and Jenny, E.: Die Plasmakonzentration und die Plasmaeiweissverbindung von Droperidol und Fentanyl waehrend der Neuroleptanalgesie beim Menschen. Proceedings of the 4th Neuroleptanalgesia Symposium, Stuttgart, Schattauer, 1969.
35. Drug information 84. American Hospital Formulary Service. Bethesda, American Society of Hospital Pharmacists, 1984.
36. Janssen, P.A.J., Niemegeers, C.J.E., Schellekens, K.H.L.: Is it possible to predict the clinical effects of neuroleptic drugs (major tranquillizers) from animal data? Part II: "Neuroleptic activity spectra" for dogs. Arzneimittelforschung, 15:1196, 1965.
37. Yelnosky, J., and Gardocki, J.F.: A study of some of the pharmacologic actions of fentanyl citrate and droperidol. Toxicol. Appl. Pharmacol., 6:48, 1964.
38. Morrison, J.D.: Neuroleptic techniques. In Intravenous Anaestheisa. Edited by J.W. Dundee and G.M. Wyant. Edinburgh, Churchill Livingstone, 1974.
39. Morrison, J.D., Loan, W.B., and Dundee, J.W.: Controlled comparison of the efficacy of fourteen preparations in the relief of postoperative pain. Br. Med. J., 3:287, 1971.
40. Morrison, J.D.: Alterations in response to somatic pain associated with anaesthesia, XIX. Studies with the drugs used in neuroleptanaesthesia. Br. J. Anaesth., 43:838, 1970.
41. Kreuscher, H.: The action of dehydrobenzperidol on the cardiovascular system in man. Acta Anaesthesiol. Scand., 9:155, 1965.
42. Yelonsky, J., Katz, R., and Dietrich, E.: A study of some of the pharmacologic actions of droperidol. Toxicol. Appl. Pharmacol., 6:37, 1964.
43. Kreuscher, H.: Der Einfluss von Dehydrobenzperidol auf die Kontraktilitaet des Herzmuskels. In Die Neuroleptanalgesie. Edited by W.F. Henschel. Berlin, Springer, 1966.
44. Schaper, W.K.A., Jagenequ, A.H.M., and Bogaard, J.M.: Haemodynamic and respiratory responses to dehydrobenzperidol (R 4749), a potent neuroleptic compound in intact anaesthetized dogs. Arzneimittelforschung, 13:316, 1963.
45. Stanley, T.H.: Cardiovascular effects of droperidol during enflurane and enflurane-nitrous oxide anaesthesia in man. Can. Anaesth. Soc. J., 25:26, 1978.
46. Muldoon, S.M., Janssen, W.J., Verbeuren, T.J., and Vanhoutte, P.M.: Alpha-adrenergic blocking properties of droperidol on isolated blood vessels of the dog. Br. J. Anaesth., 49:211, 1977.
47. Puddy, B.R.: Effects of droperidol on vasoconstriction produced by noradrenaline, histamine, sympathetic nerve stimulation and potassium ions in the isolated rabbit auricular artery. Br. J. Anaesth., 43:441, 1971.
48. Israel, J.S., Janssen, G.T., and Dobkin, A.B.: Circulatory and respiratory response to tilt with pentazocine, droperidol, droperidol-fentanyl and methotrimeprazine in normal healthy male subjects. Anesthesiology, 26:253, 1965.
49. Lawin, P., Herden, H., Badran, H., and Berta, J.: Drei Herzstillstaende bei Einleitung der

Neuroleptanalgesie Typ II bei vorbehandelten Patienten mit vasodilatorischen Medikamenten. Anaesthesist, *15*:19. 1966.

50. Au, A.S.W., Evans, D., Graco, R., and Jones, W.M.: Blood pressor effects of lower abdominal aorta surgery with particular reference to the use of morphine and droperidol in modifying the responses. Can. Anaesth. Soc. J., *24*:293, 1977.

51. Fitch, W., Barker, J., Jennett, W.B., and McDowall, D.G.: The influence of neuroleptanalgesic drugs on cerebrospinal fluid pressure. Br. J. Anaesth., *41*:800, 1969.

52. Michenfelder, J.D., and Theye, R.A.: Effects of fentanyl, droperidol and Innovar on canine cerebral metabolism and blood flow. Br. J. Anaesth., *43*:630, 1971.

53. Miller, J.D., and Barker, J.: The effect of neuroleptanalgesic drugs on cerebral blood flow and metabolism. Br. J. Anaesth., *41*:554, 1969.

54. Misfeldt, B.B., Jorgensen, P.B., Spotoft, H., and Ronde, F.: The effects of droperidol and fentanyl on intracranial pressure and cerebral perfusion pressure in neurosurgical patients. Br. J. Anaesth., *48*:963, 1976.

55. Birch, A.A., and Boyce, W.H.: Effects of droperidol-dopamine interaction on renal blood flow in man. Anesthesiology, *47*:70, 1977.

56. Faulkner, S.L., Boerth, R.C., and Graham, T.P.: Direct myocardial effects of precatheterization medication. Am. Heart. J., *88*:609, 1974.

57. Ostheimer, G.W., Shanahan, E.A., Guyton, B.S., Dagget, W.M., and Loewenstein, E.: Effects of fentanyl and droperidol on canine left ventricle performance. Anesthesiology, *42*:228, 1975.

58. Long, G., Dripps, R.D., and Price, H.L.: Measurements of anti-arrhythmic potency of drugs in man: effects of dehydrobenzperidol. Anesthesiology, *28*:318, 1967.

59. Bertolo, L., Novakovic, L., and Penna, M.: Antiarrhythmic effects of droperidol. Anesthesiology, *37*:529, 1972.

60. Bauer, H., Kreuscher, H., and Menzel, H.: Antiarrhythmic effect of dehydrobenzperidol in dogs. Acta Anesthesiol. Scand., *15*:277, 1971.

61. Carmeliet, E., Xhonneux, R., van Glabbek, A., and Renneman, R.: Electrophysiological effects of droperidol in different cardiac tissues. Arch. Pharm. (Weinheim) *293*:57, 1976.

62. Johnstone, M.: The pharmacology of drugs used in neuroleptanesthesia. Br. J. Anaesth., *42*:630, 1970.

63. Dahlgren, B.E.: Droperidol in treatment of catecholamine-induced arrhythmia during nitrous oxide-halothane anesthesia. Opuscula Medica, *15*:148, 1970.

64. Alexander, J.P.: Dysrhythmia and oral surgery. Br. J. Anaesth., *43*:773, 1971.

65. AMA Drug Evaluations. 5th Ed. New York, American Medical Association, Standard Book No. 089970-160-4, 1983.

66. Whalley, D.G., Tidnam, P.F, Tyrell, M.F., and Thompson, D.S.: A comparison of the incidence of cardiac arrhythmias during two methods of anaesthesia for dental extractions. Br. J. Anaesth., *48*:1207, 1976.

67. Prys-Roberts, C., and Kelman, G.R.: The influence of drugs used in neuroleptanalgesia on cardiovascular and ventilatory function. Br. J. Anaesth., *39*:134, 1967.

68. Corssen, G., and DeKornfeld, T.J.: Comparison of the respiratory depressant effects of phentanyl, phentanyl and droperidol, and morphine. Anesthesiology, *27*:213, 1966.

69. Tornetta, F.J., and Boger, W.P.: Liver function studies in droperidol-fentanyl anesthesia. Anesth. Analg., *43*:544, 1964.

70. Oyama, T., and Takiguchi, M.: Effect of neuroleptanaesthesia on adrenocortical function in man. Br. J. Anaesth., *42*:425, 1970.

71. Oyama, T., and Takiguchi M.: Effect of neuroleptanaesthesia on plasma levels of growth hormone and insulin. Br. J. Anaesth., *42*:1105, 1970.

72. Gemperle, M.: Herabsetzung der Sauerstoffaufnahme in Normothermie durch Neuroleptanalgesia. *In* Die Neuroleptanalgesie. Edited by W. Henschel. Berlin, Springer, 1966.

73. Aronson, H.B., Magora, F., and London, M.: The influence of droperidol on blood viscosity in man. Br. J. Anaesth., *42*:1089, 1970.

74. Corssen, G., Reves, J.G., and Carter, J.R.: Neuroleptanesthesia, dissociative anesthesia and hemorrhage. Int. Anesthesiol. Clin., *12*:145, 1974.

75. Clark, M.M.: Droperidol in preoperative anxiety. Anaesthesia, *24*:36, 1969.

76. Tasker, R.R., and Marshall, B.M.: Analgesia for surgical procedures performed on conscious subjects. Can. Anaesth. Soc. J., *12*:29, 1965.

77. DeJong, R.: Neurologic complications of drugs with primary action on nervous system. N.Y. State J. Med., *70*:1857, 1980.

78. Patton, C.M.: Rapid induction of acute dyskinesia by droperidol. Anesthesiology, *43*:126, 1975.

79. Morrison, J.D.: Drugs used in neuroleptanalgesia. *In* Newer Intravenous Anesthetics. Edited by R.S.J. Clarke. Boston, Little Brown, 1969.

80. Ellis, F.R., and Wilson, J.: An assessment of droperidol as a premedicant. Br. J. Anaesth., *44*:1280, 1972.

81. Shephard, N.W.: The Application of Neuroleptanalgesia in Anaesthetic and Other Practice. London, Pergamon Press, 1964.
82. Herr, G.P., Conner, J.T., Katz, R.L., Dorey, F., L'Armand, J., and Schehl, D.: Diazepam and droperidol as i.v. premedicants. Br. J. Anaesth., 51:537, 1979.
83. Ferrari, H.A., and Stephen, C.R.: Neuroleptanalgesia: pharmacology and clinical experiences with droperidol and fentanyl. South. Med. J., 59:185, 1966.
84. Prescott, R.J., Espley, A.J., Davie, I.T., Slawson, K.B., and Ruckley, C.V.: Double-blind clinical trial of anesthetic premedication for use in major day-surgery. Lancet, 1:1148, 1976.
85. Fozard, J.R., and Manford, M.L.M.: A controlled clinical trial of oral droperidol and droperidol plus diazepam for premedication in children. Br. J. Anaesth., 49:1147, 1977.
86. Sadove, M.S., Hatano, S., Redlin, T., Thomason, R., Arastounejad, P., and Roman, V.: Clinical study of droperidol in the prevention of the side effects of ketamine anesthesia: a progress report. Anesth. Analg., 50:526, 1971.
87. Patton, C.M., Moon, M.R., and Dannemiller, F.J.: The prophylactic antiemetic effect of droperidol. Anesth. Analg., 53:361, 1974.
88. Alsner, T., Brandt, M.R., and Sorensen, B.: The postanesthetic antiemetic effect of premedication with dehydrobenzperidol before ether anesthesia. Acta Anaesthesiol. Scand., 20:65, 1976.
89. Sloan, J.B.: Innovar as a preoperative medication. South. Med. J., 68:1407, 1975.
90. Johnson, W.H., Money, K.E., and Grayriel, A.: Airborne testing of three antimotion sickness preparations. Aviat. Space Environ. Med., 47:1214, 1976.
91. Cordingley, F.T., and O'Conner, D.T.: Neuroleptanalgesia in obstetric practice. Aust. N.Z. J. Obstet. Gynaecol., 7:108, 1967.
92. Pettit, G.P., Smith, G.A., and McLroy, W.L.: Droperidol in obstetrics: a double-blind study. Milit. Med., 141:316, 1976.
93. Kopman, A.F., Wollman, S.B., Ross, K., and Surks, S.N.: Awake endotracheal intubation: a review of 267 cases. Anesth. Analg., 54:343, 1975.
94. Gedeon, A.: Droperidol in the management of acute circulatory failure. Arzneimittelforschung, 20:674, 1970.
95. Van Leeuwen, A.J.H., Molders, J., Sterkmans, P., Mielants, P., Martens, C., Toussaint, C., Hovent, A.M., Desseils, M.F., Koch, H., Devroye, A., and Parent, M.: Droperidol in acutely agitated patients. J. Nerv. Ment. Dis., 164:280, 1977.
96. Nilsson, E.: Origin, rationale and practical use of neuroleptanalgesia. Ir. J. Med. Sci., 1:407, 1963.
97. Ingvar, D., and Nilsson, E.: Central nervous effects of neuroleptanalgesia as induced by haloperidol and phenoperidine. Acta Anaesthesiol. Scand., 5:85, 1961.
98. Gaveau, Th., and Viars, P.: Etude de l'utilisation de phenoperidine et de dehydrobenzperidol associes en chirurgie peripherique. Anaesth. Analg., 23:927, 1966.
99. Delineau, M.A., and Sabathie, M.: Interet de l'association dehydrobenzperidol-phenoperidine en chirurgie generale (a propos de 132 observations). Ann. Anesth. Franc., 7:213, 1966.
100. Lasagna, L., DeKornfeld, T., and Safar, P.: A clinical trial of dextromoramide LR 875, SKF d-5137. J. Chronic Dis., 8:689, 1958.
101. Lear, E., Tadeo, J., Chiron, A.E., Ona, V., Trinidad, C.C., and Pallin, I.M.: SKF d-5137, a new synthetic analgesic. Anesth. Analg., 37:295, 1958.
102. Keats, A.S., Telford, J., and Kurosu, Y.: Studies of analgesic drugs III. Dextromoramide and a comparison of methods of estimating pain relief in man. J. Pharmacol. Exp. Ther., 130:212, 1960.
103. Lasagna, L.: The clinical evaluation of morphine and its substitutes as analgesics. Pharmacol. Rev., 16:47, 1964.
104. Doenicke, A.: Klinische Pharmakologie. In Lehrbuch der Anaesthesiologie, Reanimation and Intensiv therapie. Edited by H. Benzer, R. Frey, W. Huegin, and O. Mayrhofer. Berlin, Springer, 1977.
105. Cass, L.J., Frederick, W.S., and Theodore, J.V.J.: Pentazocine as an analgesic. Clinical evaluation. JAMA, 188:112, 1964.
106. Duncan, S.L., Ginsburg, J., and Morris, N.F.: Comparison of pentazocine and pethidine in normal labour. Am. J. Obstet. Gynecol., 105:197, 1969.
107. Kay, B., Kearney, J.P.D., and Taylor, G.J.: Neuroleptanalgesia: a double-blind comparison of pentazocine and phenoperidine for neuroradiological investigations. Br. J. Anaesth., 42:329, 1970.
108. Foldes, F.F., Shiffman, H.P., and Kronfeld, P.P.: The use of fentanyl, meperidine or alphaprodine for neuroleptanalgesia. Anesthesiology, 33:35, 1970.
109. Foldes, F.F., Kepes, E.R., Torda, T.A.G., Bailey, R., and Wulfsohn, N.L.: Clinical-pharmacological studies with fentanyl and droperidol. Proceedings of the Third World Congress of Anesthesiology, Sao Paulo, Brazil, 1964.
110. Graves, C.L., Downs, N.H., and Browne, A.B.: Cardiovascular effects of minimal analgesic quantities of Innovar, fentanyl, and droperidol in man. Anesth. Analg., 54:15, 1975.

111. Yanagida, H., and Yamamura, H.: The site of action of Innovar in the brain. Can. Anaesth. Soc. J., *18*:522, 1971.
112. Sovijarvi, A.R.A., and Asinio, K.: Neuroleptanalgesia and the function of the auditory cortex in the cat. Anesthesiology, 37:406, 1972.
113. Doenicke, A., Kugler, J., Schellenberger, A., and Guertner, Th.: The use of electroencephalography to measure recovery time after intravenous anesthesia. Br. J. Anaesth., 38:580, 1966.
114. Sari, A., Okuda, Y., and Takeshita, H.: The effects of thalamonal on cerebral circulation and oxygen consumption in man. Br. J. Anaesth., *44*:330, 1972.
115. Adams, R.W., Gronert, G.A., Sundt, R.M., and Michenfelder, J.D.: Halothane, hypocapnia, and cerebrospinal fluid pressure in neurosurgery. Anesthesiology, 37:510, 1972.
116. Yusa, T., and Iwatsuki, K.: Effects of thalamonal on coronary circulation and cardiac efficiency. Masui., 20:377, 1971.
117. Dixon, S.H., Nolan, S.P., Stewart, S., and Morrow, A.G.: Neuroleptanalgesia: effects of Innovar on myocardial contractility, total peripheral vascular resistance and capacitance. Anesth. Analg., 49:331, 1970.
118. Stoelting, R.K., Gibbs, P.S., Creasser, C.W., and Peterson, C.: Hemodynamic and ventilatory responses to fentanyl, fentanyl-droperidol and nitrous oxide in patients with acquired valvular heart disease. Anesthesiology, 42:319, 1975.
119. Ferrari, H.A., Gorten, R.J., Talton, I.H., and Goodrich, J.K.: The action of droperidol and fentanyl on cardiac output and related hemodynamic parameters. South. Med. J., *67*:49, 1974.
120. Tarhan, S., Moffitt, E.A., Lundborg, R.O., and Frye, R.L.: Hemodynamic and blood gas effects of Innovar in patients with acquired heart disease. Anesthesiology, 34:250, 1971.
121. Zauder, H.L., Delguercio, L.R.M., Feins, N., Barton, N., and Wollman, S.: Hemodynamics during neuroleptanalgesia. Anesthesiology, 26:266, 1965.
122. Calligari, G., Allaria, B., and Citro, A.: Influence of neuroleptanalgesia II on cardiac dynamics and on the general circulation. Anaesth. Vig. Subvig., *1/2*:285, 1970.
123. Marta, J.A., Davis, H.S., and Eisele, J.H.: Vagomimetic effects of morphine and Innovar in man. Anesth. Analg., *52*:817, 1973.
124. Kettler, D., Cott, L.A., Hellige, G., Hensel, I., Martel, J., Paschen, K., and Bretschneider, H.J.: Der Sauerstoffverbrauch des linken Ventrikels bei Aether-Halothan-Ketamin-Methoxyfluran- und Piritramid- Narkose sowie bei Neuroleptanalgesie. Anasth. Intensivther. Notfallmed., 80:203, 1974.
125. Dietzel, W.: Wirkung der NLA auf den venoesen Rueckfluss. Anaesthesist, 20:446, 1971.
126. Brismer, B., Bergenwald, L., Cronestrand, R., Jorfeldt, L., and Julin-Dannfelt, A.: The cardiovascular effects of neuroleptanaesthesia. Acta Anaesthesiol. Scand., *21*:100, 1977.
127. Dietzel, W., and Massion, W.H.: The prophylactic effect of Innovar in experimental hemorrhagic shock. Anesth. Analg., *48*:968, 1969.
128. Hirasawa, H., and Yonezawa, T.: The effects of ketamine and Innovar on the renal cortical and medullary blood flow of the dog. Anaesthesist, 24:349, 1975.
129. Ivankovich, A.D., El-Etr, A.A., Janeczko, G.F., and Maronic, J.P.: The effect of ouabaine and of Innovar anesthesia on digitalis tolerance in dogs. Anesth. Analg., *54*:106, 1975.
130. Foldes, F.F.: Neuroleptanesthesia for general surgery. Int. Anesthesiol. Clin., *11*:1, 1973.
131. Kallos, T., and Smith, T.C.: The respiratory effects of Innovar given for premedication. Br. J. Anaesth., *41*:303, 1969.
132. Harper, M.H., Hickey, R.F., Cromwell, T.H., and Linwood, S.: The magnitude and duration of respiratory depression produced by fentanyl and fentanyl plus droperidol in man. J. Clin. Pharmacol. Exp. Ther., *199*:464, 1976.
133. Becker, L.D.: Biphasic respiratory depression after fentanyl-droperidol or fentanyl alone used to supplement nitrous oxide anesthesia. Anesthesiology, 44:291, 1976.
134. Kallos, T., Wyche, M.Q., and Garman, J.K.: The effects of Innovar on functional residual capacity and total chest compliance in man. Anesthesiology, 39:558, 1973.
135. Muggenburg, B.A., and Mauderly, J.L.: Cardiopulmonary function of awake, sedated and anesthetized beagle dogs. J. Appl. Physiol., 37:152, 1974.
136. Pontinen, P.J.: Respiratory effects of thalamonal and diazepam during epidural anaesthesia. Anesth. Vig. Subvig., *9*:33, 1970.
137. Gemperle, M.: Verbesserung der postoperativen Hypoxie nach Neuroleptanalgesie. *In* Die Neuroleptanalgesie. Edited by W.F. Henschel. Berlin, Springer, 1966.
138. Gergis, S.D., Hoyt, J.L., and Sokoll, M.D.: Effects of Innovar, and Innovar plus nitrous oxide, on muscle tone and "H" reflex. Anesth. Analg., 50:743, 1971.
139. Sokoll, M.D., Hoyt, J.I., and Gergis, S.D.: Studies in muscle rigidity, nitrous oxide, and narcotic analgesic agents. Anesth. Analg., *51*:16, 1972.
140. Corssen, G., Domino, E.F., and Sweet, R.B.: Neuroleptanalgesia and anesthesia. Anesth. Analg., 43:748, 1964.
141. Farb, S., and Tornetta, F.J.: Topical endoscopic anaesthesia with two new adjuncts. Ear Nose Throat J., *44*:56, 1965.

142. Martin, S.J., Murphy, J.D., Collition, R.J., and Zeffiro, R.G.: Clinical studies with Innovar. Anesthesiology, 28:458, 1967.

143. Guertner, Th.: Einfluss der Neuroleptanalgesie auf die Leberfunktion. Anesthesiol. Resusc., 18:113, 1966.

144. Canellas, J., Roquebert, J., Dumartin, A., and Courtois, P.: Action on Oddi's sphincter of guinea-pigs of an analgesic, a neuroleptic and their combination. Comot. Rand. Soc. Biol., 159:1538, 1965.

145. Gorman, H.M., and Craythorne, H.W.B.: The effects of a new neuroleptanalgesic agent (Innovar) on renal function in man. Acta Anaethesiol. Scand. [Suppl.], 24:111, 1966.

146. Finsterer, V., Brechtelsbauer, H., Prucksunand, P., Feist, H., and Kramer, K.: Natrium- und Wasserbilanz beim Hund im Wachzustand und unter verschiedenen Narkosebedingungen, III. Mitteilung: Neuroleptanalgesia. Anaesthesist, 24:483, 1975.

147. Kay, B.: Antidiuretic effects of anesthesia and neuroleptanesthesia (NLA). *In* Internationales Bremen NLA Symposium. Edited by W.F. Henschel, Stuttgart, Schattauer, 1972.

148. Clarke, R.S.J.: The hyperglycemic response to different types of surgery and anesthesia. Br. J. Anaesth., 42:45, 1970.

149. Dowdy, E.G., Goksen, N., Arnold, G.E., Moore, W.T., and Fabian, L.W.: A new treatment of Meniere's disease. Arch. Otolaryng., 82:494, 1965.

150. Dowdy, E.G., and Moore, W.T.: Droperidol and fentanyl combination: effect on the human labyrinth. Anesthesiology, 30:604, 1969.

151. Harris, I., Eviatar, A., and Goodhill, V.: Droperidol and fentanyl citrate compound as a vestibular depressant. Arch. Otolaryngol., 89:182, 1969.

152. Sturzenbecher, K., and Pascher, W.: Zur Vestibular und Hoerfunktion waehrend der Neuroleptanalgesie. *In* Die Neuroleptanalgesie. Edited by W.F. Henschel. Berlin, Springer, 1966.

153. Corssen, G.: Unpublished data.

154. Corssen, G.: Neuroleptanalgesia and anesthesia: its usefulness in poor-risk surgical cases. South. Med. J., 59:801, 1966.

155. Wiklund, R.A., and Ngai, S.H.: Rigidity and pulmonary edema after Innovar in a patient on levodopa therapy. Anesthesiology, 35:545, 1971.

156. Rivera, V.M., Keichian, A.H., and Oliver, R.E.: Persistent parkinsonism following neuroleptanalgesia. Anesthesiology, 42:635, 1975.

157. Radnay, P.A.: Hypertension during anesthesia and surgery should not be ignored. N.Y. State J. Med., 74:2193, 1974.

158. Bechtoldt, A.A., and Murray, W.J.: Innovar-induced respiratory depression. Anesth. Analg., 47:395, 1968.

159. Gieseke, A.H., Jenkins, M.T., Crout, J.R., and Collett, J.M.: Urinary epinephrine and norepinephrine during Innovar-nitrous oxide anesthesia in man. Anesthesiology, 28:701, 1967.

160. Browne, R.A., and Catton, D.V.: Awareness during anesthesia: a comparison of anesthesia with nitrous oxide-oxygen and nitrous oxide-oxygen with Innovar. Can. Anaesth. Soc. J., 20:763, 1973.

161. Doenicke, A., Kugler, J., Schellenberger, A., Guertner, Th., and Spiess, W.: Die Erholungszeit nach Narkosen mit Droperidol und Fentanyl. Arzneimittelforschung, 15:269, 1965.

162. Briggs, R.M., and Ogg, M.J.: Patients refusal of surgery after Innovar medication. Plast. Reconstr. Surg., 51:158, 1973.

163. Lee, C.M., and Yeakel, A.E.: Patient refusal of surgery following Innovar premedication. Anesth. Analg., 54:224, 1975.

164. DeOliveira, R., Melo, M.A., and Monteiro, H.: Neuroleptanalgesia in poor risk cardiac patients— Neuroleptoanalgesia em doentes cardiacos de grave risco. Rev. Bras. Anesth., 19:208, 1969.

165. Bergmann, H., and Necek, St.: Spezielle Probleme der Anaesthesieinleitung bei Risikopatienten. *In* Probleme der intravenoesen Anaesthesie. Edited by W.F. Henschel. Erlangen, Straube, 1976.

166. Teuteberg, H.W., King, J.E., and Massion, W.H.: Neuroleptanalgesia: a clinical evaluation of 106 cases. J. Okla. State Med. Assoc., April:178, 1967.

167. McKenzie, R.: Anesthesia for jejuno-ileal shunt: review of 88 cases. Anesth. Analg., 54:65, 1975.

168. Morgan, M., Lumley, J., and Gillies, I.D.S.: Neuroleptanesthesia for major surgery. Br. J. Anaesth., 46:288, 1974

169. Muenchen, I.: Erfahrungen mit der Neuroleptanalgesie in der Magenchirurgie. *In* Neuroleptanalgesie. Klinik und Fortschritte. Edited by W.F. Henschel. Stuttgart, Schattauer, 1967.

170. Aubry, U., Carignan, G., Charette, D., Keeri-Szanto, M., and Lavallee, J.: Neuroleptanalgesia with fentanyl-droperidol: an appreciation based on more than 1000 anaesthetics for major surgery. Can. Anaesth. Soc. J., 13:263, 1966.

171. Fox, J.W.C., and Fox, E.J.: Neuroleptanalgesia: a review. N.C. Med. J., 27:471, 1966.

172. Berenyi, K.J., Sakarya, I., and Snow, J.C.: Innovar-nitrous oxide anesthesia in otolaryngology. Laryngoscope, 76:772, 1966.

173. Keeri-Szanto, M., Telmosse, F., and Trop, D.: Anesthesia time/dose curves. V. Data on neuroleptic drugs and their action. Can. Anaesth. Soc. J., *10*:484, 1963.
174. Corssen, G.: Neuroleptanalgesia: a new approach to protection from surgical pain. Surg. Digest, *11*:21, 1966.
175. Menzel, T.H., Langbein, L., Liebenscheutz, F., and Henneberg, U.: Postoperative vomiting and gastric reflex following aorto-femoral bypass surgery: a comparison of halothane and neuroleptanesthesia. Anaesthetist, 26:98, 1977.
176. Mandelstam, J.P.: An inquiry into the use of Innovar for pediatric premedication. Anesth. Analg., *49*:746, 1970.
177. Corssen, G.: Proper use of ketamine and Innovar. MCV Quart., *8*:85, 1972.
178. Henschel, W.F.: Pharmakologie und Technik der Neuroleptanalgesie. *In* Fortschritte der Neuroleptanalgesie. Edited by M. Gemperle. Berlin, Springer, 1966.
179. Ferrari, H.A., and Stephen, C.R.: Bronchoscopy and esophagoscopy under neuroleptanalgesia with droperidol-fentanyl. J. Thorac. Cardiovasc. Surg., *54*:143, 1967.
180. Stoffregen, J.: Einleitungs-und Ausleitungsphase der Goettinger-NLA-Infusionsnarkose unter besonderer Beruecksichtigung kurzdauernder Eingriffe. *In* Probleme der intravenoesen Anaesthesie. Edited by W.F. Henschel. Erlangen, Straube, 1976.
181. Stoffregen, J., Opitz, A., Meyer, E., and Sonntag, H.: Die NLA-Infusions Narkose. *In* Die Neuroleptanalgesie. Spezielle Probleme, Einsatz in der nicht-operativen Medizin. Teil II. Edited by W.F. Henschel. Stuttgart, Schattauer, 1972.
182. Ferrari, H.A., Fuson, R.L., and Dent, S.J.: The relationship of the anesthetic agent to postoperative analgesic requirements. South. Med. J., *62*:1201, 1969.
183. Brebner, J., and Hadley, L.: Experiences with physostigmine in the reversal of adverse postanaesthetic effects. Can. Anaesth. Soc. J., *23*:574, 1976.
184. Bidway, A.V., Cornelius, L.R., and Stanley, T.H.: Reversal of Innovar-induced postanesthetic somnolence and disorientation with physostigmine. Anesthesiology, *44*:249, 1976.
185. Thompson, D.E.A.: Physostigmine as an adjunct to neuroleptanesthesia in neurosurgical procedures. Can. Anaesth. Soc. J., *23*:582, 1976.
186. Huse, K., Hartung, E., and Nadjmabadi, M.H.: Wirkungen von Naloxone (Narcan) auf Kreislauf und Atmung nach Neuroleptanaesthesie fuer neurochirurgische Operationen. Anaesthetist, *23*:493, 1974.
187. Foldes, F.F., Keepes, E.R., Kronfeld, P.P., and Schiffman, H.P.: A rational approach to neuroleptanesthesia. Anesth. Analg., *45*:642, 1975.
188. Corssen, G., Chodoff, P., Domino, E.F., and Kahn, D.R.: Neuroleptanalgesia and anesthesia for open heart surgery. Pharmacologic rationale and clinical experience. J. Thorac. Cardiovasc. Surg., *49*:901, 1965.
189. Morpurgo, C.V.: Die Anwendung der Neuroleptanalgesie im Kindesalter. *In* Fortschritte der Neuroleptanalgesie. Edited by M. Gemperle. Berlin, Springer, 1966.
190. Kay, B.: Neuroleptanesthesia for neonates and infants. *In* Probleme der intravenoesen Anaesthesie. Edited by W.F. Henschel. Erlangen, Straube, 1976.
191. Jones, W.M., Samis, W.D., MacDonald, and Boyes, H.W.: Neuroleptanalgesia for intraocular surgery. Can. J. Ophthalmol., *4*:163, 1969.
192. Curtis, J.L.: Innovar as preoperative medication for cataract surgery. Ann. Ophthalmol., 5:1025, 1973.
193. Sloan, J.F.: Innovar as a preoperative medication. South. Med. J., *68*:1407, 1975.
194. Tait, E.C., and Tornetta, F.J.: Neuroleptanalgesia as adjunct to local anesthesia in intraocular surgery. Am. J. Ophthalmol., *59*:412, 1965.
195. Wine, N.A.: Sedation with neuroleptanalgesia in cataract surgery. Am. J. Ophthalmol., *61*:456, 1966.
196. Jones, W.M.: Neuroleptanalgesia for intraocular surgery. Can. Anesth. Soc. J., *15*:491, 1968.
197. Jones, W.M., Samis, W.D., McDonald, D.A., and Boyes, H.W.: Neuroleptanalgesia for intraocular surgery. Can. J. Ophthalmol., *4*:163, 1969.
198. Edelman, L.B., Olson, J.A., Croll, M., and Sallee, W.T.: The effect of neuroleptanalgesia on intraocular pressure. Grace Hosp. Bull., *51*:68, 1972.
199. Sarmany, B.J.: Further investigations on the effect of anaesthetics on the intraocular pressure with special reference to neuroleptic analgesia. Anaesthetist, *18*:72, 1969.
200. Jones, W.M., Fee, G.A., Bell, R.D., and Boyes, H.W.: Neuroleptanalgesia for stapes surgery. Arch. Otolaryngol., *88*:491, 1968.
201. Shea, J.: Personal communication.
202. Leslie, N.H., and Dontinon, P.J.: Neuroleptanalgesia in ear, nose and throat surgery. N. Z. Med. J., *63*:660, 1964.
203. Hutschenreuter, K., Beerhalter, E., and Beerhalter, H.: Erfahrungen mit der Neuroleptanalgesie in der Hals-Nasenohren Heilkunde. *In* Fortschritte der Neuroleptanalgesie. Edited by M. Gemperle. Berlin, Springer, 1966.

204. Manolidis, L., Manolidou, F., and Georgopoulos, G.: Narosemethoden bei Tonsillectomien und Adenoidektomien. Anaesthetist, *19*:443, 1970.
205. Watson, R., Hughes, K., Cheney, D., and Duffey, H.: A clinical and pharmacological approach to neurolepsis and its reversal in oral surgery. J. Oral Maxillofac. Surg., *29*:633, 1971.
206. Nyberg, C.D., Samartano, J.G., and Terry, R.N.: Use of Innovar as an anesthetic adjunct in oral surgery. J. Oral Maxillofac. Surg., *28*:175, 1970.
207. Boedts, D.A.A., and Vandenhove, P.T.E.: Droperidol-fentanyl citrate in equilibratory disturbances. Arch. Otolaryngol., *89*:715, 1969.
208. Vanch, M.E., Hemenway, W.G., Spindler, J., and Block, F.D.: Suppression of alcohol-induced nystagmus by Innovar. Arch. Otolaryngol., *90*:182, 1969.
209. Anand, J.S.: Awake intubation with neuroleptanalgesia in a patient with severe respiratory obstruction. Br. J. Anaesth., *46*:413, 1974.
210. Coppen, J.E., and Fox, J.W.C.: Endotracheal intubation under neuroleptanalgesia for a patient with severe haemoptysis. Anaesth. Analg., *47*:70, 1968.
211. Tahir, A.H., and Adriani, J.: General anesthesia for a patient with a full stomach. J. Am. A.N.A., *38*:112, 1970.
212. Keller, R., Waldvogel, H., and Herzog, H.: Neuroleptanalgesia for bronchoscopy examinations. Chest, *67*:315, 1975.
213. Lebrun, H.I.: Neuroleptanalgesia in upper alimentary endoscopy. Gut, *17*:655, 1976.
214. Foldes, F.F., and Maisel, W.: Neuroleptanalgesia for peroral endoscopy. Arch. Otolaryngol., *91*:280, 1970.
215. Hargrove, R.L., and Pearce, D.J.: An anaesthetic technique for bronchoscopy. Anaesthesia, *19*:226, 1964.
216. Sporel, W.E., and Chan, W.S.: Innovar in surgical anestheisa. Can. Anaesth. Soc. J., *12*:622, 1965.
217. Egel, P.M., and Gaines, H.R.: Cooperative gastrocamera study with intravenous Innovar. I.M.J., *140*:214, 1971.
218. Takahashi, K., and Iwatsuki, K.: Effects of pentazocine and fentanyl on the pulmonary hemodynamics. Tohoku J. Exp. Med., *113*:89, 1974.
219. Graham, T.P., Atwood, G.F., and Werner, B.: Use of droperidol-fentanyl sedation for cardiac catheterization in children. Am. Heart J., *87*:287, 1974.
220. Lee, C., Barnes, A., and Nagel, E.L.: Neuroleptanalgesia for awake pronation of surgical patients. Anesth. Analg., *56*:276, 1977.
221. Bridenbough, L.D., Moore, D.C., and Bridenbaugh, P.O.: Clinical experience with Innovar as post-nerve block sedation: report of 100 patients. Bull. Mason Clin., *23*:86, 1969.
222. Kennedy, W.F.: Innovar as a supplement to regional anesthesia. Anesthesiology, *31*:574, 1969.
223. McNabb, T.G., and Goldwyn, R.M.: Blood gas and hemodynamic effects of sedatives and analgesics when used as a supplement to local anesthesia in plastic surgery. Plast. Reconstr. Surg., *58*:37, 1976.
224. Schara, J.: Zur Kombination von Neuroleptanalgesie und Lokalanesthesie. *In* Fortschritte der Neuroleptanalgesie. Edited by M. Gemperle. Berlin, Springer, 1966.
225. Brindle, G.F.: The use of neuroleptic agents in neurosurgical unit. Clin. Neurosurg., *16*:234, 1969.
226. Wolfson, B., Siker, E.S., Wible, L., and Dubnansky, J.: Pneumoencephalography using neuroleptanalgesia. Anesth. Analg., *47*:14, 1968.
227. Hill, M.E., Wortzman, G., and Mashall, M.B.: Clinical use of droperidol in pneumoencephalography. Can. Med. Assoc. J., *98*:359, 1968.
228. Maini, O.P.: Anaesthetic technique for cerebral angiography. East Afr. Med. J., *46*:382, 1969.
229. Brown, A.S.: Neuroleptanalgesia. The present position for neurosurgery. Ir. J. Med. Sci., *6*:535, 1963.
230. Wins, M.H., Gonik, B., Toledo, E., and Karny, H.: Modified neuroleptanalgesia for cerebral angiography. Acta. Anesthesiol. Scand., [Suppl.], *23*:24, 1966.
231. Orr, R.B.: The use of neuroleptanalgesia during alcohol injection for tic douloureux. Lahey Clin. Found. Bull., *18*:117, 1969.
232. Jennett, W.B., McDonald, D.G., and Barker, J.: The effect of halothane on intracranial pressure in cerebral tumors, report of two cases. J. Neurosurg., *26*:270, 1967.
233. Jennett, W.B., and Barker, J.: The effect of anaesthesia on intracranial pressure in patients with space-occupying lesions. Lancet, *1*:61, 1969.
234. Boehmert, F., Aebert, K., and Plass, N.: Erfahrungen mit der Neuroleptanalgesie in der Neurochirurgie. *In* Neuroleptanalgesie. Klinik und Fortschritte. Edited by W.F. Henschel. Stuttgart, Schattauer, 1967.
235. Shinozaki, M.: Clinical study on NLA in hypothermia for intracranial surgery with special consideration of comparison with halothane and methoxyflurane. Masui, *22*:45, 1973.
236. Kampschulte, S.: Erfahrungen mit der Neuroleptanalgesie bei neurochirurgischen Eingriffen. *In* Fortschritte der Neuroleptanalgesie. Edited by M. Gemperle. Berlin, Springer, 1966.

237. Lundberg, D.M., Kjallquist, A., and Bien, C.: Reduction of increased intracranial pressure by hyperventilation: a therapeutic aid in neurosurgery. Acta Psychiatr. Scand., *34*(Suppl. 139):1, 1959.
238. Carignan, G., Keeri-Szanto, M., Lavalle, J.P., and LePage, C.: First experiences with a new anaesthetic in a teaching hospital. Anesth. Analg., *43*:560, 1964.
239. Malatinsky, J., Sramka, M., Kadlic, T., and Nadvornik, P.: Neuroleptanalgesia in some special neurosurgical operations. Rozhl. Chir., *52*:744, 1973.
240. Miller, R., Tausk, H.C., and Stark, D.C.: Effects of Innovar, fentanyl, and droperidol on the cerebrospinal fluid pressure in neurosurgical patients. Can. Anaesth. Soc. J., *22*:502, 1975.
241. Henschel, W.F.: Neuroleptanalgesie in der Neurochirurgie. *In* Fortschritte der Neuroleptanalgesie. Edited by M. Gemperle. Berlin, Springer, 1966.
242. Lillehei, R.C., Lillehei, C.W., Grismer, J.T., and Levy, M.J.: Plasma catecholamines in open heart surgery: prevention of their pernicious effects by pretreatment with dibenzyline. Surg. Forum, *14*:269, 1963.
243. Lehmann, C.: Erfahrungen mit der Neuroleptanalgesie in der Lungenchirurgie. *In* Neuroleptanalgesie. Klinik und Fortschritte. Edited by W.F. Henschel. Stuttgart, Schattauer, 1967.
244. Fox, J.W.C., Fox, E.J., and Crandell, D.L.: Neuroleptanalgesia for heart and major surgery. Arch. Surg., *94*:102, 1967.
245. Eunike, S., and Zindler, M.: Erfahrungen mit der Neuroleptanalgesie bei Operationen von Mitralstenosen. *In* Die Neuroleptanalgesie. Edited by W.F. Henschel. Berlin, Springer. 1966.
246. Grabow, L., and L'Allemand, H.: Beobachtungen bei der Anwendung der Neuroleptanalgesie in der Chirurgie des Herzens. *In* Neuroleptanalgesie. Klinik und Fortschritte. Edited by W.F. Henschel. Stuttgart, Schattauer, 1967.
247. Horatz, K., Rittmeyer, P., and Schumann, J.: Vergleichende Untersuchungen waehrend Halothannarkosen und Neuroleptanalgesien bei Operationen am offenen Herzen. *In* Neuroleptanalgesie. Klinik und Fortschritt. Edited by W.F. Henschel. Stuttgart, Schattauer, 1967.
248. Ruegheimer, E.: Zur Anwendung der Neuroleptanalgesie bei Operationen mit der Herz-Lungen Maschine. *In* Neuroleptanalgesie. Klinik und Fortschritte. Edited by W.F. Henschel. Stuttgart, Schattauer, 1967.
249. Zindler, M.: Klinische Erfahrungen mit der Neuroleptanalgesie. Neuroleptanalgesie fuer Mitralstenose Operationen. *In* Fortschritte der Neuroleptanalgesie. Edited by M. Gemperle. Berlin, Springer, 1966.
250. Corssen, G.: Neuroleptanalgesie fuer die Chirurgie am offenen Herzen. *In* Fortschritte der Neuroleptanalgesie. Edited by M. Gemperle. Berlin, Springer, 1966.
251. Fox, J.W.C., and Fox, E.J.: Neuroleptanalgesia: technique of choice for cardiac surgery. South. Med. J., *60*:1228, 1967.
252. Radnay, P.A., Rao, D.V.S., Yun, H., and Duncalf, D.: Hemodynamic changes during induction of neuroleptanesthesia for aortocoronary by-pass surgery. Anesthesiol. Rev., *3*:13, 1977.
253. Pruszynski, J.A., and Watson, R.L.: A new anesthetic for open heart surgery. J. Am. A.N.A., *35*:340, 1968.
254. Corssen, G.: Neuroleptanalgesia und extracorporaler Kreislauf. Anaesth. Resusc., *18*:130, 1966.
255. Jacobson, E., Nagashima, H., Shah, N., and Frank, H.L.: Neuroleptanesthesia for open heart surgery: a comparative study of 400 patients. Anaesthesist, *19*:16, 1970.
256. Reves, J.G., Samuelson, P.N., Younes, H.J., and Lell, W.A.: Anesthetic considerations for coronary artery surgery. Anesthesiol. Rev. 19, August, 1977.
257. Zadeck, P.: Die Neuroleptanalgesie als Anaesthesieverfahren zur Schrittmacherimplantation. *In* Neuroleptanalgesie. Klinik und Fortschritte. Edited by W.F. Henschel. Stuttgart, Schattauer, 1967.
258. Lutz, H., and Mueller, C.: Erfahrungen mit der Neuroleptanalgesie bei Gedfaessoperationen. *In* Neuroleptanalgesie. Klinik und Fortschritte. Edited by W.F. Henschel. Stuttgart, Schattauer, 1967.
259. Corssen, G., and Chodoff, P.: Clinical management of the patient in shock: neuroleptanalgesia. Clin. Anesth., *2*:137, 1965.
260. Prinzhorn, G.: Zur Anwendung der Neuroleptanalgesie unter Katastrophen Bedingungen. *In* Neuroleptanalgesie. Klinik und Fortschritte. Edited by W.F. Henschel. Stuttgart, Schattauer, 1967.
261. Whitmann, J.G., and Russell, W.J.: The acute cardiovascular changes and adrenergic blockade by droperidol in man. Br. J. Anaesth., *43*:581, 1971.
262. Clarke, A.D., Tobias, M.A., and Challen, P.D.P.: The use of neuroleptanalgesia during surgery of pheochromocytoma. Br. J. Anaesth., *44*:1093, 1972.
263. Ogawa, R., and Fujita, T.: Neuroleptanesthesia for the surgery of pheochromocytoma. Masui, *21*:174, 1972.
264. Kaniak, J.: A case of emergency surgical removal of a phaeochromocytoma under type II neuroleptanalgesia (NLA II). Pol. Tyg. Lek., *24*:602, 1969.

265. Simone, M., Barusco, G., and Coan, B.: Impiego della NLA tipo II nel traffamento chirurgico del feocromocitoma. Acta Anesthesiologica, *19*:233, 1968.
266. Yusa, T., Hashimoto, Y., and Shima, T.: Droperidol and pheochromocytoma. Masui, 22:474, 1973.
267. Gotoh, F., Miyashita, K., and Ogawa, R.: Anesthesia for pheochromocytoma: roles of catecholamines and histamine. Masui, 22:1293, 1973.
268. Sumikawa, K., and Amakata, Y.: The pressor effect of droperidol on a patient with pheochromocytoma. Anesthesiology, *46*:359, 1977.
269. Trudnowski, R.J., Mostert, J.W., Hobika, G.H., and Rico, R.: Neuroleptanalgesia for patients with kidney malfunction. Anesth. Analg., 50:679, 1971.
270. Gutierrez, F.A., Gutierrez, J.F., and Corssen, G.: Neuroleptanesthesia for renal transplantation. Proceedings of the 6th World Congress of Anesthesiology, Mexico City, 1976.
271. Radakovic, D.: Erfahrungen mit der Neuroleptanalgesie bei Operationen an Gallenblase und Gallenwegen. *In* Neuroleptanalgesie. Klinik und Fortschritte. Edited by W.F. Henschel. Stuttgart, Schattauer, 1967.
272. Uray, E., and Kosa, C.: Wirkung der bei der Neuroleptanalgesie verwendeten Medikamente auf die Druckwerte der Gallenwege. Anaesthesist, *18*:76, 1969.
273. Kantor, E., Jakab, T., and Szabo, L.: Influence of neuroleptic-analgesia on the tonus of the sphincter of Oddi. Anaesthesist, *18*:183, 1969.
274. Hunter, J.M., Schneider, L.H., Dumont, J.D., and Erickson, J.C.: A dynamic approach to problems of hand function, using local anesthesia supplemented by intravenous fentanyl-droperidol. Clin. Orthop., *104*:112, 1974.
275. Corssen, G.: Neuroleptanalgesia and anesthesia in obstetrics. Clin. Obstet. Gynecol., *17*:241, 1974.
276. Friss, E., Schaedlich, M., Neumann, G., and Trunschke, D.: Stellenwertsbestimmung der geburtshilflichen Neuroleptanalgesie. Anaesthesiol. Reanimat., 6:115, 1981.
277. Wuller, E.G., Inmon, B.L., and Smith, B.E.: Innovar in obstetrics: preliminary report. Proceedings of the Southern Society of Anesthesiology, Houston, March, 1971.
278. Ovadia, L., and Halbrecht, I.: Neuroleptanalgesia. A new method of analgesia in normal childbirth. Harefuah, 72:143, 1967.
279. Weiss, V.: Thalamonaltropfinfusion fuer geburtshilfliche Analgesie. Anaesthesist, 20:56, 1971.
280. Larson, J.V., Barker, A., Barker, M., and Brown, R.S.: A technique combining neurolept-analgesia with local analgesia for caesarean section. S. Afr. Med. J., *45*:750, 1971.
281. Vogel, W.: Die Neuroleptanalgesia in der Langzeitbehandlung. *In* Neuroleptanalgesie. Klinik und Fortschritte. Edited by W.F. Henschel. Stuttgart, Schattauer, 1967.
282. Schorer, R., Kettler, D., und Stoffregen, J.: Erste Erfahrungen ueber die Langzeitbehandlung von Tetanuskranken mit hohen Dosen Thalamonal. *In* Die Neuroleptanalgesie. Edited by W.F. Henschel. Berlin, Springer, 1966.
283. Greiffenhagen, M., and Plass, N.: Der Einsatz von Neuroleptanalgesiesubstanzen in der Behandlung des schweren Tetanus. Anaesthesist, 20:449, 1971.
284. Bloomquist, E.R.: A synergistic danger in ketamine and Innovar. Calif. Med., *115*:64, 1971.
285. Brown, A.S.: Neuroleptanalgesia for the surgical treatment of parkinsonism. Anaesthesia, *19*:70, 1964.

Chapter 9

THE BENZODIAZEPINES

HISTORY

Through the pioneering research of Leo H. Sternbach, the benzodiazepines were introduced for synthesis and study.[1] In May of 1957, Sternbach delivered the first member of the benzodiazepine group of drugs, chlordiazepoxide (Librium), to Lowell O. Randall for pharmacologic testing. The compound elicited a broad spectrum of anxiolytic, sedative, hypnotic, amnesic, muscle relaxant, and anticonvulsant properties. Several researchers also reported a calming effect of chlordiazepoxide on anxiety and tension.[2–5]

Brandt and colleagues, the first anesthesiologists involved in the clinical evaluation of chlordiazepoxide, employed the drug as a tranquilizer as part of pre-anesthetic medication.[6] Meanwhile, Sternbach synthesized other benzodiazepines, all similar in action but different in potency. The most promising and most potent compound, diazepam (Valium), was similarly scrutinized by Randall and associates, for use in psychiatric patients. Then DuCailar, et al., and Campan and Espagno gave diazepam to surgical patients to allay preoperative apprehension.[7–10] Subsequently, the suitability of diazepam as an induction agent for general anesthesia was explored in France, Norway, England, and Canada.[11–15] Workers in France also used it in neuroleptanalgesia (NLA) both for induction and as a component of the NLA mixture.[12,16,17] Other studies of the utility of diazepam as an anxiolytic in labor and as an anticonvulsant and sedative in the management of eclampsia, status epilepticus, and tetanus rapidly followed.[18–23]

More recently, diazepam proved to be effective in "taming" the undesirable psychotomimetic side-effects of ketamine.[24] Diazepam remains the standard and most widely used benzodiazepine, despite its marked disadvantages, which include relatively slow onset and long duration of action, insolubility in water, venous irritation, and complications after bolus intravenous injections.

Understandably, many benzodiazepines have since been synthesized, tested, and for the most part discarded in the never-ending search for better drugs. Some of the survivors appear in Figure 9–1. Noteworthy among these agents are nitrazepam (Mogadon), an early discovery, and flurazepam (Dalmane), both well-established as hypnotic agents; the potent sedative lorazepam (Ativan); the anxiolytic, sedative, hypnotic, amnesic midazolam (Dobralam), a drug of special interest because it is water soluble; the short-lasting triazolam (Halcion); and the benzodiazepine metabolites desmethyldiazepam (Nadar) and oxazepam (Serax), now being clinically employed as active drugs.

Another exciting development is the synthesis of the imidazodiazepine Ro 15-1788 (Fig. 9–2), which is currently under study as a benzodiazepine antagonist.

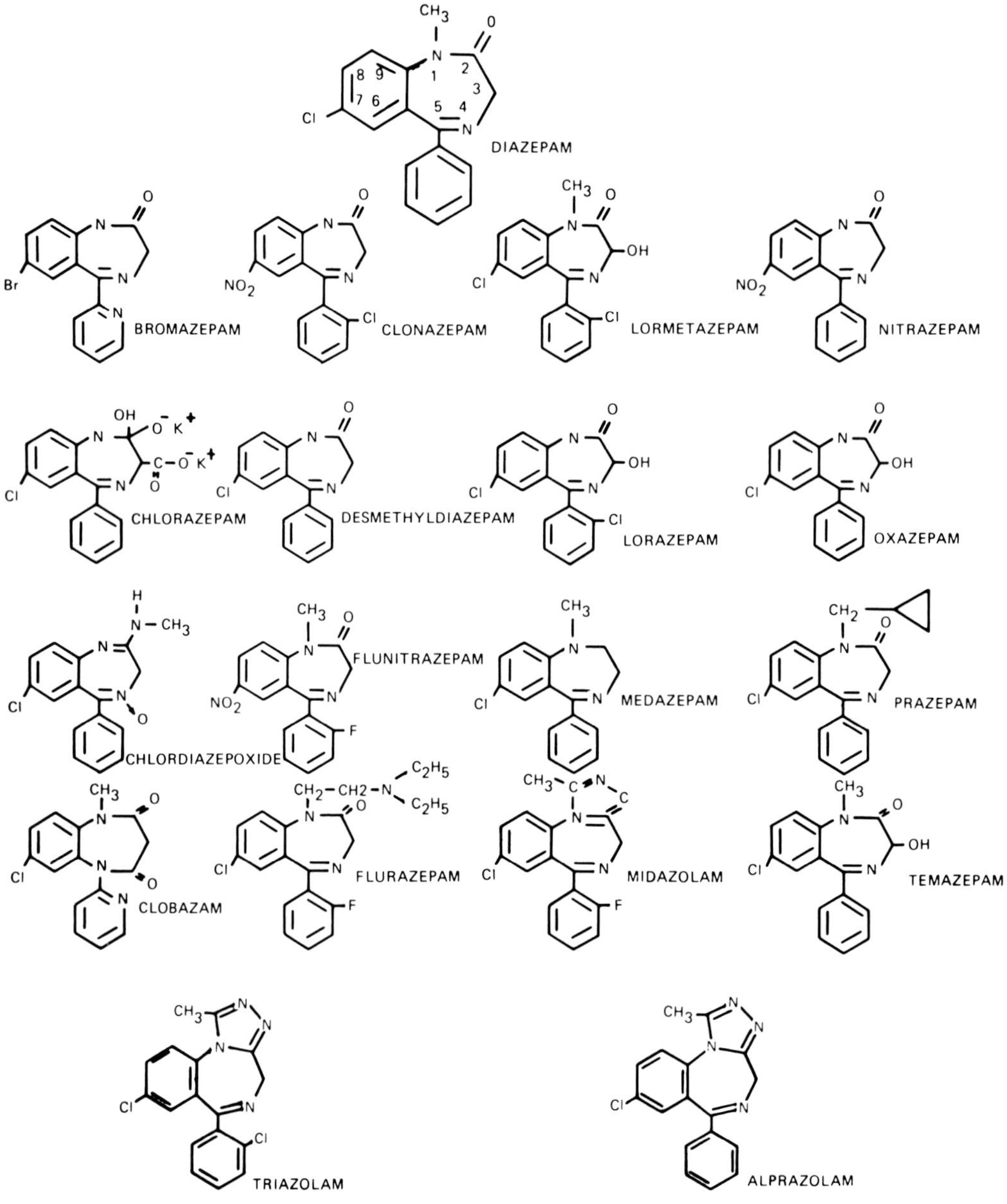

Fig. 9–1. Diazepam and 18 other diazepines.

GENERAL CONSIDERATIONS

The benzodiazepines have been termed "minor tranquilizers," but this definition is misleading. Not only do they differ markedly from the antipsychotic drugs ("major tranquilizers"), but also their use is by no means minor.[25] Chemically, the benzodiazepines share certain features: (1) the benzodiazepines ring system (numbered 1 to 9 in Fig. 9–1); (2) two nitrogen atoms in that ring, usually in positions 1 and 4 (but not always, e.g., clobazam, Fig. 9–1); (3) a phenyl group in position 5; and (4) an electronegative group (usually chlorine, occasionally

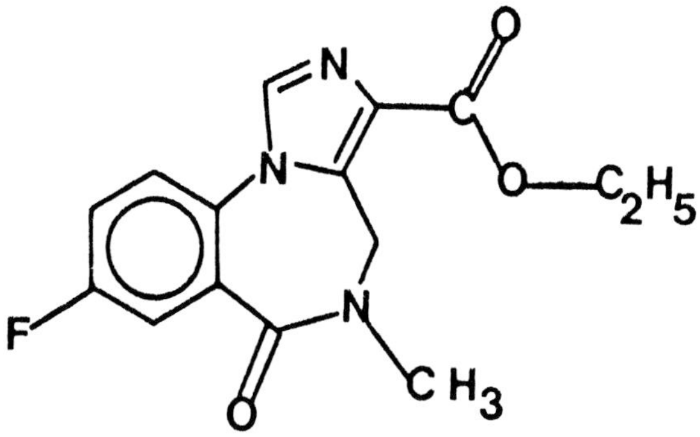

Fig. 9–2. Ro 15-1788, a benzodiazepine receptor blocker.

bromine or nitroso) in position 7.[1,26] Pharmacologically, all of the benzodiazepines exhibit the spectrum of properties mentioned previously for chlordiazepoxide.[2] They do, however, differ in potency and pharmacokinetics.

Most benzodiazepines are metabolized by hepatic microsomal enzymes, primarily by oxidation (hydroxylation), demethylation to active metabolites, or a combination of the two processes. The hydroxylated metabolites (and some of the parent benzodiazepines) undergo conjugation with either or both glucuronic and sulfuric acids. These conjugates are then excreted by the kidneys. This function is one of housekeeping, not detoxification, however, in that the conjugates are already inactive. Some inactive parent benzodiazepines, the so-called "pro-drugs" (e.g., clorazepate and prazepam), are also converted to active metabolites.[27,28]

The criterion of elimination half-life ($t\frac{1}{2}\ \beta$) enables the benzodiazepines to be classified as short-acting and long-acting drugs (Tables 9–1 and 9–2).[26] Note that a parent compound with a short half-life is classified as long-acting if it has one or more major active metabolites of long duration. In addition, the wide ranges shown in Tables 9–1 and 9–2 indicate considerable interpatient variation, so that therapeutic plasma concentrations are difficult to define.[29]

MECHANISM OF ACTION

Benzodiazepines appear to facilitate the inhibitory effect of γ-aminobutyric acid (GABA) on neuronal transmission at the limbic, thalamic, hypothalamic, and

Table 9–1.

Drug		t ½ beta (hour)	Active Metabolites	Protein Binding (%)	References
Generic Name	Trade Name				
Alprazolam		6–20	Alpha-hydroxyalprazolam	80	257
Lorazepam	Ativan	10–22	None	97	48, 211–217
Midazolam	Dobralam Dornicum	1.6–2.6	None	96	153–161 29, 75, 107
Oxazepam	Serax Lactam Serenid	3–21	None	87	29, 251, 252
Temazepam	Restoril	10–21	None	96–98	29, 256
Triazolam	Halcion	1.7–3.0	None	90	29, 254, 255

Table 9–2.

Drug		t ½ beta (hour)	Active Metabolites	Protein Binding (%)	References
Generic Name	Trade Name				
Chlordiaze-poxide	Librium	18–18	Demoxepam Desmethylchlordiazepoxide Desmethyldiazepam Oxazepam	94–97	29, 240–245
Clonazepam	Clonopin	18–50	None	47	29
Clorazepate	Trapene	30–200	Desmethyldiazepam (chlorazepate is pro-drug)	97	29
Desmethyl-diazepam	Nordiazepam Nadar	30–200	None	97	29, 249, 250
Diazepam	Valium	30–60	Desmethyldiazepam 3-Hydroxydiazepam Oxazepam	96–99	25, 43–45, 47–51 65, 66, 125
Flunitrazepam	Rohypnol	14–19	7-Amino, 3-hydroxyl, N-Desmethyl flunitrazepam	80	196–201
Flurazepam	Dalmane	203	Desalkylflurazepam	88	29, 200, 201, 253
Nitrazepam	Mogadone	24–31	None	88–97	233, 234
Prazepam	Centrax	30–200	Hydroxyprazepam Desmethyldiazepam (pro-drug) Oxazepam	90	29

spinal levels of the central nervous system (CNS).[30–34] (Previous observations of benzodiazepine inhibition of the specific binding of tritiated strychnine, a glycine antagonist, to glycine receptors suggested a glycine-mimetic action of the drugs at brain stem synapses.[35] When results of electrophysiologic studies were non-confirmatory, the glycine hypothesis was abandoned).[36]

The benzodiazepine-GABA interaction is depicted in Figure 9–3 as a complex of proteins, GABA receptor (GABA-R protein), benzodiazepine receptor (BDZ-R protein), and chloride channel proteins, respectively.[37] Each of these proteins in turn contains a binding domain for GABA agonists and antagonists, benzodiazepine agonists and antagonists (BDZ), and barbiturates (BABB); the barbiturate domain also binds picrotoxin and the convulsant benzodiazepine Ro 5-3663. The large, heavy arrow (1) indicates that activation of the GABA receptor leads to opening of the chloride channel, a process involving the benzodiazepine receptor as a putative coupling protein. The coupling function and resultant channel opening are enhanced by benzodiazepine agonists (2) and are impaired by inverse agonists (3); pure competitive antagonists do not affect coupling but do block the effects of both direct and inverse agonists. Arrows 4 and 5 indicate, respectively, that benzodiazepine agonists enhance GABA binding and that GABA agonists increase the binding of benzodiazepine agonists. Barbiturates enhance the coupling process (1) near or at the chloride channel (6), and when present in sufficiently high concentrations open the channel directly (7); they also enhance GABA binding (8).[37]

Benzodiazepine receptor proteins have been visualized autoradiographically by

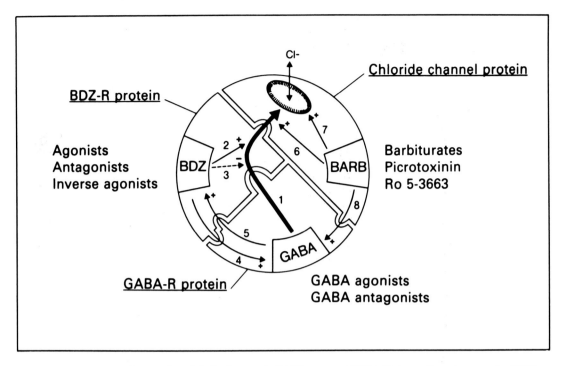

Fig. 9–3. Proposed model of subsynaptic GABA receptor (GABA-R)-benzodiazepine receptor (BDZ-R)-chloride channel complex.(From Polc, P., Bonetti, E.P., Schaffner, R., and Haefely, W.: A three-state model of the benzodiazepine receptor explains the interactions between the benzodiazepine antagonist Ro 15-1788, benzodiazepine tranquilizers, B = carbolines, and phenobarbitone. Naunyn. Schmiedebergs. Arch. Pharmacol., *321*:260, 1982.)

using an electron microscope. Under the influence of ultraviolet radiation, in a process termed photoaffinity labeling, the receptor proteins are coupled to benzodiazepine ligands (e.g., clonazepam and flunitrazepam) containing a nitro group in position 7 (Fig. 9–1).[38] When photoaffinity labeling with ³H-flunitrazepam was combined with immunocytochemical demonstration of the GABA-synthesizing enzyme GAD (glutamic acid decarboxylase), the benzodiazepine binding sites were localized at GABA-ergic synapses.[39]

Specific benzodiazepine binding sites have been demonstrated with the use of the tritiated benzodiazepine receptor blocker Ro 15-1788 (Fig. 9–2) in various areas of rat brain by means of light-microscope autoradiography (Fig. 9–4).[40–42] Although these sites are not necessarily identical to the binding domains of pharmacologically active benzodiazepine receptors, the likelihood of a close similarity is great.[42] Thus, benzodiazepines that are active in vivo inhibit the binding of ³H-diazepam to a CNS membrane preparation, whereas inactive pro-drugs or metabolites do not. Overall, the correlation between in vivo potency of benzodiazepine tranquilizers and their in vitro affinity for specific binding sites is good.[42]

The speculation arises that the existence of specific receptors for benzodiazepines (and barbiturates) might correspondingly imply the existence of naturally occurring ligands that mediate sedation and other useful physiologic functions (cf. the opiate receptors and the endorphins). To date none has been identified.

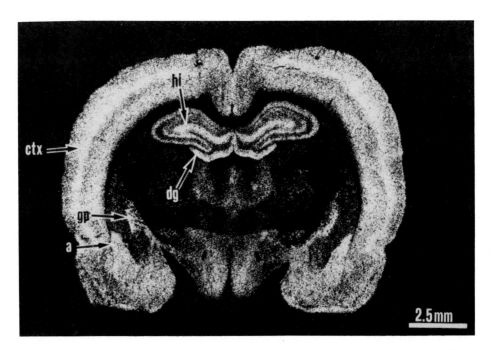

Fig. 9–4. Benzodiazepine binding sites in rat brain. Slide-mounted cryostat sections were incubated with tritiated Ro 15-1788 for 40 minutes at 4°C, washed, rapidly dried, then exposed to LKB ultrafilm 10 to 14 days at 4°C. *White areas,* binding sites in cerebral cortex (ctx), hippocampus (hi), dentate gyrus (DG), globus pallidus (gp), and lateral amygdala (a).

DIAZEPAM (VALIUM)

Chemistry and Physical Properties

Diazepam (7-chloro-1, 3-dihydro-1-methyl-5-phenyl-2*H*-1, 4-benzodiazepine-2-one) (Fig. 9–1) is insoluble in water but is highly lipid soluble, with an octanol-water partition coefficient of 840.[43,44] The injectable solution, the pH of which is about 6.6, contains diazepam compounded with propylene glycol and ethyl alcohol as solvents, sodium benzoate and benzoic acid as buffers, and benzyl alcohol as a preservative. All such contents irritate the veins, so that a bolus intravenous injection is painful. Dilution in a syringe or infusion flask with other solutions produces a cloudy emulsion of small particulate matter.

Pharmacokinetics

BIOTRANSFORMATION

Diazepam is metabolized by microsomal enzymes in the liver. The drug is demethylated to desmethyldiazepam or is hydroxylated to 3-hydroxydiazepam, which is then demethylated to oxazepam (Fig. 9–1).[45,46] All of these metabolites are pharmacologically active and are commercially available as drugs in their own right.

Diazepam has a relatively long distribution half-life (t½ α) of 30 to 60 minutes, whereas its elimination half-life (t½ β) ranges from 20 to 50 hours, with total clearance of only 0.24 to 0.53 ml/kg/minute.[25] The drug has a moderate volume of distribution (V_d) (0.7 to 1.7 L/kg), but it is widely distributed into body tissue.

Diazepam is extensively protein bound (96 to 99%), but this high degree of protein binding may be reduced by instituting competitive binding, e.g., with pentazocine.[45,46]

Diazepam and all of its active metabolites have long half-lives. Indeed, its primary active metabolite, desmethyldiazepam, has the lowest clearance and the longest half-life of any benzodiazepine currently employed (Table 9–2). Consequently, large quantities of these compounds accumulate with chronic ingestion. Diazepam is well absorbed from the gastrointestinal tract; peak plasma levels are achieved within 30 to 90 minutes of ingestion.[47,48] Concurrent therapy with cimetidine, a hepatic enzyme inhibitor, prolongs the hypnotic effect of diazepam.[49] Note that the administration of heparin, such as for use during cardiopulmonary bypass, displaces diazepam from protein, significantly increasing the free (active) diazepam fraction in plasma. Interestingly, after diazepam (10 or 20 mg intravenously) was administered to volunteers, plasma levels of the drug declined rapidly during the first 20 minutes, but then rose to a second peak 6 to 8 hours later.[50] The rise is attributed to enterohepatic recirculation.[51]

ABSORPTION

For reasons that are not entirely clear, absorption of diazepam after an intramuscular injection may occasionally be poor and erratic, with subsequent plasma concentrations that are only 50 to 60% of those attained after the administration of an equivalent oral dose.[44,47,48] This disparity may be due in part to the precipitation of diazepam at the site of intramuscular injection as the organic solvents are absorbed;[52] this action also may contribute to persistent pain at the injection site. The site of injection and the associated muscle activity may also influence the kinetics of absorption. After drug injection into the gluteal muscles, plasma levels are invariably lower than those after injection into the vastus lateralis or deltoid muscles; in both of the latter locations, exercise augments drug absorption.[53]

BLOOD LEVELS AND NEUROPHARMACOLOGIC ACTIVITY

Minimal clinical effects of sleepiness, amnesia, blurred vision, impaired mental function, and lack of coordination are observed in patients with blood levels of diazepam below 400 µg/L. Sleep occurs at levels of approximately 1000 µg/L, but individual responses vary widely, e.g., at the same blood level, one patient may be difficult to arouse while another remains wide awake.

PLACENTAL TRANSFER

The highly lipid-soluble diazepam rapidly crosses the placenta, so that equilibrium between maternal and umbilical cord blood occurs within minutes.[18,54–56] Because of enhanced plasma protein binding of diazepam in the fetus, concentrations of the drug in fetal blood usually exceed those in the mother.[54,57] Interestingly, the high levels of diazepam observed in two neonates, whose eclamptic mothers had received large doses of the drug during labor, continued to rise for 40 hours after birth before declining, and remained detectable for almost 1 week.[58]

CONDITIONS AFFECTING PHARMACOKINETICS OF DIAZEPAM

Age. Increasing age influences the $t\frac{1}{2}\beta$ of diazepam almost linearly, the range extending from 20 hours at age 20 years to 90 hours at age 80 years.[44,59]

Gender. The $t\frac{1}{2}$ β, V_d, and clearance of diazepam are all greater in female patients than in male patients.[45,60]

Race. The V_d and clearance of diazepam are greater in Caucasians than in Orientals, suggesting genetic differences in the biotransformation of the drug.[61]

Liver Disease. In patients with alcoholic cirrhosis, the $t\frac{1}{2}$ β of diazepam may be markedly increased; plasma clearance may be correspondingly decreased. These effects are attributed to decreased liver blood flow and diminished drug exposure to hepatic microsomal enzymes.[59] Binding to plasma proteins is also significantly decreased, resulting in an increase in V_d.[59]

Hepatic Enzyme Induction and Inhibition. Diazepam is an inducer of hepatic microsomal enzyme activity, thereby increasing the rate of its own biotransformation.[59] Cimetidine, a hepatic enzyme inhibitor, significantly impairs the metabolism of diazepam by prolonging its $t\frac{1}{2}$ β and reducing plasma clearance of the drug.[49] Curiously, in one study, the administration of diazepam to patients on "subchronic" diazepam therapy markedly increased $t\frac{1}{2}$ β and significantly decreased total clearance.[62] These effects, attributed to the inhibition of oxidation caused by accumulation of the oxidative metabolite desmethyldiazepam, were not reproduced in other studies.[63]

Renal Disease. The pharmacokinetics of diazepam may be altered by chronic renal disease.[64]

Pharmacology

The pharmacologic effects of diazepam are dose related: the larger the dose, the greater, more rapid, and longer-lasting is the response. Rapid intravenous injection, undesirable for its irritant effects on veins, results in presentation of higher drug concentrations to the brain, tantamount to larger dosage; the effect, however, is transient. The effects of chronic diazepam therapy are cumulative, because of its $t\frac{1}{2}$ β.[65] The effect is aggravated by the concomitant accumulation of its active metabolites, all long in action (Table 9–2).[65,66]

CENTRAL NERVOUS SYSTEM (CNS)

Diazepam can cause all degrees of CNS depression, from mild sedation to deep coma, presumably by facilitating the inhibitory effect of GABA on neuronal transmission.[30] Prime sites of action are the reticular facilitatory and limbic systems.[67–71] The thalamus and hypothalamus are also involved.[29] The amygdala, concerned with emotional influences on cortical activity, appears to be particularly affected.[72] Diazepam reduces anxiety and aggression, in both animals and man. Consequently, the drug is widely used in the treatment of psychiatric disorders, to provide preanesthetic sedation, to induce anesthesia in patients at risk from cardiovascular disease, and to reduce the undesirable side-effects of phencyclidine derivatives.[8,13,24,73,74]

Patients vary considerably in their response to diazepam, especially when it is combined with other CNS depressants, such as opiates and barbiturates.[75] Consequently, there are specific plasma benzodiazepine thresholds for the multiple pharmacodynamic effect of benzodiazepines, as illustrated in Figure 9–5.[75] Recovery from the diazepam-induced hypnotic effects occurs because of rapid redistribution of the drug. A patient awakening from an acute administration of the drug, however, may be amnesic for certain events during recovery, because blood levels still exceed the amnesic therapeutic blood level. The amnesia pro-

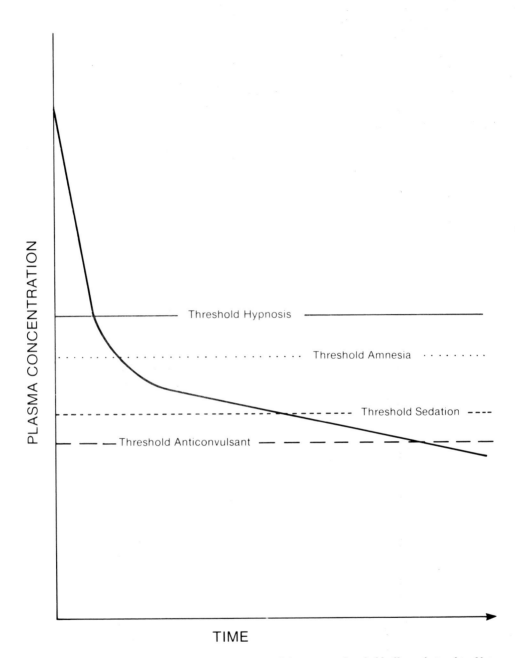

Fig. 9–5. Benzodiazepine plasma concentration and therapeutic threshold effect relationship. Note each pharmacodynamic effect has a different plasma drug concentration threshold. Each benzodiazepine has a specific plasma decay curve and therapeutic threshold. (From Reves, J.G.: Benzodiazepines. *In* Pharmacokinetics of Anesthesia. Edited by C. Prys-Roberts and C.C. Hug. Oxford, Blackwell, 1984.

duced by diazepam has been studied extensively relative to use of the drug in dentistry, cardioversion, endoscopy, and during recovery from open-heart surgery.[76-80]

The route of administration is important. The vagaries of absorption from an intramuscular depot render this route unreliable, which may explain conflicting reports of nearly total or minimal (less than 5%) preoperative amnesia after doses of 10 to 20 mg delivered intramuscularly.[81,82] With the intravenous administration of diazepam, however, antegrade, but not retrograde, amnesia is readily achieved.[83-85] Even with the preferred intravenous route, however, the onset of action is slower (2 to 3 minutes) than with the use of anesthetic barbiturates.[13] The dose-dependent effects (2.5 to 20 mg intravenously) produce levels of anxiolysis and sedation that increase linearly; interestingly, amnesia itself seems not to occur until large doses (10 to 20 mg intravenously) are administered.[86]

Diazepam is not an analgesic drug, although it may provide slight relief from the experimental pain of tibial pressure.[87] It has no antanalgesic effects.[87]

Chronic tolerance (i.e., habituation) to the CNS depressant effects of diazepam may develop with continued oral therapy.[88,89] Acute tolerance (i.e., after a single large dose) has also been observed after attempted suicide with diazepam (oral dose of 0.5 to 2.0 g); recovery occurred within 2 to 3 days despite initial plasma levels 100 times greater than those usually observed.[90]

CARDIOVASCULAR SYSTEM

Studies of diazepam use conducted in animals revealed no significant cardiovascular effects.[7] Augmented myocardial contractility observed in dogs was attributed to increased coronary blood flow and transiently decreased systemic vascular resistance, the latter probably explaining the light hypotensive response (-24 mm Hg) observed after diazepam (8 to 15 mg/kg) was given intravenously over a 3-hour period.[91,92] Correspondingly, diazepam does not significantly alter cardiovascular homeostasis in man, thus rendering the drug particularly useful for sedation and induction of anesthesia in patients with severe cardiopulmonary disease.[75,93-108] A further contribution made by diazepam to such patients is a nitroglycerine-like action on the coronary vessels, which preserves coronary blood flow and cardiac index despite decreases in systemic perfusion pressure.[99] Total myocardial oxygen consumption is markedly reduced after diazepam therapy, because of the decrease in the heart rate-systolic blood pressure product.[99] Nevertheless, the potential for hemodynamic depression does exist in patients with ischemic or valvular heart disease and in other individuals receiving diazepam with narcotics intravenously.[109] This reaction may reflect the sympatholytic action of such a combination.[110] Cardiovascular collapse and ventricular arrhythmias have been reported to be related to the use of diazepam, but these sequelae are most unusual.[111,112]

MUSCULOSKELETAL SYSTEM

Diazepam-induced relaxation of skeletal muscle is produced by inhibition of afferent spinal polysynaptic (and possibly monosynaptic) pathways.[29] This inhibition may occur directly at the level of the spinal cord. In one study conducted in unanesthetized cats, diazepam produced marked enhancement of the dorsal root reflex, presynaptic inhibition, and prolongation of synaptic recovery time.[113]

Other investigators attribute the effect to descending inhibition from supraspinal structures, e.g., the reticular facilitatory and limbic systems.[68–71]

Diazepam is capable of controlling muscle rigidity and spasm due to tetanus, low-back pain, or neurologic disorders.[29,114,115] The drug does not appreciably add to the action of neuromuscular blocking agents.[13,116]

RESPIRATORY SYSTEM

Diazepam, when delivered intravenously, may cause moderate respiratory depression, with decreases in tidal and minute volumes of 20 to 30%.[13] These effects are clinically unimportant, although severe depression of respiratory function, including apnea, has been reported with the use of diazepam.[117] This result, however, is exceptional. Neither arterial blood gas determination nor the respiratory response to CO_2 challenge is significantly altered by diazepam given in usual doses.[118–121] Other parameters, e.g., peak expiratory flow and airway resistance, remain unaffected, rendering diazepam a useful sedative for patients receiving ventilator therapy for status asthmaticus.[122] Combinations of diazepam and narcotic analgesics given intravenously for general anesthesia often cause profound respiratory depression, occurring predominantly after initiation of preanesthetic medication with these drugs.[109,123] Similar potentiation of diazepam-induced respiratory depression by barbiturates has been observed during treatment of prolonged seizure activity.[124]

Toxicity and Side-Effects

In dogs, repeated administration of diazepam (ten 20-mg injections over a period of 2 weeks) did not result in severe toxic reactions, with the exception of local irritation at the site of injection when administered intramuscularly.[125] In subacute toxicity studies, also conducted in dogs, no gross pathologic changes were recorded. When diazepam was administered to dogs in very large doses over a period of 22 months, no abnormalities in liver or kidney function or hematologic and histopathologic tests were recorded.[125]

The most important undesirable side-effect associated with the intravenous use of diazepam is venous irritation. An intravenous bolus injection of diazepam is painful ("that burns"). This irritation is caused by the solvents contained in the injectable solution, namely propylene glycol, benzyl and ethyl alcohols, sodium benzoate, and benzoic acid, components that irritate veins with attendant hazzards of thrombosis, phlebitis, and sclerosis. The warnings from the manufacturer state, "The solution should be injected slowly. . . .do not use small veins, such as those on the dorsum of the hand or wrist. . . .if it is not feasible to administer Valium directly IV, it may be injected slowly through the infusion tubing as close as possible to the vein insertion."[126]

The "puff technique" for the administration of diazepam is somewhat at variance with these warnings, but nevertheless is uniquely designed to obviate the hazards.[127] A 22-gauge needle attached to a syringe containing the drug is inserted into the most proximal (i.e., farthest from the patient) injection port of a rapidly flowing intravenous line. After commenting to the patient, "This may feel slightly warm at the hand (or wrist)," the anesthesiologist holds the barrel of the syringe in one hand and proceeds to tap rapidly and forcefully with the index or middle finger of the other hand on the plunger of the syringe. Because of the viscosity of the solution and the deliberately chosen small bore of the needle, only an infinitesimal amount of diazepam is extruded with each tap, perceptible in the infusion solution as a tiny opalescent cloud (the "puff") quickly swept along in the flowing stream. Indeed, the individual puffs are so small that at first the plunger appears immobile. Only after repeated puffs does its slow advance become perceptible. Several minutes of this tapping are required to deliver the desired dose, maximally diluted, with minimal discomfort to the patient (the slight warmth at the hand or wrist sites is usually absent if larger veins in the forearm or antecubital fossa are used) and minimal incidence of undesirable sequelae.

Clinical Applications

All benzodiazepines exhibit the spectrum of anxiolytic, sedative, hypnotic, amnesic, muscle relaxant, anticonvulsant effects first noted with chlordiazepoxide.[2] Pharmacokinetic differences may influence the choice of drug. Limiting factors of diazepam are its insolubility in water and the long duration of action of both the parent drug and the metabolites. Varying individual responses to the drug should be taken into consideration, as well as the route of administration. Thus, for rapid and dependable action, diazepam should be given orally (gastrointestinal absorption is complete) or intravenously rather than intramuscularly, because its absorption from an intramuscular depot is slow and less reliable.[44] Dosage should be reduced in elderly patients, in individuals with kidney and liver disease, and in patients taking the hepatic enzyme inhibitor, cimetidine.[44,49,59,60,63]

PREANESTHETIC MEDICATION

The amnesic and tranquilizing actions of diazepam in the preoperative period are beneficial to the anxious patient. The drug may be administered in doses of 5 to 20 mg intramuscularly well in advance of surgical procedures (60 to 90 minutes) to allow for the vagaries of absorption.[123,128] Alternatively, it may be given orally with a teaspoon of water (30 to 45 minutes in advance) or, if time is too short, it may be delivered intravenously, preferably using the aforementioned puff technique, as soon as an intravenous line has been established.

SUPPLEMENTATION OF LOCAL ANESTHESIA

Diazepam administered preoperatively is similarly a useful adjuvant to local, regional, or topical anesthesia, e.g., for endoscopy, conservative dentistry, and indeed for any operation during which the patient is awake.[76,79] An important caveat is that the regional or topical procedure must be meticulously performed; diazepam is intended to provide only light sedation and amnesia, and not to eliminate the deficits of inadequate anesthesia.

Other applications include dissociative anesthesia, in which premedication with diazepam significantly reduces the incidence and severity of the psychotomimetic side-effects of ketamine (see Chapter 7), and psychiatry, for which diazepam is used as a preinterview medication (suggested dosages are 10 to 30 mg intravenously).[129]

INDUCTION OF ANESTHESIA

Despite a slower onset of action, with slight to moderate respiratory depression, a lack of flexibility as compared to the anesthetic barbiturates, and irritant effects on the venous wall often associated with pain during injection, the cardiovascular stability observed with diazepam renders it a useful induction agent for severely ill cardiac patients and other individuals at high risk of complications.[15,104,105] An added bonus is the excellent pre- and postoperative amnesia associated with its use.[13,75] Note that, with hypovolemia and cardiac tamponade, hypotension and reduced cardiac output may follow induction with diazepam.[105]

Diazepam dosage for induction of anesthesia ranges from 0.3 to 0.6 mg/kg intravenously. Bolus injection of such doses is more predictable with regard to the hypnotic effect, but it may produce either or both undesirable hypotension and apnea.[104–106] Delivery of these divided doses of 5 mg at approximately 1-minute intervals until the patient is asleep is recommended by some clinicians.

Sedation and slurring of speech usually precede full onset of sleep. Larger doses (up to 70 mg), although still maintaining cardiovascular stability, may result in a prolonged (as many as 24 hours) recovery, which is undesirable in ambulatory patients and in most surgical patients.[87]

ENDOSCOPY

Diazepam is a useful supplement to topical anesthesia for endoscopic procedures because of its amnesic and modest muscle relaxant effects; the former ensures patient acceptance of a repeat procedure.[79,130,131] Pulmonary aspiration, reported with esophagogastroscopy, may be avoided by meticulous adherence to preprocedural fasting precautions.[132,133]

SOMNOANALGESIA

A mixture of the sedative diazepam (30 mg) and the analgesic pentazocine (90 mg), diluted with glucose or saline (250 ml), is termed "pentazepam," and may be administered by infusion to produce a state of "somnoanalgesia."[134,135] Pentazepam is a useful supplement to regional or topical anesthesia for such surgical procedures as inguinal herniorrhaphy, bronchoscopy, laparoscopy, and tubal ligation.[135] In patients at risk with a full stomach, somnoanalgesia offers the added advantage of maintaining intact laryngeal function in the patient who must be awake during intubation.

Initially, pentazepam may be infused fairly rapidly, e.g., 30 to 50 ml/minute, until somnoanalgesia is established. The patient appears to sleep but obeys commands and tolerates pinprick stimulation. The infusion is then slowed to 4 ml/minute until signs of discomfort or arousal return, when additional pentazepam (10 to 25 ml) is administered to re-establish somnoanalgesia. Diazepam dosage may be reduced if its delivery is preceded by pentazocine administration; the latter inhibits the binding of diazepam to plasma proteins, thereby increasing the level of free drug in plasma. A smaller dose of diazepam is then effective. Note that diazepam or other benzodiazepines used in combination with any narcotic should be employed with caution in geriatric or high-risk patients because of the possibility of potentiation of respiratory and cardiovascular depressant effects of the latter preparation.

DENTISTRY

Diazepam is useful both orally and intravenously, as a premedicant for apprehensive dental patients and as a supplement to local anesthesia.[76,136,137] With the use of small intermittent doses of as much as 5 mg intravenously, 10 to 15 mg is usually sufficient to obtain adequate sedation, characterized by drowsiness and slurring of speech while maintaining responsiveness to commands. Indeed, a single intravenous dose of 0.2 mg/kg may be adequate.[137] The process may be expedited by a prior small dose of methohexital (50 to 60 intravenously), but use of this drug is not routinely required. An antisialogogue, e.g., atropine or glyco-pyrrolate, given at conventional doses intravenously before the administration of diazepam is also beneficial. The amnesic action of diazepam is of particular benefit during prolonged dental procedures, which the patients perceive as lasting only a few minutes.[137] Its muscle relaxant action has also been exploited to treat trismus after dental extraction.[138]

In summary, diazepam given intravenously is a useful alternative to general anesthesia in dentistry, e.g., for the anxious or mentally handicapped child, unless the act of intravenous injection itself proves too upsetting.[76,139,140]

To safeguard against the possibility of a rebound phenomenon, outpatients should be discharged only when accompanied by a responsible adult, even when all depressant effects of diazepam have apparently dissipated and the patient is considered to be clinically safe.

CARDIOVERSION

Diazepam-induced amnesia is also beneficial for patients receiving direct-current electroshock therapy for cardioversion.[78,79,141,142] Indeed, diazepam appears the drug of choice because of its accompanying characteristics of cardiovascular stability, amnesia, tranquility, and somnolence. Whereas some clinicians consider premedication with diazepam intramuscularly as fully adequate for the procedure, most physicians prefer to deliver diazepam intravenously in doses of 10 to 20 mg (approximately 0.3 mg/kg). Alternatively, the two methods may be combined: premedication with intramuscular administration of diazepam to prepare the patient for subsequent intravenous delivery of diazepam.[78] Because of the relative safety of diazepam so utilized, many cardiologists perform cardioversions without an anesthesiologist in attendance, although such an individual is instantly available in the event of any adverse response.

CARDIAC CATHETERIZATION

Again, the amnesic-tranquilizing effects of diazepam, with minimal respiratory and cardiovascular depression, render the drug ideal for use in adults. Its use is less advantageous in uncooperative children, for whom ketamine given intramuscularly appears more suitable.[143,144]

OBSTETRICS

Although its placental transfer is rapid, diazepam in doses of 10 mg intravenously usually produces amnesia and tranquility during labor and delivery. The mother remains cooperative, and the infant shows no evidence of depression.[145] The drug may also be used during episiotomy and perineal repair.[146,147] In eclampsia, its anticonvulsant action is therapeutic, although the doses required may be depressant to the fetus.[58]

MISCELLANEOUS

The amnesic effect of diazepam, which is clinically present with doses of 10 to 20 mg intravenously, has been particularly beneficial in patients recovering from open-heart surgery.[80,148] When employed in intensive care units for patients requiring prolonged sedation, repeated doses of 10 mg intravenously every 4 hours usually provide satisfactory sedation, despite the resultant high plasma concentration.[66] In the treatment of tetanus, diazepam provides not only sedation but also muscle relaxation; however, considerably larger doses (20 mg/hour) are often required.[22,23,149] Other applications of diazepam include treatment of hallucinations and other psychomotor disturbances caused by LSD, delirium tremens, or ketamine use, as noted in Chapter 7.[150,151]

MIDAZOLAM (DORMICUM, DOBRALAM, AND VERSED)

Midazolam, the newest benzodiazepine, was synthesized in 1975 by Walser.[152]

Chemistry and Physical Properties

Midazolam is 8-chloro-6(2-fluorophenyl-1-methyl)-4H-imidazo [1,5a] [1,4] benzodiazepine (Fig. 9–1). Note that the attachment of a 5-membered ring atop the benzodiazepine nucleus of midazolam alters the numbering sequence. The important halogenated position 7 of the normal benzodiazepine system now becomes position 8. This change also occurs with the benzodiazepine antagonist Ro 15-1788 (Fig. 9–4).[153]

Because it is water soluble, requires no irritating solvents, and is short-acting with no active metabolites, midazolam offers the possibility of avoiding the major disadvantages associated with diazepam and other congeners in current use.[154]

Unique among the chemical properties of midazolam is its pH-dependent solubility. At a pH of less than 4.0, midazolam exists in an open-ring, water-soluble configuration (Fig. 9–6).[48] At pH values above 4.0, however, the ring closes and the drug becomes highly lipid soluble. The drug is formulated in aqueous solution buffered to a pH of approximately 3.5. Because its pKa is 6.0, at the physiologic pH of 7.4, midazolam is largely un-ionized, as well as highly lipid soluble, and thus rapidly crosses the blood-brain and other blood-tissue barriers.

Pharmacokinetics

Midazolam is broken down in the liver to 4 inactive metabolites.[155] The drug differs from other benzodiazepines in its juxtaposition of water solubility and rapid elimination half-life, $t\frac{1}{2} \beta$, of 1.7 to 2.6 hours (Table 9–1) (diazepam has a $t\frac{1}{2} \beta$ of 30 to 60 hours). Its only rival, triazolam, with $t\frac{1}{2} \beta$ of 1.7 to 3.0 hours (Table 9–1), is poorly soluble in water.[29] The total body clearance of midazolam is correspondingly short, 6 to 8 ml/kg/minute.[48,156–160] Approximately 96% of the total quantity of midazolam in blood is bound to protein, presumably albumin.[75] This high protein binding may affect the rapidity of onset and especially the intensity of CNS depression produced by midazolam. Marked hypoalbuminemia increases both parameters, because more unbound, free drug is available to cross the blood-brain barrier.[161]

Midazolam is well absorbed from the gastrointestinal tract.[162] Depending upon the dosage, the time of onset of action after 10 mg are given orally ranges from 10 minutes with an oral suspension to 28 minutes with a tablet. Unlike most other benzodiazepines, the intramuscular absorption of midazolam is reliable.[163] Interestingly, midazolam exhibits a significant first-pass effect; the liver extracts approximately one third of an oral dose before it reaches the general circulation.

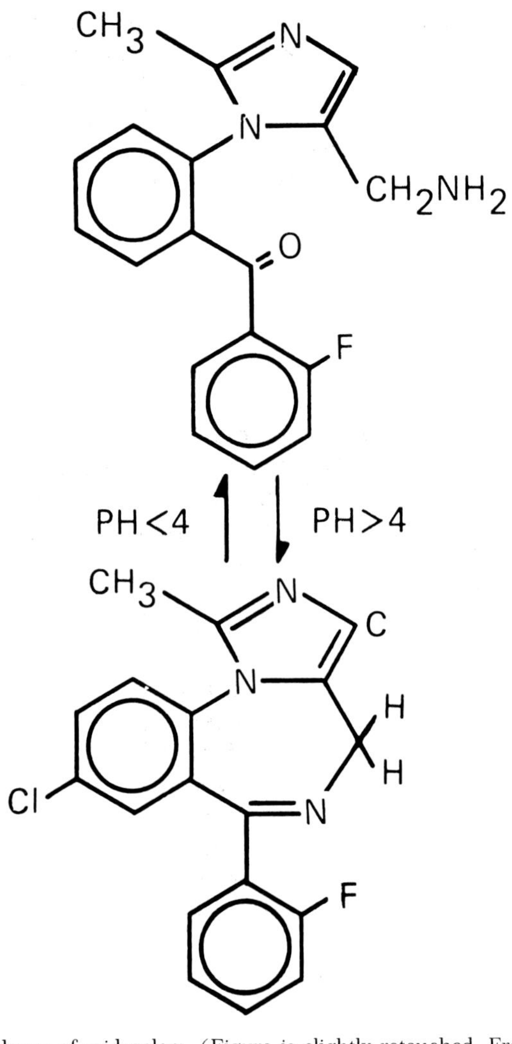

Fig. 9–6. pH dependence of midazolam. (Figure is slightly retouched. From Stanski, D.R., and Watkins, W.D.: Drug Disposition in Anesthesia. New York, Grune and Stratton, 1982.)

Effects of Midazolam

CENTRAL NERVOUS SYSTEM (CNS)

As with other benzodiazepines, midazolam produces in dose-related fashion anxiolytic, sedative, hypnotic, amnesic, muscle relaxant, and anticonvulsant effects, all presumably due to facilitation of the inhibitory action of GABA on neuronal transmission.[30] Use of midazolam decreases cerebral blood flow and oxygen consumption in man.[164,165] Midazolam is somewhat more potent than diazepam and is claimed to have a five-fold greater affinity for CNS receptors.[166] Midazolam raises the seizure threshold in mice exposed to toxic doses of local anesthetics.[167]

CARDIOVASCULAR SYSTEM

Cardiovascular stability is reasonably well maintained by the administration of midazolam over a wide dose range in animals and man.[142,144,168–171] Slight decreases in systemic blood pressure and modest increases in heart rate observed in man are considered to be clinically insignificant, but they are more pronounced than those that occur in association with diazepam. Midazolam decreases pulmonary artery pressure, which is beneficial for patients with elevated pulmonary artery occluded pressure.[170] It also decreases systemic vascular resistance, stroke index, and left ventricular stroke work index.[105,171] The combination of nitrous oxide and midazolam does not cause increased cardiovascular depression, which is in contrast to the additive depression of nitrous oxide and most narcotic analgesics.[105,172]

RESPIRATORY SYSTEM

As with diazepam, midazolam causes modest respiratory depression.[173,174] Although apnea may occur in some patients, its incidence is less than that associated with thiopental.[165,175]

GENITOURINARY SYSTEM

Glomerular filtration rate, renal blood and plasma flow, and renal vascular resistance are not significantly altered by midazolam.[176]

MUSCULOSKELETAL SYSTEM

Midazolam affects neither neuromuscular transmission nor the action of myoneural blocking agents.[177]

MISCELLANEOUS

Intraocular pressure is unaffected by midazolam.[178]

Toxicity and Side-Effects

Midazolam is minimally irritant to tissue; hence it causes little or no pain at intramuscular or intravenous injection sites.[179,180] The incidence of venous complications, such as phlebitis, thrombosis, or sclerosis, is much lower with midazolam use than with diazepam use.

Clinical Applications

Being released for clinical use, midazolam will presumably gain widespread acceptance because of its double advantages of water solubility and short duration of action. When compared to diazepam, midazolam is easier to administer and is more easily controlled pharmacologically.

PREMEDICATION

Midazolam is effective whether given orally, intramuscularly, or intravenously.[181] Anxiolytic effects appear about 15 minutes after midazolam administration (0.07 mg/kg intramuscularly), and peak sedative effects occur in 30 to 60 minutes.[182] No adverse reactions have been encountered prior to anesthesia.

INDUCTION OF ANESTHESIA

Midazolam is safe and effective for the induction of general anesthesia, especially in high-risk patients, e.g., persons with severe cardiovascular disease, for whom the use of anesthetic barbiturates may be undesirable.[179,183,184] In healthy, unpremedicated patients, approximately 0.2 mg/kg administered intravenously is considered to be a reasonable induction dose.[173,179] Indeed, probit analysis established this dose as the ED_{95} and a 0.23 mg/kg dose as the ED_{99}.[184] The dose should, of course, be modified to accommodate the effects of premedication, age, physical state, and disease. Individual differences in drug response are reportedly less with midazolam than with diazepam.[185]

Midazolam applied rectally (0.5 mg/kg) has been employed for induction of general anesthesia in infants and children as old as 6 years of age.[186] Unlike diazepam, which proved to be unsatisfactory with this mode of administration because of lack of sedation and occurrence of various undesirable psychic alterations, midazolam provided satisfactory hypnotic effects and was also associated with marked postoperative antegrade amnesia.

BALANCED ANESTHESIA

Midazolam, itself nonanalgesic, may be combined with narcotics or inhalation anesthetics to produce balanced anesthesia. Although induction with thiopental may be faster and less variable, maintenance of anesthesia with midazolam requires fewer supplemental doses. The amnesic effects assure lack of recall when used as a component in balanced anesthesia.[154]

RECOVERY

Awakening from anesthesia with midazolam is relatively rapid, depending on whether the dosage was single or multiple. Age, physical status, and concurrent drug administration can also influence recovery time. Awakening after a single dose may occur within 20 minutes, but it can be considerably delayed after multiple doses or in patients with renal disease.[183,187] When using midazolam for induction and maintenance of anesthesia in outpatients, "street fitness" is usually re-established within 4 hours.[188] Emergence after midazolam is usually uneventful, with persistent antegrade amnesia.[189] The incidence of postoperative nausea and vomiting varies with the site of operation and the adjunctive agents employed, but it seems to be lower with midazolam than with thiopental.

CONVULSANT STATES

The relatively minor effects of midazolam on cardiopulmonary function, and its reasonably short period of CNS depression, may offer advantages over the use of barbiturates and diazepam, respectively, in treating seizure activity, irregardless of cause. The drug may also be useful as a component of premedication in working against the occurrence of convulsions related to the local anesthetics used for surgical procedures.[167]

OBSTETRICS

Because of its short half-life in both the maternal and the fetal circulation, midazolam may be superior to other benzodiazepines in the anesthetic management of obstetric patients.[190]

OPHTHALMOLOGY

Midazolam does not increase intraocular pressure; hence it may be useful in ophthalmic surgery.[180] An exception is the presence of an open globe, because the drug does not prevent rises in intraocular tension caused by succinylcholine or by the placement of an endotracheal tube.

NEUROSURGERY

Midazolam may offer protection to patients with elevated intracranial pressure resulting from trauma or other causes, because it decreases cerebral blood flow, oxygen consumption, and intracranial pressure.[165]

FLUNITRAZEPAM (ROHYPNOL)

History

Flunitrazepam became available for human pharmacologic and clinical trials in the early 1970s in Europe, South America, and South Africa. After initial studies of the hypnotic properties of the drug, its suitability was explored for preanesthetic medication, reduction of the psychotomimetic side-effects of ketamine, and induction of anesthesia.[191–199] Flunitrazepam is not yet available for clinical investigation and use in the United States.

Chemistry

Flunitrazepam is 7-nitro-5-(2-fluorophenyl)-1,3-diahydro-1-methyl-2H-1,4-benzodiazepin-2-one (Fig. 9–1).

Pharmacokinetics

Flunitrazepam has a relatively rapid $t\frac{1}{2}$ α; two thirds of the drug disappear from the plasma within 60 minutes. The $t\frac{1}{2}$ β ranges from 14 to 19 hours after a single oral dose.[200] Given intravenously, its clearance is 1.9 ml/kg/minute. Protein binding amounts to only 80%, a low value for a benzodiazepine. The drug is transformed in the liver to active metabolites with relatively long $t\frac{1}{2}$ β values.[200] Thus, the effects of repeated administration are cumulative, especially in the elderly patient and in patients with liver disease. After oral or intramuscular administration of flunitrazepam, plasma levels are almost identical, but peak concentrations are more rapidly achieved after intramuscular injection.[201]

Effects of Flunitrazepam

CENTRAL NERVOUS SYSTEM (CNS)

Flunitrazepam resembles diazepam in its CNS effects, except that its onset of action is slightly more rapid and more predictable after intravenous administration.[201]

CARDIOVASCULAR SYSTEM

Unlike diazepam, flunitrazepam relaxes vascular smooth musculature, increasing vessel diameter by about 15%.[202] After induction doses of 0.015 to 0.03 mg/kg intravenously, the determinations of systolic, diastolic, ventricular filling, and pulmonary artery pressures, as well as of systemic and pulmonary vascular resistance, all decrease, whereas heart rate is either unaffected or slightly increased.[203–205]

Because flunitrazepam decreases afterload without directly depressing the myocardium, it may be useful for patients in congestive heart failure.[206] Conversely, the drug should be used with caution in patients with hypovolemia, because it lowers mean arterial blood pressure and systemic vascular resistance.[206]

Toxicity and Side-Effects

Flunitrazepam given intravenously causes less burning at the site of injection and a lower incidence of venous complications than is noted with diazepam.[207]

Clinical Applications

An intravenous anesthetic technique that involves a combination of flunitrazepam, meperidine, and muscle relaxants, but excludes nitrous oxide, has proved suitable for use in adults undergoing a variety of surgical procedures.[208]

LORAZEPAM (ATIVAN)

Chemistry and Physical Properties

Lorazepam is 7-chloro-5-(*o*-chlorophenyl)1,3-dihydro-3-hydroxy-2*H*-1,4-benzodiazepin-2-one (Fig. 9–1). The drug is insoluble in water, but is fairly lipid soluble: its octanol-water partition coefficient is 240 (compared to 840 for diazepam).[43]

POTENCY

Lorazepam ranks among the more potent benzodiazepines: doses of 2 to 4 mg orally, intramuscularly, or intravenously need not be exceeded.

Pharmacokinetics

ABSORPTION AND DISTRIBUTION

More than 90% of an oral dose of lorazepam is absorbed, with peak plasma levels occurring within 2.5 hours.[209,210] This rate is somewhat slower than that of 30 to 90 minutes required by diazepam.[48] After intramuscular injection, lorazepam, unlike diazepam, is dependably, extensively, and rapidly absorbed, with plasma concentrations peaking within 60 minutes. Intramuscular injection of the drug causes minimal discomfort.[211] Given intravenously, lorazepam has a fairly rapid distribution half-life (t½ α) of 15 to 20 minutes.[212] Its t½ β ranges from 10 to 22 hours (Table 9–1), apparently irrespective of dose, route of administration, or age; its elimination half-life is markedly prolonged by liver disease.[212–214] The volume of distribution varies from 0.8 to 1.3 L/kg (0.7 to 1.7 L/kg for diazepam), whereas its protein binding of 80 to 92% is somewhat lower than that of most other benzodiazepines.[214] Despite its shorter t½ β relative to that of diazepam, lorazepam at equipotent doses provides significantly longer amnesic activity.[215,216] This ability may be a reflection of its lesser lipid solubility, with slower transit across the blood-brain barrier.[217]

METABOLISM

Unlike diazepam, lorazepam is metabolized to pharmacologically inactive compounds, primarily to glucuronide; hence lorazepam is short-acting (Table 9–1).[210,218] Although 65 to 75% of the administered dose is accounted for in the excretion of the glucuronide, this is merely a housekeeping function that rids the body of inert debris; in no way does the kidney contribute to the termination of the action of lorazepam.

Effect of Lorazepam

Sedation is the most outstanding effect achieved by the use of lorazepam. This drug renders patients calm, relaxed, and seemingly asleep, yet they are fully responsive to questioning—an ideal preoperative state.[205,211,219–231] Usual clinical doses do not significantly alter cardiorespiratory function.[225]

Toxicity and Side-Effects

Chronic tolerance to the CNS effects of lorazepam may develop with prolonged oral administration.[212] Concomitant use with scopolamine is not advisable because such a combination may lead to increased sedation, hallucinations, or irrational behavior.[232]

Clinical Applications

Lorazepam (2 to 4 mg or 0.05 mg/kg intramuscularly or intravenously) produces anxiolytic, sedative, and amnesic effects in dose-related fashion. At the lower edge of the dose range, a 2-mg dose given intramuscularly or intravenously provides adequate preoperative tranquility for most patients but does not consistently suppress preanesthetic recall. With the higher dose (4 mg), most patients remain responsive to the spoken voice, but have no recall of preoperative events. As with any fixed dose regimen, some persons may be more heavily sedated than necessary, e.g., more soundly asleep, but this is not a serious complication.

For supplementation of local or regional anesthesia, lorazepam (0.02 mg/kg intravenously) usually suffices to produce a sedated, yet fully cooperative, patient. Note that, although sedation and anxiolysis are observed within minutes after intravenous delivery of lorazepam and approximately 30 minutes after an intramuscular dose, the onset of lack of recall is delayed about 20 minutes with the former route and 2 to 3 hours with the latter route. These delays may be reduced by the addition of an oral dose of lorazepam (e.g., 4 mg) to be administered the night before the surgical procedure.

Combinations of narcotic analgesics and lorazepam for use in premedication usually enhance sedation and anxiolysis but do not affect amnesia. Because of its prolonged action, lorazepam offers little as an agent for the induction of anesthesia.

NITRAZEPAM (MOGADON)

Nitrazepam (7-nitro-1,3-dihydro-5-phenyl-2*H*-1,4-benzodiazepin-2-one) (Fig. 9–1) is a long-established benzodiazepine. The drug has a $t\frac{1}{2}\ \beta$ of 24 to 31 hours (Table 9–2), but has no long-acting metabolite (Table 9–2).[233,234] Its large volume of distribution is markedly increased with advancing age.[234] Total clearance values range from 0.9 to 1.0 mg/kg/minute and protein binding ranges from 88 to 97%.[235]

Nitrazepam is primarily employed as a hypnotic at bedtime.[236] Given orally for preanesthetic medication, it provides sedation and reportedly prevents the vasoconstrictive reaction to fear in the immediate preoperative period[237] Nitrazepam (10 mg) in combination with droperidol (20 mg), when orally administered prior to ketamine anesthesia, proved to be effective in reducing to acceptable limits the incidence of unpleasant emergence delirium reactions to ketamine.[238] This observation has not been confirmed by other investigators.[239]

CHLORDIAZEPOXIDE (LIBRIUM)

Chlordiazepoxide (7-chloro-2-methylamino-5-phenyl-3H-1,4-benzodiazepine-4-oxide) (Fig. 9–1) was the first psychotropic agent in the benzodiazepine class. Its t½ α is rapid (10 minutes).[240,241] Unlike most benzodiazepines, chlordiazepoxide is soluble in water.[29] When given orally, chlordiazepoxide is rapidly and completely absorbed; pharmacologic effects are detectable within 10 minutes.[242] Absorption of chlordiazepoxide administered intramuscularly is slow but complete, although somewhat unpredictable.[243] Plasma concentrations are maximal at approximately 8 hours.[243] Absorption and disposition of the drug are slower in elderly persons and in patients with parenchymal liver disease.[244,245] Although its t½ β of 8 to 18 hours is in the intermediate category, the drug is classified as a long-acting benzodiazepine because 2 of its active metabolites, demoxepan and desmethyldiazepam, are long-acting (Table 9–2). The V_d of chlordiazepoxide is small (0.3 to 0.6 L/kg); total clearance values range from 0.21 to 0.56 ml/kg/minute, and the degree of protein binding is relatively high (94 to 97%).[246]

Clinically, chlordiazepoxide remains useful for preanesthetic medication because of its anxiolytic and sedative properties.[6] The drug is also used to treat withdrawal symptoms of acute alcoholism.[247] In persons with proven drug addiction, the use of chlordiazepoxide is not recommended, because development of physical and psychologic dependence and withdrawal symptoms after discontinuation of this drug have been reported.[248]

DESMETHYLDIAZEPAM (NORDIAZEPAM AND NADAR)

Desmethyldiazepam (7-chloro-1,3-dihydro-5-phenyl-2H-1,4-benzodiazepin-2-one) (Fig. 9–1) is a pharmacologically active metabolite of diazepam, chlordiazepoxide, and several other benzodiazepines, including the inactive parent or pro-drugs, clorazepate and prazepam (Table 9–1). The drug is slightly less potent than its active parent compounds.[249] Of the benzodiazepines now available, desmethyldiazepam has the lowest rate of clearance and the longest half-life (Table 9–2). It is approximately 97% bound to plasma protein.[250]

Although the metabolites of chlordiazepoxide and diazepam, including desmethyldiazepam, are claimed not to be responsible for the pharmacologic effects of their parent compounds, the occasional prolonged drowsiness experienced with the use of diazepam conceivably may be related to concentrations of desmethyldiazepam that continue to rise for as many as 24 hours after diazepam administration before beginning to decline.[48,249] The prolonged t½ β of this metabolite (30 to 200 hours in contrast to 20 to 50 hours for diazepam) (Table 9–2) doubtless contributes to the occasional prolonged drowsiness after diazepam use, although other authors do not concur.[249]

OXAZEPAM (LACTAM, SERAX, AND SERENID)

Oxazepam (7-chloro-3-hydroxy-5-phenyl-2H-1,4-benzodiazepin-2-one) (Fig. 9–1) is another active metabolite of chlordiazepoxide and diazepam. Its t½ β of 3 to 21 hours (Table 9–1) is shorter than that of most other benzodiazepines; there is no knowledge of active metabolites.[251,252] The drug is 87 to 97% protein bound. Oxazepam is used as an anxiolytic agent and in acute alcohol withdrawal.[25] Although not available in solution, it has been given orally for preanesthetic medication. Fewer side-effects are claimed with oxazepam use than with the administration of diazepam or chlordiazepoxide.[67]

FLURAZEPAM (DALMANE)

Flurazepam (7-chloro-1-diethylaminoethyl-5-(2-fluorphenyl)-2*H*-1,4–benzodiazepine) (Fig. 9–1) is well known as a sedative and hypnotic agent. Despite its short t½ β of 2 to 3 hours (Table 9–2), flurazepam is categorized as long-acting because of the long t½ β (47 to 100 hours) of its active metabolite, desalkylflurazepam (Table 9–2). In anesthetic practice, flurazepam is used primarily to control insomnia, both pre- and postoperatively.[253]

TRIAZOLAM (HALCION)

Triazolam (8-chloro-6-(*o*-chlorophenyl)-1-methyl-4*H*-5-triazolo-(4, 3-α-1, 4 benzodiazepine) (Fig. 9–1) is an hypnotic with a t½ β of 2 to 3 hours. The drug is rapidly absorbed when given orally; peak plasma concentrations occur at 1.3 hours. Its metabolites are presumably inactive.[254] Because of its strong hypnotic action, the drug is used primarily in the short-term management of insomnia characterized by difficulty in falling asleep and frequent nocturnal awakenings. The effective dose range for adults is 0.25 to 0.5 mg orally at bedtime. In elderly and debilitated patients, the administration of triazolam should be initiated at a dose of 0.125 mg to decrease the possibility of oversedation, dizziness, or impaired coordination. The drug should not be given to pregnant women. Hallucinations have been reported after the administration of triazolam.[255]

TEMAZEPAM (RESTORIL)

Temazepam (7-chloro-1,3-dihydro-3-hydroxy-1-methyl-5-phenyl-2*H*-1,4-benzodiazepin-2-one) (Fig. 9–1) is another recently introduced hypnotic agent that is absorbed within 20 to 40 minutes of delivery and reaches a peak concentration 2 to 3 hours after oral administration. No active metabolites have been identified.[256] The drug is effective in the relief of insomnia by prolonging total sleeping time and reducing the number of nocturnal awakenings with a minimum of residual medication effects (hangover). The recommended adult dose is 30 mg orally before retiring, but a 15-mg oral dose may be sufficient in elderly individuals or patients at risk. Its use in pregnant women is contraindicated.

ALPRAZOLAM (XANAX)

Alprazolam (8-chloro-1-methyl-6-phenyl-4*H*-5-triazolo (4,3 α)1,4-benzodiazepine) (Fig. 9–1) is useful in the management of anxiety disorders and depression.[257] The drug reaches its peak plasma concentration after oral administration within 1 to 2 hours; its t½ β is 12 to 15 hours. Its 2 metabolites are α-hydroxyalprazolam, the biologic activity of which is one-half that of alprazolam, and a benzophenone derivative of alprazolam, which is inactive. Safe and effective doses for the short-term relief of the symptoms of anxiety and depression range from 0.25 to 0.5 mg given orally three times daily, with a maximum total daily dose of 4 mg given in divided doses. Its use is contraindicated in pregnant women and in patients with acute narrow angle glaucoma.

PRAZEPAM (CENTRAX)

Prazepam (7-chloro-1-(cyclopropylmethyl)-1,3-dihydro-5-phenyl-2*H*-1,4-benzodiazepin-2-one) (Fig. 9–2) is another useful anxiolytic drug. Prazepam is slowly absorbed over a prolonged period. Its major metabolite, norprazepam, has a t½

Δ of 63 to 70 hours.[258] Before elimination from the body, most of the prazepam is metabolized to 3-hydroxyprazepam and oxyazepam. For the relief of anxiety and tension, the drug is effective orally in divided doses ranging from 20 to 60 mg daily, in accordance with the response of the patient. In elderly and debilitated patients, the daily dose of prazepam may be reduced to 10 to 15 mg.

RO 15-1788

History

The imidazodiazepine Ro 15-1788 (ethyl-9-fluoro-5,6-dihydro-5-methyl-6-oxo-4H-imidazo[1,5-a] [1,4] benzodiazepine-3-carboxylate) was synthesized by Hunkeler, et al., and was studied in animals, human volunteers, and patients who were in deep coma from benzodiazepine (diazepam, clonazepam, and flunitrazepam) overdose and in whom the administration of Ro 15-1788 (10 mg at a rate of 2.5 mg/minute intravenously) reversed the effects of the benzodiazepines.[259–266]

Chemistry

As with midazolam (see *Midazolam: Chemistry and Physical Properties*), the fluorosubstituent is at position 8, but corresponds to the position 7 of diazepam and other "normal" benzodiazepines (Fig. 9–1).[153]

Pharmacokinetics

This water-soluble compound has a $t\frac{1}{2}$ β of 100 to 150 minutes, with a total plasma clearance of 450 mg/kg/minute.[267]

Effects of Ro 15-1788

In animals, Ro 15-1788 is virtually devoid of pharmacologic activity in doses that selectively antagonize many behavioral, electrophysiologic, and biochemical effects of diazepam and other active benzodiazepines.[33,34,36,42,260,261,268]

Ro 15-1788 is not an antagonist for barbiturates, meprobamate, alcohol, GABA mimetics, or opioids.[33] The drug precipitates withdrawal symptoms in animals made dependent by chronic administration of high doses of benzodiazepines.[262] The number of binding sites (B_{max}) for Ro 15-1788 in the CNS is identical to the B_{max} for clorazepate, which binds to the central, but not to the peripheral, benzodiazepine receptors.[269] Indeed, the topographic distribution of Ro 15-1788 is indistinguishable from that of ^{3}H-clorazepate.[33,34]

In human volunteers, Ro 15-1788, given orally or intravenously, is a potent benzodiazepine antagonist.[263–265,267] In the absence of benzodiazepines, the compound seems pharmacologically inert at small to moderate doses.[33,34] Several patients, comatose from benzodiazepine overdoses, awakened promptly after receiving a few milligrams of Ro 15-1788.

As a specific benzodiazepine antagonist, the practical implications of this compound for the anesthesiologist are in the controlled termination of the effects of benzodiazepines used in anesthesia and in the treatment of overdose.

REFERENCES

1. Sternbach, L.H.: The benzodiazepine story. *In* Drug Research. Vol. 22. Edited by E. Jucker. Basel, Birkhauser, 1978.

2. Randall, L.O., Schallek, W., Heise, G.A., Keith, E.F., and Bagdon, R.E.: The psychosedative properties of methaminodiazepoxide. J. Pharmacol. Exp. Ther., *129*:163, 1960.

3. Tobin, J.M., Bird, I.F., and Beyle, D.E.: Preliminary evaluation of Librium (Ro5-0690) in the treatment of anxiety reactions. Dis. Nerv. Syst., *21*(Suppl. 3):11, 1960.

4. Kinross-Wright, J., Cohe, I.M., and Knight, J.A: The management of neurotic and psychotic states with Ro5-0690 (Librium). Dis. Nerv. Syst., *21*(Suppl. 3):23, 1960.

5. Harris, T.H.: Methaminodiazepoxide. JAMA, *172*:1162, 1960.

6. Brandt, A.L., Liu, S.C.Y., and Briggs, B.D.: Trial of chlordiazepoxide as a preanesthetic medication. Anesth. Analg., *41*:557, 1962.

7. Randall, L.O., Heise, G.A., Schallek, W., Bagdon, R.E., Banziger, R., Boris, A., Moe, R.A., and Abrams, W.B.: Pharmacological and clinical studies on Valium, a new psychotherapeutic agent of the benzodiazepine class. Curr. Ther. Res., *3*:405, 1961.

8. Towler, M.L.: The clinical use of diazepam in anxiety states and depression. J. Neurol. Neurosurg. Psychiatry, *3*(Suppl. 1):568, 1962.

9. DuCailar, J., Rious, J., Bellanger, A., and Grolleau, D.: Utilisation du diazepam (Valium) en premedication. Ann. Anesth. Franc., *5*:706, 1964.

10. Campan, L., and Espagno, M. Th.: Note sur le diazepam en anesthesiologie. Ann. Anesth. Franc., *5*:711, 1964.

11. Blondeau, P.: Diazepam et anesthesie generale. Cah. Anesthesiol., *13*:207, 1965.

12. Du Cailar, J., Gestin, Y., and Galibert, A.M.: Utilisation du diazepam (Valium) comme agent narcotique d'induction au cours de narco-ataralgesie. Ann. Anesth. Franc., *7*:203, 1966.

13. Stovner, J., and Andresen, R.: Diazepam in intravenous anesthesia. Lancet, *2*:1298, 1965.

14. Cushman, R.P.A.: Diazepam in intravenous anaesthesia. Lancet, *1*:1042, 1966.

15. McClish, A.: Diazepam as an intravenous induction agent for general anaesthesia. Can. Anaesth. Soc. J., *13*:562, 1966.

16. Huguenard, J., and Margelidon, J.B.: Two special indications for injectable diazepam. Ann. Anesth. Franc., *5*:731, 1964.

17. Aguado-Matorras, A., and Aquerreta, M-L.E.: Neuroleptanalgesie avec Valium-Palfium (neuroleptanalgesia with Valium plus dextromoramide). Ann. Anesth. Franc., *5*:722, 1964.

18. Bepko, F., Lowe, E., and Waxman, B.: Relief of the emotional factor in labor with parenterally administered diazepam. Obstet. Gynecol., *26*:852, 1965.

19. Lean, T.H., Ratnam, S.S., and Sivasamboo, R.: Use of benzodiazepines in the management of eclampsia. Br. J. Obstet. Gynaecol, *75*:856, 1968.

20. Gastaut, H., Naquet, R., Pire, R., and Tassinari, C.A.: Treatment of status epilepticus with diazepam (Valium). Epilepsia, *6*:167, 1965.

21. Lombroso, C.T.: Treatment of status epilepticus with diazepam. Neurology, *16*:629, 1966.

22. Shershin, P.H., and Katz, S.S.: Diazepam in the treatment of tetanus—report of a case following tooth extraction. Clin. Med., *71*:362, 1964.

23. Weinberg, W.A.: Control of the neuromuscular and convulsive manifestations of severe systematic tetanus: case report with a new drug. Valium (diazepam). Clin. Pediatr. (Phila.), *3*:226, 1964.

24. Coppel, D.L., Bovill, J.G., and Dundee, J.W.: The taming of ketamine. Anaesthesia, *28*:293, 1973.

25. British National Formulary. London, British Medical Association and Pharmaceutical Society of Great Britain, 1983, p. 123.

26. Greenblatt, D.J., and Shader R.I.: Benzodiazepines in Clinical Practice. New York, Raven Press, 1974.

27. Shader, R.I., Georgotas, A., Greenblatt, D.J., Harmatz, J.S., and Allen, M.D.: Impaired absorption of desmethyldiazepam for clorazepate by magnesium aluminium hydroxide. Clin. Pharmacol. Ther., *24*:308, 1978.

28. Smith, M.T., Evans, L.E.J., and Eadie, M.J.: Pharmacokinetics of prazepam in man. Eur. J. Clin. Pharmacol., *16*:141, 1979.

29. Drug Information 86. American Hospital Formulary Service. Bethesda, American Society of Hospital Pharmacists, 1986.

30. Richter, J.J.: Current theories about the mechanisms of benzodiazepines and neuroleptic drugs. Anesthesiology, *54*:66, 1981.

31. Bertillson, L.: Mechanisms of action of benzodiazepines—GABA hypothesis. Acta Psychiatr. Scand. [Suppl.], *274*:19, 1978.

32. Costa, E., and Giudotti, A.: Molecular mechanisms in the receptor actions of benzodiazepines. Annu. Rev. Pharmacol. Toxicol., *19*:531, 1979.

33. Haefely, W.: The biological basis of benzodiazepine actions. J. Psychoactive Drugs, *15*:19, 1983.

34. Haefely, W., Pieri, L., Polc, P., and Schaffner, R.: General pharmacology and neuropharmacology of benzodiazepine derivatives. *In* Handbook of Experimental Pharmacology. Vol. 55/II. Edited by F. Hoffmeister and G. Stille. Berlin, Springer, 1981.

35. Snyder, S.H., and Enna, S.J.: The role of central glycine receptors in the pharmacologic actions of benzodiazepines. Adv. Biochem. Psychopharmacol., *14*:81, 1975.
36. Haefely, W.: Alleviation of anxiety—the benzodiazepine saga. *In* Discoveries in Pharmacology. Vol. 1. Psycho- and Neuropharmacology. Edited by M.J. Parnham and J. Bruinvels. Amsterdam, Elsevier, 1983.
37. Polc, P., Bonetti, E.P., Schaffner, R., and Haefely, W.: A three-state model of the benzodiazepine receptor explains the interactions between the benzodiazepine antagonist Ro 15-1788, benzodiazepine tranquilizers, B-carbolines, and phenobarbitone. Naunyn. Schmiedebergs Arch. Pharmacol., *321*:260, 1982.
38. Moehler, H., Battersby, M.K., and Richards, J.G.: Benzodiazepine receptor protein identified and visualized in brain tissue by a photoaffinity label. Proc. Natl. Acad. Sci. U.S.A., 77:1666, 1980.
39. Moehler, H., Wu, J.-T., and Richards, J.G.: Benzodiazepine receptors: autoradiographical and immunocytochemical evidence for their localization in regions of GABAergic synaptic contacts. *In* GABA and Benzodiazepine Receptors. Edited by E. Costa and G. DiChiari. New York, Raven Press, 1981.
40. Richards, J.G., Moehler, H., and Haefely, W.: Benzodiazepine binding sites: receptors or acceptors? Trends Pharmacol. Sci., *3*:233, 1982.
41. Young, W.S., and Kuhar, M.J.: Autoradiographic localization of benzodiazepine receptors in rat brain. J. Pharmacol. Exp. Ther., *212*:337, 1980.
42. Haefely, W., Kulcsar, A., Moehler, H., Pieri, L., Polc, P., and Schaeffer, R.: Possible involvement of GABA in the central actions of benzodiazepines. *In* Mechanism of Action of the Benzodiazepines. Edited by E. Costa and P. Greengard. New York, Raven, 1975.
43. Ritschel, W.A., and Hammer, G.V.: Prediction of the volume of distribution from in vitro data and use for estimating the absolute extent of absorption. Int. J. Clin. Pharmacol. Res., *18*:298, 1980.
44. Mandelli, M., Tognoni, G., and Garattini, S.: Clinical pharmacokinetics of diazepam. Clin. Pharmacokinet., *3*:72, 1978.
45. Greenblatt, D.J., Allen, M.D., Harmatz, J.S., and Shade, R.: Diazepam disposition determinants. Clin. Pharmacol. Ther., *27*:301, 1980.
46. Yamamoto, K., Kuze, S., Murakami, S., and Tsuji, A.: Pentazocine-diazepam-N_2O anesthesia: influence of pentazocine on protein binding and distribution of diazepam. *In* Trends in Intravenous Anesthesia. Edited by J.A. Aldrete and T.H. Stanley. Miami, Symposia Specialists, 1980.
47. Hillestad, L., Hansen, T., and Melsom, H.: Diazepam metabolism in normal man. I. Serum concentrations and clinical effects after intravenous, intramuscular, and oral administration. Clin. Pharmacol. Ther., *16*:479, 1974.
48. Stanski, D.R., and Watkins, W.D.: Drug Disposition in Anesthesia. New York, Grune and Stratton, 1982.
49. Klotz, U., and Reimann, I.: Delayed clearance of diazepam due to cimetidine. N. Engl. J. Med., *302*:1012, 1980.
50. Baird, E.S., and Hailey, D.H.: Delayed recovery from a sedative: correlation of the plasma levels of diazepam with clinical effects after oral and intravenous administration. Br. J. Anaesth., *44*:803, 1972.
51. Van der Kleijn, E., Van Rossum, J.M., Muskens, E.T.J.M., and Risntijes, N.V.M.: Pharmacokinetics of diazepam in dogs, mice and humans. Acta Pharmacol. Toxicol. (Copenh.), *29*(Suppl. 3):109, 1971.
52. Greenblatt, D.J., and Koch-Weser, J.: Intramuscular injection of drugs. N. Engl. J. Med., *295*:542, 1976.
53. Korttila, K., and Linnoila, M.: Absorption and sedative effects of diazepam after oral administration and intramuscular administration into the vastus lateralis muscle and the deltoid muscle. Br. J. Anaesth., *47*:857, 1975.
54. Kerkkola, R., and Kangas, L.: The transfer of diazepam across the placenta during labor. Acta Obstet. Gynecol. Scand., *52*:167, 1973.
55. Cavanagh, D., and Condo, C.S.: Diazepam—a pilot study of drug concentrations in maternal blood, amniotic fluid, and cord blood. Curr. Ther. Res., *6*:122, 1964.
56. DeSilva, J.A.F., D'Arconte, L., and Kaplan, L.: The determination of blood levels and the placental transfer of diazepam in humans. Curr. Ther. Res., *6*:115, 1964.
57. Idanpaan, H.J.E., Jouppila, P.I., Poulakka, J.O., and Vorne, M.S.: Placental transfer and fetal metabolism of diazepam in early human pregnancy. Am. J. Obstet. Gynecol., *109*:1011, 1971.
58. McCarthy, G.T., O'Connell, B., and Robinson, A.E.: Blood levels of diazepam in infants of two mothers given large doses of diazepam during labor. Br. J. Obstet. Gynecol., *80*:349, 1973.
59. Klotz, U., Avant, G.R., Hoyumpa, A., Schenker, S., and Wilkinson, G.R.: The effects of age and liver disease on disposition and elimination of diazepam in adult man. J. Clin. Invest., *55*:347, 1975.

60. MacLeod, S.M., Giles, H.G., Bengert, B., Liu, F.F., and Sellers, E.M.: Age- and gender-related differences in diazepam pharmacokinetics. J. Clin. Pharmacol., *19*:15, 1979.
61. Ghoneim, M.M., Korttila, K., and Chiang, C.K.: Diazepam effects and kinetics in caucasians and orientals. Clin. Pharmacol. Ther., *29*:749, 1981.
62. Klotz, U., Anonin, K.H., and Bieck, P.R.: Comparison of the pharmacokinetics of diazepam after single and subchronic doses. Eur. J. Clin. Pharmacol, *10*:121, 1976.
63. Abernethy, D.R., and Greenblatt, D.J.: Effects of desmethyldiazepam on diazepam kinetics: a study of effects of a metabolite on parent drug disposition. Clin. Pharmacol. Ther., *29*:757, 1981.
64. Kangas, L., Kanto, J., and Forsstrorn, J.: The protein binding of diazepam and N-desmethyl-diazepam in patients with poor renal function. Clin. Nephrol., *5*:114, 1976.
65. Kaplan, S.A., Jack, M.L., Alexander, K., and Weinfeld, R.E.: Pharmacokinetic profile of diazepam in man following single intravenous and oral and chronic oral administrations. J. Pharm. Sci., *62*:1789, 1973.
66. Gamble, J.A.S., Dundee, J.W., and Gray, R.C.: Plasma diazepam concentrations following prolonged administration. Br. J. Anaesth., *48*:1087, 1976.
67. Dundee, J.W., and Haslett, W.H.K.: The benzodiazepines. A review of their actions and uses relative to anesthetic practice. Br. J. Anaesth., *42*:217, 1970.
68. Parkes, M.W.: The pharmacology of diazepam. *In* Diazepam in Anaesthesia. Edited by F.P. Knight and C.G. Burgess. Bristol, Wright, 1967.
69. Ngai, S.H., Tseng, D.T.C., and Wang, S.C.: Effect of diazepam and other central nervous system depressants on spinal reflexes in cats: a study of site of action. J. Pharmacol. Exp. Ther., *153*:344, 1966.
70. Nakanishi, T., and Morris, F.H.: Effect of diazepam on rat spinal reflexes. J. Neurol. Sci., *13*:189, 1971.
71. Himwich, H.E., Morillo, A., and Steiner, W.G.: Drugs affecting rhinencephalic structures. J. Neuropsych., *4*(Suppl. 1):515, 1962.
72. Papex, J.W.: A proposed mechanism of emotion. Arch. Neurol., *38*:725, 1937.
73. Svenson, S.E., and Gordon, L.E.: Diazepam: a progress report. Curr. Ther. Res., *7*:367, 1965.
74. Knapp, R.B., and Dubow, H.S.: Diazepam as an induction agent for patients with cardiopulmonary disease. South. Med. J., *63*:1451, 1970.
75. Reves, J.G.: Benzodiazepines. *In* Pharmacokinetics of Anesthesia. Edited by C. Prys-Roberts and C.C. Hug. Oxford, Blackwell, 1984.
76. Brown, P.R.H., Main, D.M.G., and Lawson, J.I.M.: Diazepam in dentistry. Br. Dent. J., *125*:498, 1968.
77. Kahler, R.L., Burrow, G.N., and Felig, P.: Diazepam-induced amnesia for cardioversion. JAMA, *200*:997, 1967.
78. Vinge, L.N., Wyant, G.M., and Lopez, J.F.: Diazepam in cardioversion. Can. Anaesth. Soc. J., *18*:166, 1971.
79. Rogers, W.K., Waterman, D.H., Domm, S.E., and Sunay, A.: Efficacy of a new psychotropic drug in bronchoscopy. Dis. Chest, *47*:280, 1965.
80. McClish, A., Andres, D., and Tetreault, L.: Intravenous diazepam for psychiatric reactions following open-heart surgery. Can. Anaesth. Soc. J., *15*:63, 1968.
81. Steen, S.N., and Hahl, D.: Controlled evaluation of parenteral diazepam as preanesthetic medication. Anesth. Analg., *48*:459, 1969.
82. Pandit, S.K., and Dundee, J.W.: Preoperative amnesia: the incidence following the intramuscular injection of commonly used premedicants. Anaesthesia, *25*:493, 1970.
83. Clarke, P.R.F., Eccersley, P.S., Frisby, J.P., and Thornton, J.A.: The amnesic effect of diazepam (Valium). Br. J. Anaesth., *42*:690, 1970.
84. Dundee, J.W., and Pandit, S.K.: Anterograde amnesic effects of pethidine, hyoscine, and diazepam in adults. Br. J. Pharmacol., *44*:140, 1972.
85. Pandit, S.K., Dundee, J.W., and Keilty, S.R.: Amnesia studies with intravenous premedication. Anaesthesia, *26*:421, 1971.
86. Conner, J.T., Belleville, J.W., Wender, R.H., Wapner, S., and Katz, R.L.: Evaluation of intravenous diazepam as a surgical premedicant. Anesth. Analg., *56*:211, 1977.
87. Brown, S.S., and Dundee, J.W.: Clinical studies of induction agents. XXV. Diazepam. Br. J. Anaesth., *40*:108, 1968.
88. Hillestad, L., Hansen, T., and Melsom, H.: Diazepam metabolism in normal man. II. Serum concentrations and clinical effects after oral administration and cumulation. Clin. Pharmacol. Ther., *16*:485, 1974.
89. Greenblatt, D.J., and Shader, R.I.: Dependence, tolerance and addiction to benzodiazepines: clinical and pharmacokinetic considerations. Drug Metab. Rev., 8:13, 1978.
90. Greenblatt, D.J., Woo, E., Allen, M.D., Orsulak, P.J., and Shader, R.I.: Rapid recovery from massive diazepam overdose. JAMA, *240*:1872, 1978.
91. Abel, R.M., Staroscik, R.M., and Reis, R.L.: Effects of diazepam (Valium) on left ventricular function and systemic vascular resistance. J. Pharmacol. Exp. Ther., *173*:364, 1970.

92. Abel, R.M., Reis, R.L., and Staroscik, R.N.: The pharmacologic basis of coronary and systemic vascular dilator action of diazepam (Valium). Br. J. Pharmacol., *39*:261, 1970.

93. Katz, J., Finestone, S.C., and Pappas, M.T.: Circulatory response to tilting after intravenous diazepam in volunteers. Anesth. Analg., *46*:243, 1967.

94. Rao, S., Sherbaniuk, R.W., Prasad, K., Lee, J.K., and Spoule B.J.: Cardiopulmonary effects of diazepam. Clin. Pharmacol. Ther., *14*:182, 1973.

95. Knapp, R.B., and Dubow, H.: Comparison of diazepam with thiopental as an induction agent in cardiopulmonary disease. Anesth. Analg., *49*:722, 1970.

96. D'Amelio, G., Volta, S.D., Stritoni, P., Chioin, R., and Menozzi, L.: Acute cardiovascular effects on diazepam in patients with mitral valve disease. Eur. J. Clin. Pharmacol., *6*:61, 1973.

97. Ikram, H., Rubin, A.P., and Jewkes, R.F.: Effects of diazepam on myocardial blood flow of patients with and without coronary artery disease. Br. Heart J., *35*:626, 1973.

98. Stanley, T.H., Bennett, G.M., Loeser, E.A., Kavamura, R., and Sentker, C.R.: Cardiovascular effects of diazepam and droperidol during morphine anesthesia. Anesthesiology, *44*:255, 1976.

99. Cote, P., Gueret, P., and Bourassa, M.G.: Systemic and coronary hemodynamic effects of diazepam in patients with normal and diseased coronary arteries. Circulation, *50*:1210, 1974.

100. Clarke, R.S.J., and Lyons, S.M.: Diazepam and flunitrazepam as induction agents for cardiac surgical operations. Acta Anaesthesiol. Scand., *21*:282, 1977.

101. Jackson, A.P.F., Dhadphale, P.R., Callaghan, M.L., and Alseri, S.: Haemodynamic studies during induction of anaesthesia for open-heart surgery using diazepam and ketamine. Br. J. Anaesth., *50*:375, 1978.

102. Stanley, T.H., and Webster, L.R.: Anesthetic requirements and cardiovascular effects of fentanyl-oxygen and fentanyl-diazepam oxygen anesthesia in man. Anesth. Analg., *57*:411, 1978.

103. McCammon, R.L., Hilgenberg, J.C., and Stoelting, R.K.: Hemodynamic effects of diazepam and diazepam-nitrous oxide in patients with coronary artery disease. Anesth. Analg., *59*:438, 1980.

104. Samuelson, P.N., Lell, W.A., Kouchoukos, N.T., Strong, S.D., and Dole, K.M.: Hemodynamics during diazepam induction of anesthesia for coronary artery bypass grafting. South. Med. J., *73*:332, 1980.

105. Samuelson, P.N., Reves, J.G., Kouchoukos, N.J., Smith, L.R., and Dole, K.M.: Hemodynamic responses to anesthetic induction with midazolam or diazepam in patients with ischemic heart disease. Anesth. Analg., *60*:802, 1981.

106. Prakash, R., Thurer, R., and Vargas, A.: Cardiovascular effects of diazepam induction in patients for aortocoronary saphenous vein bypass grafts. Abstracts of Scientific Papers, American Society of Anethesiologists Annual Meeting, San Francisco, 1976.

107. Reves, J.G., and Kissin, I.: Intravenous anesthetics. *In* Cardiac Anesthesia. Vol. II. Cardiovascular pharmacology. Edited by J.A. Kaplan. New York, Grune and Stratton, 1983.

108. Stanley, T.H., and Webster, L.R.: Anesthetic requirements and cardiovascular effects of fentanyl-oxygen and fentanyl-diazepam-oxygen anesthesia in man. Anesth. Analg., *57*:411, 1978.

109. Stanley, T.H.: Pharmacology of intravenous narcotic anesthetics. *In* Anesthesia. Edited by R.D. Miller. New York, Churchill Livingstone, 1981.

110. Liu, W.S., Bidwai, A.V., Lunn, J.K.L., and Stanely, T.H.: Urine catecholamine excretion after large doses of fentanyl, fentanyl and diazepam, and fentanyl, diazepam and pancuronium. Can. Anaesth. Soc. J., *24*:371, 1977.

111. Rollason, W.N.: Diazepam as an intravenous induction agent for general anaesthesia. *In* Diazepam in Anaesthesia. Edited by P.F. Knight and C.G. Burgess. Bristol, John Wright and Sons, 1968.

112. Barrett, J.S., and Hey, E.B.: Ventricular arrhythmias associated with the use of diazepam for cardioversion. JAMA, *214*:1323, 1970.

113. Schlosser, L.: Action of diazepam on the spinal cord. Arch. Int. Pharmacodyn. Ther., *194*:93, 1971.

114. Olafson, R.A., Mulder, D.W., and Howard, F.H.: "Stiffman" syndrome: a review of the literature, report of three additional cases and discussion of pathophysiology and therapy. Mayo Clin. Proc., *39*:131, 1964.

115. Nathan, P.W.: The action of diazepam in neurological disorders with excessive motor activity. J. Neurol. Sci., *10*:33, 1970.

116. Hunter, A.R.: Diazepam (Valium) as a muscle relaxant during general anaesthesia: a pilot study. Br. J. Anaesth., *39*:633, 1967.

117. Buskop, J.J., Price, M., and Molnar, I.: Untoward effect of diazepam. N. Engl. J. Med., *277*:316, 1967.

118. Dalen, J.E., Evans, G.L., Banas, J.S., Brooks, H.L., Paraskos, J.A., and Dexter, L.: The hemodynamic and respiratory effects of diazepam (Valium). Anesthesiology, *30*:259, 1969.

119. Healy, T.E.J.: Intravenous diazepam for cardiac catheterisation. Anaesthesia, *24*:537, 1969.

120. Steen, S.N., Weitzner, S.W., Amaha, K., and Martinez, L.R.: The effect of diazepam on the respiratory response to carbon dioxide. Can. Anaesth. Soc. J., *13*:374, 1966.

121. Sadove, M.S., Balagot, R.C., and McGrath, J.M.: Effects of chlordiazepoxide and diazepam on the influence of meperidine on the respiratory response to carbon dioxide. J. New Drugs, *5*:121, 1965.

122. Heinonen, J., and Muittari, A.: The effect of diazepam on airway resistance in asthmatics. Anaesthesia, *27*:37, 1972.

123. Dundee, J.W., Haslett, W.H.K., Keilty, S.R., and Pandit, S.K.: Studies of drugs given before anaesthesia. XX. Diazepam-containing mixtures. Br. J. Anaesth., *42*:143, 1970.

124. Prensky, A.L., Raff, M.C., Moore, M.J., and Schwab, R.S.: Intravenous diazepam in the treatment of prolonged seizure activity. N. Engl. J. Med., *276*:770, 1967.

125. Dundee, J.W., and Wyant, G.M.: Intravenous Anaesthesia. Edinburgh, Churchill Livingstone, 1974.

126. Package insert, Valium injectable (diazepam/Roche). Nutley, N.J., Hoffman-La Roche, May 1983.

127. Mark, L.C.: The "puff technic" for IV diazepam (letter to the editor). Anesthesiology, *61*:631, 1984.

128. Brandt, A.L., and Oakes, F.D.: Preanesthesia medication. Double blind study of a new drug, diazepam. Anesth. Analg., *44*:125, 1965.

129. Farb, H.H.: Intravenous diazepam as pre-interview medication (a clinical note). Dis. Nerv. Syst., *24*:233, 1963.

130. Davidau, A.: La premedication pour les malades difficiles: ou sur les seances de soir tres longues. Rev. Stomatol. Chir. Maxillofac., *67*:589, 1966.

131. Waterman, D.H., Domm, S.W., Rogers, W.K., and Borrell, J.L.: The effective use of bronchoscopy in chronic bronchitis. Ann. Otol. Rhinol. Laryngol., *78*:499, 1969.

132. Taylor, P.A., Cotton, P.B., Tovey, R.M., and Gent, A.E.: Pulmonary complications after oesophagogastroscopy using diazepam. Br. Med. J., *1*:660, 1972.

133. Prout, B.J., and Metreweli, C.: Pulmonary aspiration after fiber-endoscopy of the upper gastrointestinal tract. Br. Med. J., *4*:269, 1972.

134. Aldrete, J.A., Tan, S.T., Carron, D.J., and Watts, M.K.: Pentazepam (pentazocine and diazepam) supplementing local analgesia for laparoscopic sterilisation. Anesth. Analg., *55*:177, 1976.

135. Aldrete, J.A.: Somnoanalgesia with pentazepam. *In* Trends in Intravenous Anesthesia. Edited by J.A. Aldrete and T.H. Stanley. Miami, Symposia Specialists, 1980.

136. Baird, E.S., and Curson, I.: Orally administered diazepam in conservative dentistry. Br. Dent. J., *128*:26, 1970.

137. Healy, T.E.J., Robinson, J.S., and Vickers, M.D.: Physiological responses to intravenous diazepam as a sedative for conservative dentistry. Br. Med. J., *3*:10, 1970.

138. Sorabjee, S.E.: A case of trismus following dental extraction treated with diazepam. East Afr. Med. J., *44*:186, 1967.

139. Healy, T.E.J., and Hamilton, M.: Intravenous diazepam in the apprehensive child. Br. Dent. J., *130*:25, 1972.

140. Healy, T.E.J., Edmondson, H.D., and Hall, N.: The use of intravenous diazepam during dental surgery in the mentally handicapped patient. Br. Dent. J., *128*:22, 1970.

141. Orko, R.: Anaesthesia for cardioversion. Br. J. Anaesth., *48*:257, 1976.

142. Nutter, D.O., and Massumi, R.A.: Diazepam in cardioversion. N. Engl. J. Med., *273*:650, 1965.

143. Healy, T.E.J.: Intravenous diazepam for cardiac catheterisation. Anesthesia, *24*:537, 1969.

144. Samuelson, P.N.: Anesthesia for pediatric cardiac catheterisation. Symposium of Cardiac Anesthesia. American Academy of Pediatrics, Maui, Hawaii, March, 1982.

145. Rouchy, R., Blondeau, P., Cannelier, R.L., Creze, J., and Grosieux, P.: Diazepam by the intravenous route in obstetrics. Presse Med., *74*:312, 1966.

146. Stoeri, P.R., and Bossart, H.: Sedation centrale per le Valium intraveineux pour la suture de l'episiotomie. Gynaecologia, *167*:324, 1969.

147. Blanc, B., and Milani, P.: Utilisation du Valium en obstetrique. Gynecol. Obstetrique, *18*:296, 1966.

148. Conner, J.T., Katz, R.L., Pagano, R.R., and Graham, C.W.: Ro 21-3981 for intravenous surgical premedication and induction of anesthesia. Anesth. Analg., *57*:1, 1978.

149. Femi-Pearse, D.: Experience with diazepam in tetanus. Br. Med. J., *2*:862, 1966.

150. Levy, R.M.: Diazepam for LSD intoxication. Lancet, *1*:1297, 1971.

151. Thompsen, W.L., Johnson, A.D., and Maddry, W.L.: Diazepam and paraldehyde for treatment of severe delirium tremens. Ann. Intern. Med., *82*:175, 1975.

152. Walser, A.: Literature review of Ro 21-3981. Basel, Roche Laboratories, Hoffmann-LaRoche, 1977–78.

153. Sternbach, L.: Personal communication to Lester C. Mark.

154. Reves, J.G.: Midazolam compared with thiopentone as a hypnotic component in balanced anaesthesia: a randomized, double-blind study. Can. Anaesth. Soc. J., *26*:42, 1979.

155. Woo, G.K., Kolis, S.J., and Schwartz, M.A.: In vitro metabolism of an imidazobenzodiazepine. Pharmacologists, *19*:164, 1977.
156. Sarnquist, F.H., Mathers, W.D., and Blaschke, T.F.: Steady-state pharmacokinetics of midazolam maleate. Anesthesiology, *51*:S41, 1971.
157. Allonen, H., Anttila, V., and Klotz, U.: Effect kinetics of midazolam, a new hypnotic benzodiazepine derivative. Arch. Pharmacol., *316*:R74, 1981.
158. Puglisi, C.V., Meyer, J.C., D'Arconte, L., Brooks, M.A., and DeSilva, A.F.: Determination of water soluble imidazo1,4-benzodiazepines in blood by electron-capture, gas-liquid chromatography and in urine by differential pulse polarography. J. Chromatogr., *145*:81, 1978.
159. Brown, C.R., Sarnquist, F.H., Canup, C.A., and Pedley, T.A.: Clinical electroencephalographic, and pharmacokinetic studies of water-soluble benzodiazepine, midazolam maleate. Anesthesiology, *50*:467, 1979.
160. Greenblatt, D.J., Locniskar, A., Ochs, H.R., and Lauven, P.M.: Automated gas chromatography for studies of midazolam pharmacokinetics. Anesthesiology, *55*:176, 1981.
161. Reves, J.G., Newfield, P., and Smith, L.R.: Influence of serum protein, serum albumin concentrations, and dose on midazolam anaesthesia induction times. Can. Anaesth. Soc. J., *28*:556, 1981.
162. Smith, M.T., Eadie, M.J., O'Rourke, T., and Brophy, T.: The pharmacokinetics of midazolam in man. Eur. J. Clin. Pharmacol., *19*:271, 1981.
163. Crevoisier, P.C., Eckert, M., and Heizmann, P.: Relation entre l'effect clinique et pharmacocinetique du midazolam apres administration i.v. et i.m. Arzneimittelforschung, *31*:2211, 1981.
164. Forster, A., Juge, O., and Morel, D.: Effects of midazolam on cerebral blood flow in human volunteers. Anesthesiology, *55*:A263, 1981.
165. Nugent, M., Artru, A.A., and Michenfelder, J.D.: Cerebral effects of midazolam and diazepam. Anesthesiology, *53*:5, 1980.
166. Moehler, H., and Okada, T.: Benzodiazepine receptor: demonstration in the central nervous system. Science, *198*:849, 1977.
167. DeJong, R.H., and Bonin, J.D.: Benzodiazepines protect mice from local anesthetic convulsions and death. Anesth. Analg., *60*:385, 1981.
168. Reves, J.G., Mardis, M., and Strong, S.: Cardiopulmonary effects of midazolam. Ala. J. Med. Sci., *15*:347, 1978.
169. Jones, D.J., Stehling, L.D., and Zauder, H.L.: Cardiovascular responses to diazepam and midazolam maleate in the dog. Anesthesiology, *51*:430, 1979.
170. Reves, J.G., Samuelson, P.N., and Linnan, M.: Effects of midazolam maleate in patients with elevated pulmonary artery occluded pressure. *In* Trends in Intravenous Anesthesia. Edited by J.A. Aldrete and T.H. Stanley. Miami, Symposia Specialists, 1980.
171. Reves, J.G., Samuelson, P.N., and Lewis, S.: Midazolam maleate induction in patients with ischaemic heart disaease: haemodynamic observations. Can. Anaesth. Soc. J., *26*:402, 1979.
172. Lappas, D.G., Buckley, M.J., and Laver, M.B.: Left ventricular performance and pulmonary circulation following addition of nitrous oxide to morphine during coronary artery surgery. Anesthesiology, *43*:61, 1975.
173. Reves, J.G., Corssen, G., and Holcomb, C.: Comparison of two benzodiazepines for anaesthesia induction: midazolam and diazepam. Can. Anaesth. Soc. J., *25*:211, 1978.
174. Forster, A., Gardaz, J.P., Suter, P.M., and Gemperle, M.: Respiratory depression by midazolam and diazepam. Anesthesiology, *53*:494, 1980.
175. Sarnquist, F.H., Mathers, W.D., Brock-Utne, J., Carr, B., Camup, C., and Brown, C.R.: A bioassy of water-soluble benzodiazepine against sodium thiopental. Anesthesiology, *52*:149, 1980.
176. Lebonitz, P.W., Cote, M.E., Daniels, A.L., and Benventre, J.V.: Comparative renal effects of midazolam and thiopental in man. Anesthesiology, *59*:381, 1983.
177. Dundee, J.W.: Benzodiazepines in anesthesia. *In* Trends in Intravenous Anesthesia. Edited by J.A. Aldrete and T.H. Stanley. Miami, Symposia Specialists, 1980.
178. Fragen, R.J., and Hauch, T.: The effect of midazolam maleate and diazepam on intraocular pressure in adults. *In* Trends in Intravenous Anesthesia. Edited by J.A. Aldrete and T.H. Stanley. Miami, Symposia Specialists, 1980.
179. Pagano, R.R., Graham, C.W., Galligan, M., Conner, J.T., and Katz, R.L.: Histopathology of veins after intravenous lorazepam and Ro 21-3981. Can. Anaesth. Soc. J., *25*:50, 1978.
180. Fragen, R.J., Gahl, F., and Caldwell, N.: A water-soluble benzodiazepine, Ro 21-3981, for induction of anesthesia. Anesthesiology, *49*:41, 1978.
181. Fragen, R.J., Funk, D.I., and Avram, M.J.: Midazolam versus hydroxyzine as intramuscular premedicants. Anesthesiology, *55*:278, 1981.
182. Reves, J.G., Vinik, H.R., and Wright, D.: Midazolam efficacy for intramuscular premedication: a double-blind placebo, hydroxyzine, controlled study. Abstracted at the Annual Meeting of the American Society of Anesthesiologists, Las Vegas, 1982.
183. Reves, J.G., Samuelson, P.N., and Vinik, H.R.: Midazolam. *In* Contemporary Anesthesia Practice. Edited by B.R. Brown. Philadelphia, Davis, 1980.

184. Reves, J.G., Kissin, I., and Smith, L.R.: The effective dose of midazolam. Anesthesiology, 55:82, 1981.

185. Dundee, J.W., Samuel, I.O., Tomer, W., and Howard, P.J.: Midazolam: a water-soluble benzodiazepine. Anaesthesia, 35:454, 1980.

186. Kretz, F.J., Liegl, M., Heinemeyer, G., and Eyrich, K.: Die rektale Narkoseeinleitung bei Kleinkindern mit Diazepam und Midazolam. Anaesth. Intensemed., 26:343, 1985.

187. Vinik, R., Reves, J.G., Nixon, D., Whelehel, J., and McFarland, L.: Midazolam induction and emergence in renal failure patients. Anesthesiology, 55:A262, 1981.

188. Fragen, R.J., and Caldwell, N.J.: Recovery from midazolam used for short operations. Anesthesiology, 53:S11, 1980.

189. Forster, A., Gardaz, J.P., Suter, P.M., and Gemperle, M.: I.V. midazolam as an induction agent for anaesthesia: a study in volunteers. Br. J. Anaesth., 52:907, 1980.

190. Graham, C.W., Conklin, K.A., Katz, R.L., and Brinkman, C.R.: A new psychotropic agent for women during labor and delivery. Abstracted at the Annual Meeting of the American Society of Anesthesiologists, 1977.

191. Monti, J.M., and Altier, H.: Flunitrazepam (Ro 5-4200) and sleep cycle in normal subjects. Psychopharmacologia, 32:343, 1973.

192. Monti, J.M., Trenchi, H.M., Morales, F., and Monti, L.: Flunitrazepam (Ro 5-4200) and sleep cycle in insomniac patients. Psychopharmacologia, 35:371, 1974.

193. Freuchen, I., Ostergaard, J., Kuhl, J.B., and Mikkelsen, B.O.: Reduction of psychotomimetic side effects of Ketalar (ketamin) by Rohypnol (flunitrazepam). Acta Anaesthesiol. Scand., 20:97, 1976.

194. Vega, D.E.: Induccion del sueno anesthesico con un nuevo derivado benzodiazepinico. Comunicacion preliminar. Rev. Urug. Anest., 5:41, 1971.

195. Stovner, J., Endresen, R., and Osterud, A.: Intravenous anaesthesia with a new benzodiazepine Ro 5-4200. Acta Anaesthesiol. Scand., 17:163, 1973.

196. Ungerer, M.J., and Erasmus, F.R.: Evaluation of a new benzodiazepine, flunitrazepam (Ro 5-4200) as an anesthetic induction agent. S. Afr. Med. J., 47:787, 1973.

197. Wickstrom, E.: Flunitrazepam (Ro 5-4200)—a new hypnotic. Tidsskr. Nor. Laegeforen, 93:1494, 1973.

198. Wickstrom, E.: Double-blind study of flunitrazepam (Ro 5-4200) and mandrax. Anaesthesist, 23:90, 1974.

199. Freuchen, I., Ostergaarol, J., and Nickelson, B.O.: Flunitrazepam (Rohypnol) compared with enibomal (Narcodorm) as an anaesthetic induction agent: a controlled clinical trial. Curr. Ther. Res., 20:36, 1976.

200. Boxenbaum, H.G., Posmanter, H.N., Macasieb, T., Geitner, K.A., Weinfeld, R.E., Moore, J.D., Darragh, A., O'Kelly, D.A., Weissman, I., and Kaplan, S.A.: Pharmacokinetics of flunitrazepam following single- and mutiple-dose oral administration to healthy human subjects. J. Pharmacokinet. Biopharm., 6:283, 1978.

201. Clarke, R.S.J., Dundee, J.W., McGowan, W.A.W., and Howard, P.J.: Comparison of the subjective effects and plasma concentrations following oral and i.m. administration of flunitrazepam in volunteers. Br. J. Anaesth., 52:437, 1980.

202. Pasch, T., and Bugsch, L.A.: Beeinflussung der glatten Muskulatur kleiner Arterien durch Analgetika, Droperidol, Diazepam und Flunitrazepam. Anaesthesist, 28:283, 1979.

203. Mattila, M.A.K., and Larni, H.M.: Flunitrazepam: a review of its pharmacological properties and therapeutic use. Drugs, 20:353, 1980.

204. Coleman, A.J., Downing, J.W., Moyes, D.G., and O'Brien, A.: Acute cardiovascular effects of Ro 5-4200: a new anaesthetic induction agent. S. Afr. Med. J., 47:382, 1973.

205. Seitz, W., Hempelmann, G., and Piepenbrock, S.: Zur kardiovaskulaeren Wirkung von Flunitrazepam (Rohypnol, Ro 5-4200). Anaesthesist, 26:249, 1977.

206. Haldermann, G., Hoessli, G., and Schaer, H.: Die Anaesthesie mit Rohypnol (Flunitrazepam) und Fentanyl, beim geriatrischen Patienten. Anaesthesist, 26:168, 1977.

207. Korttila, K., and Aromaa, U.: Venous complications after intravenous injection of diazepam, flunitrazepam, thiopentone and etomidate. Acta Anaesthesiol. Scand., 24:227, 1980.

208. Castanos, C.C.: Intravenous anesthesia with flunitrazepam-meperidine. *In* Trends in Intravenous Anesthesia. Edited by J.A. Aldrete and T.H. Stanley. Miami, Symposia Specialists, 1980.

209. Greenblatt, D.J., Comer, W.H., Elliott, H.W., Shader, R.I, Knowles, J.A., and Reulius, H.W.: Clinical pharmacokinetcs of lorazepam. III. Intravenous injection. Preliminary results. J. Clin. Pharmacol., 17:490, 1977.

210. Greenblatt, D.J., Shader, R.I., Franke, K., MacLaughlin, D.S., Harmatz, J.S., Allen, M.D., Werner, A., and Woo, E.: Pharmacokinetics and bioavailability of intravenous, intramuscular and oral lorazepam in humans. J. Pharm. Sci., 68:57, 1979.

211. Verschraegen, R., and Rolly, G.: Intra-muscular premedication with lorazepam (Temesta). Acta Anaesthesiol. Belg., 25:68, 1974.

212. Greenblatt, D.J., Knowles, J.A., Comer, W.H., Shader, R.I., Harmatz, J.S., and Ruelius, H.W.:

Clinical pharmacokinetics of lorazepam. IV. Long-term oral administration. J. Clin. Pharmacol., 17:495, 1977.

213. Greenblatt, D.J., Allen, M.D., Locniskar, A., Harmatz, J.S., and Shader, R.I.: Lorazepam kinetics in the elderly. Clin. Pharmacol. Ther., 26:103, 1979.

214. Kraus, J.W., Desmond, P.V., Marshall, J.P., Johnnson, R.F., Schenker, S., and Wilkinson, G.R.: Effects of aging and liver disease on disposition of lorazepam. Clin. Pharmacol. Ther., 24:411, 1978.

215. George, K.A., and Dundee, J.W.: Relative amnesic actions of diazepam, flunitrazepam and lorazepam in man. Br. J. Clin. Pharmacol., 4:45, 1977.

216. Dundee, J.W., McGowan, W.A.W., Lilburu, J.K., McKay, A.C., and Hegarty, J.E.: Comparison of the actions of diazepam and lorazepam. Br. J. Anaesth., 51:439, 1979.

217. Aaltonen, L., Kanto, J., and Sado, M.: Cerebrospinal fluid concentrations and serum protein binding of lorazepam and its conjugate. Acta Pharmacol. Toxicol. (Copenh.), 46:156, 1980.

218. Elliott, H.W.: Metabolism of lorazepam. Br. J. Anaesth., 48:1017, 1976.

219. Hedges, A., Turner, P., and Harry, T.V.A.: Preliminary studies on the central effects of lorazepam, a new benzodiazepine. J. Clin. Pharmacol., 11:423, 1971.

220. Norris, W., and Wallace, P.G.M.: Wy 4036 (lorazepam): a study of its use in premedication. Br. J. Anaesth., 43:785, 1971.

221. Harry, T.V.A., and Richards, D.J.: Lorazepam—a study in psychomotor depression. Br. J. Clin. Pract., 26:371, 1972.

222. Powell, W.F., and Comer, W.H.: Controlled comparison of lorazepam and pentobarbital as hypnotics for pre-surgical patients. Anesth. Analg., 52:267, 1973.

223. Nanivadekar, A.S., Wig, N.N., Khorana, A.B., and Kulkarni, S.S.: A multicenter investigation of lorazepam in anxiety neurosis. Curr. Ther. Res., 15:500, 1973.

224. Cremonesi, E., Nunes de Silva, L.F., Curras, J.S., Cavalcanti, A.H., Moraes, R., and Sartoretto, J.N.: Evaluation of lorazepam as an oral preanesthetic medication. A comparative double-blind study with diazepam and placebo. Curr. Med. Res., 2:244, 1974.

225. Knapp, R.B., and Fierro, L.: Evaluation of the cardiopulmonary safety and effects of lorazepam as a premedicant. Anesth. Analg., 53:122, 1974.

226. Coleman, A.J., and Bees, L.T.: Double-blind comparative trial of parenteral lorazepam and papaveretum in premedication. S. Afr. Med. J., 48:862, 1974.

227. Heisterkamp, D.V., and Cohen, P.J.: The effect of intravenous premedication with lorazepam (Ativan), pentobarbitone or diazepam on recall. Br. J. Anaesth., 47:79, 1975.

228. Conner, J.T., Parson, N., Katz, R.L., Wapner, S., and Belleville, J.W.: Evaluation of lorazepam and pentothal as surgical premedicants. Clin. Pharmacol. Ther., 19:24, 1976.

229. Conner, J.T., Katz, R.I., Belleville, J.W., Graham, C., Pagano, R., and Dorey, F.: Diazepam and lorazepam for intravenous surgical premedication. J. Clin. Pharmacol., 18:285, 1978.

230. Hewitt, J.M., and Barr, A.M.: Premedication with lorazepam for bronchoscopy and general anaesthesia. Br. J. Anaesth., 50:1149, 1978.

231. Aleniewkis, M.I., Bulas, B.J., Maderazo, L., and Mendoza, C.: Intramuscular lorazepam vs. pentobarbital premedication: a comparison of patient sedation, anxiolysis and recall. Anesth. Analg., 56:489, 1977.

232. Physician's Manual. Ativan (Lorazepam) Injection for Preanesthetic Medication. Philadelphia, Wyeth Laboratories, September, 1980.

233. Kangas, L., Iisalo, E., Kanto, J., Lehtinen, V., Pynnoenen, S., Salminen, J., Sillanpaeae, M., and Syvaelahti, E.: Human pharmacokinetics of nitrazepam: effect of age and diseases. Eur. J. Clin. Pharmacol., 15:163, 1979.

234. Iisalo, E., Kangas, L., and Ruikka, I.: Pharmacokinetics of nitrazepam in young volunteers and aged patients. Br. J. Clin. Pharmacol., 4:646, 1977.

235. Kangas, L., Allonen, H., and Lammintausta, R.: Pharmacokinetics of nitrazepam in saliva and serum after a single oral dose. Acta Pharmacol. Toxicol. (Copenh.), 45:20, 1979.

236. Kangas, L., Kanto J., and Lehtinen, V.: Long-term nitrazepam treatment in psychiatric outpatients with insomnia. Psychopharmacology (Berlin), 63:63, 1979.

237. Johnstone, M.: The effects of oral sedatives on the vasoconstrictive reaction to fear. Br. J. Anaesth., 43:380, 1971.

238. Johnstone, M.: Psychoses and ketamine. Br. Med. J., 1:442, 1972.

239. Abajian, J.D., Page, P., and Morgan, M.: Effects of droperidol and nitrazepam on emergence delirium reactions following ketamine anesthesia. Anesth. Analg., 52:385, 1973.

240. Schwartz, M.A., Postma, E., and Gaut, Z.: Biological half-life of chlordiazepoxide and its metabolite, demoxepam, in man. J. Pharm. Sci., 60:1500, 1971.

241. Boxenbaum, H.G., Geitner, K.A., Jack, M.L., Dixon, W.R., Spiegel, H.E., Symington, J., Christian, R., Moore, J.D., Weissman, L., and Kaplan, S.A.: Pharmacokinetic and biopharmaceutic profile of chlordiazepoxide HC1 in healthy subjects: single-dose studies by the intravenous, intramuscular, and oral routes. J. Pharmacokinet. Biopharm., 5:3, 1977.

242. Greenblatt, D.J., Shader, R.I., MacLeod, S.M., Sellers, E.M., Franke, K., and Giles, H.G.: Absorption of oral and intramuscular chlordiazepoxide. Eur. J. Clin. Pharmacol., *13*:267, 1978.

243. Greenblatt, D.J., Shader, R.I., and Koch-Weser, J.: Slow absorption of intramuscular chlordiazepoxide. N. Engl. J. Med., *291*:116, 1974.

244. Shader, R.I., Greenblatt, D.J., Harmatz, J.S., Franke, K., and Koch-Weser, J.: Absorption and disposition of chlordiazepoxide in young and elderly male volunteers. J. Clin. Pharmacol., *17*:709, 1977.

245. Roberts, R.K., Wilkinson, G.R., Branch, R.A., and Schenker, S.: Effects of age and parenchymal liver disease on the disposition and elimination of chlordiazepoxide (Librium). Gastroenterology, *75*:479, 1978.

246. Greenblatt, D.J., Shader, R.I., and MacLeod, S.M.: Clinical pharmacokinetics of chlordiazepoxide. Clin. Pharmacokinet., *3*:381, 1978.

247. Kissen, M.D.: Cited in Ban, T.A., Lehmann, H.E., Matthews, V., and Donald, M.: Comparative study of chlorpromazine and chlordiazepoxide in the prevention and treatment of alcohol withdrawal symptoms. Clin. Med., *72*:59, 1960.

248. Holister, L.E., Motzebecker, P., and Degan, R.O: Withdrawal reactions from chlordiazepoxide ("Librium"). Psychopharmacologia, *2*:63, 1961.

249. Randall, L.O., Scheckel, C.L., and Banzinger, R.F: Pharmacolgy of the metabolites of chlordiazepoxide and diazepam. Curr. Ther. Res., *7*:590, 1965.

250. Curry, S.H., and Whelpton, R.: Pharmacokinetics of closely related benzodiazepines. Br. J. Clin. Pharmac., *8*:15S, 1979.

251. Alvan, G., Siwers, B., and Vessman, J.: Pharmacokinetics of oxazepam in healthy volunteers. Acta Pharmacol. Toxicol. (Copenh.), *40*:40, 1977.

252. Alvan, G., and Cederlof, O.: The pharmacokinetic profile of oxazepam. Acta Psychiatr. Scand., *274*:47, 1978.

253. Kales, J.D., Kales, A., Bixler, E.O., and Slye, E.S.: Effects of placebo and flurazepam on sleep patterns in insomniac subjects. Clin. Pharmacol. Ther., *12*:691, 1971.

254. Eberts, F.S. Philopoulos, Y., Reineke, L.M., and Vliek, R.W.: Triazolam disposition. Clin. Pharmacol. Ther., *29*:81, 1981.

255. Einarson, T.R., Moschitto, L.J., Greenblatt, D.J., Divoll, M., Abernathy, D.R., Smith, R.B., and Shader, R.I.: Hallucinations from triazolam. Drug Intell. Clin. Pharm., *14*:714, 1980.

256. Heel, R.C., Brogden, R.N., Speight, T.M., and Avery, G.S.: Temazepam: a review of pharmacological properties and therapeutic efficacy as an hypnotic. Drugs, *21*:321, 1981.

257. Moschitto, L., Greenblatt, D.J., and Divoll, M.: Alprazolam kinetics in the elderly: relation to antipyrine disposition. Clin. Pharmacol. Ther., *29*:267, 1981 (Abstr.).

258. Allen, M.D., Greenblatt, D.J., Harmatz, J.S., and Shader, R.I.: Desmethyl-diazepam kinetics in the elderly after oral prazepam. Clin. Pharmacol. Ther., *28*:196, 1980.

259. Hunkeler, W., Moehler, Pieri, L., Polc, P., Bonetti, E.P., Cumin, R., Schaffner, R., and Haefely, W.: Selective antagonists of benzodiazepines. Nature, *290*:514, 1981.

260. Polc, P., Laurent, J.-P., Scherschlicht, R., and Haefely, W.: Electrophysiological studies on the specific benzodiazepine antagonist Ro 15-1788. Naunyn. Schmiederbergs. Arch. Pharmacol., *316*:317, 1981.

261. Bonetti, E.P., Pieri, L., Cumin, R., Schaffner, R., Pieri, M., Gamzu, E.R., Muller, R.K.M., and Haefely, W.: Benzodiazepine antagonist Ro 15-1788: neurological and behavioural effects. Psychopharmacology (Berlin), *78*:8, 1982.

262. Cumin, R., Bonetti, E.P., Scherschlicht, R., and Haefely, W.: Use of the specific benzodiazepine antagonist, Ro 15-1788, in studies of physiological dependence on benzodiazepines. Experientia, *38*:833, 1982.

263. Lauven, P.M., Stoeckel, H., Schwilden, R., Arendt, R., Greenblatt, D.J., and Schuttler, J.: Application of a benzodiazepine antagonist (Ro 15-1788) under steady state conditions of midazolam. Anesthesiology, *57*:A325, 1982.

264. Darragh, A., Lambe, R., Kenny, M., Brick, I., Taafe, W., and O'Boyle, L.: Ro 15-1788 antagonizes the central effect of diazepam in man without altering diazepam bioavailability. Br. J. Clin. Pharmacol., *14*:677, 1982.

265. Ziegler, W.H., and Schalch, E.: Antagonism of benzodiazepine-induced sedation in man. *In* Sleep 1982. Edited by W.P. Koella. Basel, Karger, 1983.

266. Scollo-Lavizzari, G.: First clinical investigation of the benzodiazepine antagonist Ro 15-1788 in comatose patients. Eur. Neurol., *22*:7, 1983.

267. Schwilden, H., Stoeckel, H., Lauven, P.M., and Schuettler, J.: Action of a benzodiazepine antagonist during midazolam infusion in a steady-state: quantitative EEG studies. Anesthesiology, *57*:A326, 1982.

268. Moehler, H., Burkard, W.P., Keller, H.H., Richards, J.G., and Haefely, W.: Benzodiazepine antagonist Ro 15-1788: binding characteristics and interaction with drug-induced changes in dopamine turnover and cerebellar GMP levels. J. Neurochem., *37*:714, 1981.

269. Schoemaker, H., Bliss, M., and Yamamura, H.I.: Specific high-affinity saturable binding of [^{3}H] Ro 5-4864 to benzodiazepine binding sites in the rat cerebral cortex. Eur. J. Pharmacol., *71*:173, 1981.

Chapter 10

PROPANIDID

HISTORY

The observation that eugenol (1-vinyl-3-methoxy-4-hydroxybenzene) (Fig. 10–1), derived from oil of clover and cinnamon, exhibits anesthetic properties when given intravenously prompted Thuillier and Domenjoz in Basel, Switzerland, to explore the suitability of some of its congeners for use as intravenous anesthetics.[1] The most promising of these congeners, designated G 29505 (1-vinyl-3-methoxy-4-N-diethylcarbamoylmethoxybenzene) (Fig. 10–1), epitomizes the group in causing respiratory stimulation and in lasting for an extremely short time period. The insolubility of these congeners in water was a serious drawback. A related eugenol, propinal, in which a 1-propyl group replaced the 1-vinyl of G 29505, was briefly described by researchers from Japan.[2] Clinical studies with G 29505 in Europe and the United States were soon terminated because the drug frequently caused serious venous complications.[3,4] This difficulty was largely overcome in another derivative, propanidid (Epontol and Fabantol) (3-methoxy-4-(N-diethylcarbamoyl-methoxy)-phenylacetic-n-propylester) (Fig. 10–1), which was introduced in Germany by Hiltmann, et al.[5]

CHEMISTRY AND PHYSICAL PROPERTIES

Propanidid is a faintly yellowish oil that is insoluble in water (Fig. 10–1). For clinical use, propanidid is dissolved by a solubilizing compound, Oleum ricini polyoxyethylat Elb, Tensid ORPE or Tensid, for short, which incorporates propanidid molecules into its micelles to form a colloidal solution, itself soluble in water.[6] Each 10-ml ampule contains a stable mixture (shelf life of 2 years) of 500 mg of propanidid, 1600 mg of Tensid, and 70 mg of sodium chloride in water. This highly viscous solution should be diluted with saline immediately before use.[7] Note that Tensid has replaced Cremophor EL, another polyoxylated castor

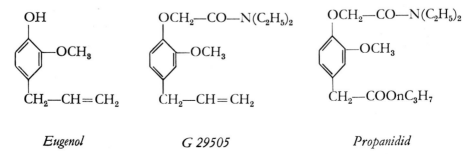

Fig. 10–1. Structural formula of propanidid as compared to eugenol and G 29505.

oil, which was the initial solubilizing agent. In most of the early studies, propanidid formulated with Cremophor EL was used.

PHARMACOKINETICS

Propanidid is rapidly broken down by a nonspecific esterase in the bloodstream (Fig. 10–2).[8–12] Pseudocholinesterase is the same plasma enzyme that inactivates procaine, succinylcholine, and any other foreign substances containing an ester linkage (see Chapter 15). This nonspecific esterase should not be confused with true cholinesterase, a highly specific enzyme found in tissues, which hydrolyzes acetylcholine and practically nothing else. Blood levels reveal a short $t\frac{1}{2}$ α (about 3 minutes), which actually involves the distribution and the metabolism of the drug. Indeed, tissue distribution is rapid and extensive, because of high lipid solubility. The $t\frac{1}{2}$ β is somewhat longer (about 10 minutes) when considering metabolism alone.[9]

Two steps in the biotransformation of propanidid have been elucidated: (1) ester hydrolysis to the main metabolite, 3-methoxy-4-(N-diethylcarbamoyl-methoxy)-phenylacetic acid, and n-propyl alcohol, and (2) deamination of the main metabolite to 3-methoxy-4-acetoxy-phenylacetic acid and diethylamine (Fig. 10–2). Speedy metabolism is further confirmed by the appearance of 50 to 75% of the metabolites in the urine within 2 hours of administration.[10] Because these metabolites are pharmacologically inert, the rapidity of their production is a controlling factor in terminating the action of propanidid.[12]

As with thiopental, both dosage and speed of injection of propanidid are important: the initial depth of sleep is greater when propanidid is intravenously administered rapidly rather than slowly. Curiously, the time of recovery is essentially the same with both routes of administration. This fact does not indicate acute tolerance, as was suggested elsewhere, because the same dose, injected rapidly, should have resulted in shorter duration of sleep if acute tolerance had developed.[13] Doenicke, et al., observed a transient inhibition (20%) of pseudocholinesterase activity after the rapid intravenous administration of propanidid (7 mg/kg over a period of 5 seconds) that is promptly reversed as the drug disappears from the circulation.[11] This finding suggests that propanidid injected rapidly initially produces high drug levels, while simultaneously enhancing initial rates of enzymatic breakdown. The result is a more rapid disappearance of propanidid from the bloodstream. Because propanidid and succinylcholine are both esters, and hence compete for hydrolysis by the same enzyme, pseudocholines-

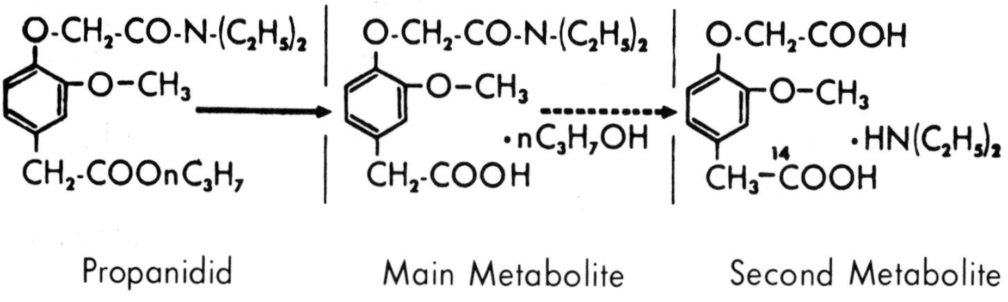

Propanidid   Main Metabolite   Second Metabolite

Fig. 10–2. Metabolic breakdown of propanidid. (From Puetter, J.: Uber den fermentativen Abbau des Propanidid. *In* Die intravenose Kurznarkose mit dem neuen Phenoxyessigsaurederivat Propanidid (Eponotol). Edited by K. Horatz, R. Frey, and M. Zindler. Berlin, Springer, 1965).

terase, it is not surprising that propanidid enhances the duration of apnea produced by succinylcholine.[14–17]

Approximately 40% of the total amount of propanidid in plasma is bound to protein, presumably albumin.[6] Because pharmacologic activity varies with the concentration of drug lying free in plasma water, hypoalbuminemia should enhance and prolong the effects of propanidid. This enhanced and prolonged drug effect also occurs in debilitated or elderly patients with low plasma levels of pseudocholinesterase. The rapid distribution of propanidid into tissues, especially richly perfused organs, may play an important role in terminating drug action.[18]

PHARMACOLOGY

Central Nervous System (CNS)

An adequate intravenous dose of propanidid produces loss of consciousness in one arm-brain circulation time. The onset of unconsciousness is reflected in electroencephalographic (EEG) changes similar to those observed with the anesthetic barbiturates, i.e., a transition to high voltage, slow waves (4 to 5 Hz), together with 12- to 14-Hz spindles and irregular 1- to 2-Hz activity as sleep deepens.[19,20] Return of rapid activity signals emergence from CNS depression.[7,19] Because of its truly ultra-short duration of action, frequent incremental doses of propanidid are required to maintain anesthesia; this requirement is indicative of minimal accumulation of this drug, unlike the correspondingly lipid-soluble barbiturates.

Potency

Propanidid is reportedly about one-fourth to one-fifth as potent as methohexital. Because methohexital is about two to three times as potent as thiopental, it seems reasonable to rate propanidid as one-half as potent as thiopental.[18,20–22] This proposed rate is confirmed by the generally accepted dose range of propanidid (5 to 10 mg/kg) compared to the "standard" sleep of thiopental (4 mg/kg).[23–26] The relationship between the dose of propanidid and the duration of sleep induced is not linear, i.e., larger doses do not prolong sleep proportionately. A higher initial blood level of propanidid is not followed by a proportionately longer duration of sleep, apparently because of the more rapid enzymatic destruction of the drug at high plasma levels, as previously discussed. When studying the relationship between the dose and the duration of sleep in 150 patients receiving between 0.5 and 15.5 mg/kg of propanidid, Clarke found the prediction of a specific dose required to produce anesthesia for 4 to 5 minutes impracticable because the doses ranged from 225 to 1000 mg, or 3.8 to 17.6 mg/kg.[27] Clarke suggested that the longest duration of sleep likely to be provided after a safe, single intravenous dose of propanidid is approximately 6 minutes. Similar findings were recorded on the basis of studies concerned with recovery from propanidid when used for minor operations.[28]

Analgesia

Propanidid produces no clinically useful level of analgesia, despite reported findings to the contrary in a study of dental patients and in experimental findings in rabbits (electric stimulation of tooth pulp) and man (tibial pressure).[8,29–32] Propanidid also does not exert any antanalgesic action.[32]

Recovery

Rapid recovery is the hallmark of anesthesia with propanidid, the only intravenous "anesthetic" the effects of which are truly terminated by its ability to be rapidly metabolized. Patients awaken faster after propanidid use than after receiving the anesthetic barbiturates; also, once awake, they tend to remain alert rather than to relapse into sleep if undisturbed, as noted with the barbiturates, with the exception of methohexital.[19,22,28,33,34] Confirmatory EEG studies during this period show prompt restoration of patterns of wakefulness without relapse after propanidid use; frequently, characteristic sleep patterns are noted for as long as 24 hours after the intravenous delivery of barbiturates.[34] Similarly, the level of "street fitness" returns to normal within 30 minutes of regaining consciousness after propanidid, as does simulated driving ability; the latter remains significantly impaired, however, after barbiturate administration (6 to 8 hours).[35,36] The operation of a motor vehicle or other machinery should be prohibited for at least 2 hours after propanidid use and probably for as long as 24 hours after anesthesia with barbiturates.[36] Interestingly, even after 12 hours, the barbiturate residuum in the body enhances the sedative effects of 500 ml of beer; this enhancement does not occur with propanidid.[34]

Cardiovascular System

Propanidid causes transient dose-related hypotension with compensatory tachycardia in animals and man.[8,13,24,37–46] These effects are usually transient because of the speedy decline in plasma concentrations of propanidid caused by the rapid metabolism of the drug, as previously noted. Decreased myocardial contractility and peripheral vasodilatation were both observed in studies in the dog, as was histamine release induced by the solubilizing agent.[39] In man, however, digital plethysmography shows compensatory vasoconstriction, not dilatation.[47] Propanidid-induced hypotension is thus attributable solely to transient cardiac depression, as evidenced by deepening and widening of the S waves and even short-lasting A-V block.[47] These effects suggest that propanidid should not be used in patients with congestive heart failure, ventricular hypertrophy, conduction disorders, or valvular heart disease. Severe cardiovascular depression, including two instances of asystole after propanidid use, was reported in adults and children.[48–53]

Propanidid seems to prevent cardiac arrhythmias that may result from stimulation of laryngoscopy and endotracheal intubation and may also correct ventricular arrhythmias during light anesthesia.[47] These effects are probably mediated by the diethylamino configuration of the substituent in position 4 of the molecule (Fig. 10–1), a structural feature shared by the antiarrhythmic drugs, quinidine and procaine amide.[54]

Respiratory System

Propanidid exerts a biphasic effect on respiration that is characterized by hyperventilation starting with the loss of consciousness and lasting about 30 seconds, followed by a short period of hypoventilation, periodic breathing, or apnea.[55] The overall changes in arterial blood gases are not of essential clinical significance; the exception is a further lowering in arterial oxygen tension in patients who already have a decreased value and in patients after prolonged apnea or hypoventilation. In these individuals, and probably in all high-risk patients, it seems advisable to provide oxygen by mask and to assist or control ventilation.

The hyperventilatory response related to propanidid use has been ascribed to the stimulation of carotid chemoreceptors by the drug; injection of these chemoreceptors with lidocaine prevented the response in cats, whereas vagotomy did not.[56] More pronounced hyperventilation after use of the eugenol derivative, G 29505, could also be due, in part, to an action on peripherally located receptors.[57] Lung biopsy specimens obtained from dogs at the peak of G 29505-induced hyperventilation showed multiple fat droplets that presumably were remnants of the oil-water emulsion in the walls of the alveoli, thereby implicating that the drug may also be found in this region. Arterial hypotension and desensitization of pulmonary stretch receptors have also been suggested as playing a role in the hyperventilatory response to propanidid.[37]

The biphasic respiratory response to propanidid is not significantly altered by premedication with sedative drugs, but narcotics do reduce respiratory stimulation and prolong apnea.[55,58] The incidence of apnea seems more proportionate to the dose of propanidid than to the degree of hyperventilation, thus eliminating hypocarbia as a major factor.[13,55]

Note that propanidid-induced hyperventilation enhances the uptake of inhalational anesthetics, which can be further augmented by vigorous manual ventilation during the period of apnea. The hyperventilation may also expedite "blind" nasotracheal intubation.[59] Conversely, PaO_2 levels may fall significantly during the secondary hypoventilation phase, thus necessitating manual assistance with oxygen.[58]

Interaction with Succinylcholine

The duration of neuromuscular blockade and apnea after succinylcholine use is lengthened by several minutes with prior administration of propanidid.[14–17,60] As mentioned previously, this relationship is not surprising. Because the two drugs are inactivated by the same enzyme (pseudocholinesterase) in the plasma, they compete for available binding sites on the same enzyme protein. The sites occupied by propanidid, injected first, are not accessible to succinylcholine until the propanidid molecules are hydrolyzed. Because this reaction occurs swiftly, the hindrance to metabolism of succinylcholine is short-lived. Meanwhile, succinylcholine molecules bind to the many free sites remaining, so that their inactivation proceeds with its usual rapidity. Consequently, the muscle-relaxant effect is only briefly prolonged. For some unknown reason, the incidence and severity of succinylcholine-induced postoperative muscle pains are reduced by the administration of propanidid.[15]

Interaction with Other Relaxants

Propanidid also prolongs the muscle-relaxant action of decamethonium, presumably by the same mechanism.[60] Conversely, requirements for tubocurarine in man are reportedly higher with propanidid use than with thiopental use; the putative mechanism, a minor degree of neuromuscular block by thiopental or reduction in cholinesterase by propanidid that potentiates endogenous acetylcholine, may be disputable.[13,15,61] Although the high plasma concentrations of thiopental briefly present during induction of anesthesia may produce transient muscular relaxation, the effect is negligible at ordinary anesthetic levels. Also, the interaction between propanidid and pseudocholinesterase in plasma does not involve true cholinesterase at the myoneural junction. The latter enzyme is highly specific for acetylcholine and is totally unaffected by propanidid.

Metabolism

Blood glucose levels rise slightly in patients undergoing operations during propanidid-nitrous oxide anesthesia.[62] Those patients who are so anesthetized, but who do not undergo surgery, do not experience such an increase, which suggests that the hyperglycemia is the result of surgical trauma rather than of propanidid use.

Other Systems

Propanidid does not adversely affect hepatorenal or hematopoietic function in man.[8,63–66]

TOXICITY AND SIDE-EFFECTS

Results of acute toxicity studies in animals show that the LD_{50} of propanidid given intravenously approximates that of hexobarbital and is 25 to 50% that of thiopental. Decreasing the speed of injection markedly reduces the toxic effects.

Local Irritation

In view of the high incidence of intravascular complications noted with the eugenol derivative, G 29505, this aspect of propanidid requires clarification. Studies of tissue damage (edema and necrosis) in rabbits, cats, and rats after intraarterial injection of various intravenous drugs showed that propanidid (at 2.5%) is less irritative than a corresponding solution of thiopental.[67] Cremophor EL, the initial solubilizing agent for propanidid, proved innocuous; presumably the current solubilizer, Tensid, is equally innocuous.[67] Comparable studies in man are necessarily limited, but no vascular complications followed intra-arterial injections of propanidid in six patients awaiting limb amputation, or in two other individuals who received it so inadvertently.[13,68,69] The incidence of venous complications (phlebitis and thrombosis) after direct intravenous injection of propanidid was reported to vary from 4 to 15.2%.[70–72] Dilution of the commercially available 5% propanidid solution to 3.5% with saline solution or administration of the drug into the tubing of a freely running infusion reduces the overall incidence of venous sequelae to less than 6%.[70,72]

Excitatory Phenomena

The incidence of excitatory phenomena during propanidid anesthesia, including involuntary muscle movements, shivering, tremor, cough, hiccoughs, and laryngospasm, is about 10% (8% in one study, 11% in another); corresponding figures with thiopental and with methohexital are 9 and 24%, respectively.[42,73] The severity of these side-effects is enhanced by increasing the dosage of propanidid.[13] These phenomena are also affected by preanesthetic medication, increasing with the use of scopolamine and antinauseants (e.g., cyclizine and promethazine) and decreasing after the delivery of opiates.[74]

Nausea and Vomiting

The reported incidence of vomiting after propanidid administration varies from 0 to 40%, and is independent of the rate of administration.[42,73,75] Premedication with antiemetic drugs does reduce vomiting, but at the cost of the aforementioned motor side-effects; atropine has no effect.[73,76] The addition of nitrous oxide increases the incidence of vomiting after propanidid use, whereas halothane reduces the incidence.[77]

Hypersensitivity

Flushing and a precipitous fall in blood pressure level are the most frequent anaphylactoid responses to propanidid. Other reactions include erythema, skin rashes, urticaria, abdominal pain, bronchospasm, moderate to severe hypotension, and cardiovascular collapse.[46,49–53,78–88] Among these responses, flushing or hypotension alone is most probably due to the drug itself, rather than to a hypersensitivity reaction caused by the release of histamine.

A histamine reaction is most likely to occur in the one half of that group of patients who react adversely after receiving propanidid for the second time.[43] But anaphylaxis that occurs after propanidid use is not necessarily caused by the administration of that drug. In one case report, a woman received propanidid (8.5 mg/kg) and cyclizine (50 mg) before undergoing dilatation and cauterization of the cervix; urticaria, bronchospasm, and hypotension followed. Subsequent skin testing elicited a marked reaction to cyclizine, but not to propanidid.[89]

Severe histamine reactions to propanidid require aggressive therapy with vasopressors, steroids, and even cardiac massage.[79,82,87] Nevertheless, in view of their relative infrequency, the suggestion for routine prophylactic premedication with an antihistamine drug or corticosteroids hardly seems warranted.[90]

CLINICAL APPLICATIONS

After initial clinical trials by various European and Canadian investigators, propanidid was released for general use. The drug rapidly gained popularity as a suitable anesthetic for minor diagnostic and surgical procedures performed in ambulatory patients.[18,24,25,29–31,35,42,63,64,69,80,91,92]

Outpatient Dentistry

In pediatric outpatient dentistry, propanidid proved to be particularly suitable when the procedure involved extraction of a few teeth and did not exceed the duration of anesthesia provided by a single intravenous injection at a dose of approximately 8 mg/kg.[30,93,95] In adult patients, an average single dose of 5 to 7 mg/kg is sufficient to perform brief dental manipulations. Intermittent intravenous injections of propanidid may be required if the procedure outlasts the anesthesia produced by a single injection.[96,97]

In one investigative series, satisfactory results were reported with the intermittent administration of propanidid to 13,500 dental outpatients.[98] The author of this study considered the use of propanidid in dentistry contraindicated in patients with poorly controlled epilepsy. Another researcher used propanidid as the sole anesthetic and also for the induction of nitrous oxide-halothane anesthesia in 650 operative procedures in dentistry. In this report, stress was placed on the need for close cooperation between the dental surgeon and the anesthesiologist to assure optimal results.[99] Anesthesia with propanidid, nitrous oxide, and halothane for prolonged dental procedures may be less satisfactory because recovery may be quicker when propanidid is used alone. The more rapid restoration of mental clarity and "street fitness" after propanidid use is the main reason for its preference over thiopental and methohexital in dentistry.[100] In one study, incremental subanesthetic doses of propanidid were administered intravenously to dental outpatients who were premedicated with diazepam (5 mg intravenously); adequate operating conditions were obtained with a total dose of 0.22 mg/kg.[101]

Cardioversion

Propanidid is highly suitable for use during cardioversion.[102] Because only a few seconds of anesthesia are required to protect the patient from experiencing pain during application of the electric current, injection of a low individual dose of propanidid (3 to 5 mg/kg) is recommended. The dose should be injected slowly over a period of 40 to 60 seconds, and oxygen should be administered by mask during the hypoventilation phase. Allergic patients may be given an antihistaminic preparation for premedication. In the presence of hypokalemia, digitalis intoxication, and beta-receptor blockade, the use of propanidid is contraindicated.

Obstetrics

Propanidid has been successfully employed for vaginal delivery and cesarean section. Although the drug rapidly crosses the placental barrier, no significant depressant effects on the fetus have been observed. One researcher reported clinical experience with the use of propanidid in obstetric analgesia-anesthesia in 1600 parturients for uncomplicated vaginal delivery, vacuum or forceps extraction, duplex and breech delivery, repair of obstetric trauma, exploration of the uterus, and induction of analgesia-anesthesia for cesarean section.[103] The intravenous dose of propanidid ranged from 250 to 750 mg, depending on the weight and physical status of the patient. The advantages of the use of propanidid in obstetrics include quick induction of anesthesia with the patient remaining supine for a minimum of time to reduce the possibility of the development of supine hypotensive syndrome, good oxygenation during hyperventilation, no depressant effects on the infant, no uterine relaxation, smooth awakening, and no postoperative "hangover" feeling. These favorable results, especially related to use of the drug for cesarean section, were confirmed by other investigators.[104] Propanidid is particularly advantageous when employed as an anesthetic for cesarean section performed in primitive surroundings because of the minimal amount of equipment needed.[105]

Propanidid has also been administered in a continuous slow-drip intravenous infusion for lengthy obstetric procedures.[106] With a 1% propanidid solution (10 mg/ml), anesthesia is induced with 2 to 5 ml/minute for an average total dose of 12.5 to 62.5 mg of propanidid. During maintenance of anesthesia, the drip rate varies from 2 to 3 ml/minute during uterine contractions to 1 ml/minute during pauses between contractions. If required during special obstetric manipulations, the drip can be increased briefly to a maximum of 15 ml/minute. Although periods longer than 20 minutes are rarely needed for the delivery process, anesthesia with the slow-drip infusion technique can of necessity be maintained for longer periods. The administration of propanidid by continuous intravenous infusion occasionally fails to provide adequate analgesia, even when given in a dose as great as 100 mg/minute (approximately 15 mg/kg). One researcher cautions against the routine application of propanidid by this method, and recommends that the slow-drip infusion of propanidid be discontinued at the time of ligation of the umbilical cord.[107]

Use of propanidid, in contrast to thiopental, for induction of anesthesia in cesarean section does not seem to offer any particular advantage over the use of the barbiturates.[108]

Prolonged Surgical Procedures

Good results have been reported with the use of propanidid in more than 1000 patients undergoing prolonged surgical and obstetric procedures with the drug administered either by continuous intravenous infusion or by fractional intravenous application.[109] In most cases, nitrous oxide-oxygen mixtures were added to the propanidid anesthesia. A 1- to 2-g amount, and rarely more than a 3-g amount, of propanidid was required to induce and maintain adequate anesthesia for 20 to 60 minutes. The maximal dose administered for a 90-minute orthopedic procedure in a 24-year-old man was 10 g. The use of propanidid for prolonged operations requires special vigilance and increased work load for the anesthesiologist. Decisive advantages of propanidid in prolonged procedures are lack of drug-induced organ toxicity and prompt, complete restoration of the preoperative state of consciousness.[109]

With a 2% propanidid infusion, administered in combination with nitrous oxide-oxygen for anesthesia in prolonged surgical procedures, satisfactory results were reported. One exception was a 4% incidence of cyanosis, which was thought to be related to an allergic response and seemed to be unrelated to the dose of propanidid used.[110]

Miscellaneous Applications

Propanidid was employed successfully in the anesthetic management of children undergoing tonsillectomy and adenoidectomy with an unobstructed airway secured by the placement of a nasotracheal tube.[111] Propanidid is suitable as an anesthetic in patients with myasthenia gravis undergoing thymectomy without using neuromuscular blocking agents.[112] Other procedures for which propanidid has been safely employed include bronchoscopy, laryngoscopy, and diagnostic angiography.[113–115] Propanidid is a safe alternative anesthestic for patients with porphyria in whom the use of barbiturates is contraindicated.[116]

Employing propanidid anesthesia during certain neurosurgical procedures has proved valuable when prompt restoration of alertness is desired to rule out postoperative disturbance of consciousness, possibly caused by the neurosurgical intervention.[117]

The use of propanidid in patients subjected to electroconvulsive therapy was evaluated.[118] After propanidid administration, patients awakened within 8 minutes and were ambulatory after 15 minutes; after thiopental delivery, the awakening time was 18.5 minutes and patients were not ambulatory until after 90 minutes. No problems were encountered in connection with the potentiation of action of succinylcholine by propanidid. Excellent results have also been reported with the use of propanidid (7 to 8 mg/kg intravenously) mixed with gallamine (20 to 30 mg) as anesthetic agents during electroconvulsive therapy.[119] The hiccoughs that frequently occur after the electric discharge were not encountered.

In summary, propanidid is a useful short-acting intravenous anesthetic that is particularly suitable for brief diagnostic and therapeutic procedures. Unfortunately, side-effects, including hypotension and hypersensitivity reactions, cloud the clinical future of propanidid use.

REFERENCES

1. Thuillier, M.J., and Domenjoz, R.: Zur Pharmakologie der intravenoesen Kurznarkose mit 2-Methoxy-4-Allylphenoxyessigsaeure-N, N-diathylamide (G 29, 505). Anaesthesist, *6*:163, 1957.
2. Nishimura, N.: On propinal (2-M-4-P): a new intravenous nonbarbiturate anesthetic agent. Anesth. Analg., *41*:265, 1962.
3. Wright, D.A., and Payne, J.P.: A clinical study of intravenous anaesthesia with a eugenol derivative G 29505. Br. J. Anesth., *34*:379, 1962.
4. Riding, J.E., Dundee, J.W., Rajagopalan, M.S., Hamilton, R.C., and Bascett, P.J.F.: Clinical studies of induction agents. VI: Miscellaneous observations with G 29505. Br. J. Anaesth., *35*:480, 1963.
5. Hiltmann, R., Wollweber, H., Wirth, and Hoffmeister, F.: Neue estergruppenhaltige Phenoxyessigsaeureamide mit narkotischer Wirksamkeit. *In* Die intravenoese Kurznarkose mit dem neuen Phenoxyessigsaeurederivat Propanidid (Epontol). Edited by K. Horatz, R. Frey, and M. Zindler, Berlin, Springer, 1965.
6. Scholtan, W., and Lie, S.Y.: Kollid-chemische Eigenschaften eines neuen Kurznarkotikums. Arzneimittelforschung, *16*:679, 1966.
7. Conway, C.M., and Ellis, D.B.: Propanidid. Br. J. Anaesth., *42*:249, 1970.
8. Wirth, W., and Hoffmeister, F.: Pharmakologische Untersuchungen mit Propanidid (3-methoxy-4(N,N-diathylcarbamoylemethoxy)-phenylessigsaure-n-propylester). *In* Die intravenoese Kurznarkose mit dem neuen Phenoxyessigsaeurederivat Propanidid (Epontol). Edited by K. Horatz, R. Frey, and M. Zindler. Berlin, Springer, 1965.
9. Puetter, J.: Uber den fermentativen Abbau des Propanidid. *In* Die intravenoese Kurznarkose mit dem neuen Phenoxyessigsaeurederivat Propanidid (Eponotol). Edited by K. Horatz, R. Frey, and M. Zindler. Berlin, Springer, 1965.
10. Duhm, B., Maul, W., Medenwald, H., Patschke, K., and Wegner, L.A.: Tierexperimentelle Untersuchungen mit Propanidid 14C. *In* Die intravenoese Kurznarkose mit dem neuen Phenoxyessigsaurederivat Propanidid (Epontol). Edited by K. Horatz, R. Frey, and M. Zindler. Berlin, Springer, 1965.
11. Doenicke, A., Krumley, I., Kugler, J., and Klempa, J.: Experimental studies of the breakdown of Epontol determinations of propanidid in human serum. Br. J. Anaesth., *40*:415, 1968.
12. Doenicke, A.: General pharmacology of propanidid. *In* Intravenous Anaesthesia for Outpatients. Acta Anaesthesiol. Scand. [Suppl.], *17*:21, 1965.
13. Clarke, R.S.J.: The Eugenols. *In* Intravenous Anaesthesia. Edited by J.W. Dundee and G.M. Wyant. Edinburgh, Churchill Livingstone, 1974.
14. Clarke, R.S.J., Dundee, J.W., and Daw, R.H.: Clinical studies of induction agents. XI: The influence of some intravenous anaesthetics on the respiratory effects and sequelae of suxamethonium. Br. J. Anaesth., *36*:307, 1964.
15. Clarke, R.S.J., Dundee, J.W., and Hamilton, R.C.: Interactions between induction agents and muscle relaxants. Anaesthesia, *22*:235, 1967.
16. Ellis, F.R.: The neuromuscular effects of propanidid. Br. J. Anaesth., *39*:515, 1967.
17. Ellis, F.R.: The neuromuscular interaction of propanidid with suxamethonium and tubocurarine. Br. J. Anaesth., *40*:818, 1968.
18. Wyant, G.M., and Zoerb, D.L.: Propanidid—a new nonbarbiturate intravenous anaesthetic. Can. Anaesth. Soc. J., *12*:569, 1965.
19. Doenicke, A., Kugler, J., Schellenberger, A., and Guertner, T.: The use of electroencephalography to measure recovery time after intravenous anaesthesia. Br. J. Anaesth., *38*:580, 1966.
20. Doenicke, A., Gurtner, Th., Kugler, J., Schellenberger, A., and Spiess, W.: Experimentelle Untersuchungen ueber das Ultra-kurznarkoticum Propanidid mit Serumcholinesterasebestimmungen, EEG, psychodiagnostischen Tests und Kreislaufanalysen. *In* Die intravenoese Kurznarkose mit dem neuen Phenoxyessigaeurederivat Propanidid (Epontol). Edited by K. Horatz, R. Frey, und M. Zindler. Berlin, Springer, 1965.
21. Clarke, R.S.J., Dundee, J.W., Barron, D.W., and McArdle, P.J.: Clinical studies of induction agents. XXVI: The relative potencies of thiopentone, methohexitone and propanidid. Br. J. Anaesth., *40*:593, 1968.
22. Howels, T.H., Harnik, E., Kellner, G.A., and Rosenoer, V.M.: Propanidid and methohexitone: their comparative potency and narcotic action. Br. J. Anaesth., *39*:31, 1967.
23. Goldman, V.: Method of administration and dose of propanidid. Acta Anaesthesiol. Scand. [Suppl.], *17*:32, 1965.
24. Radnay, P.A.: Method of administration and dose of propanidid. Acta Anaesthesiol. Scand. [Suppl.], *17*:32, 1965.

25. Zindler, M.: Method of administration and dose of propanidid. Acta Anesthesiol. Scand. [Suppl.], 17:32, 1965.
26. Wulfson, N.L., and Joshi, C.W.: Thiopentone dosage based on lean body mass. Br. J. Anaesth., 41:516, 1969.
27. Clarke, R.S.J.: Clinical studies of induction agents. XXVII: The relationship between dosage of propanidid and duration of anaesthesia. Br. J. Anaesth., 40:781, 1968.
28. Swerdlow, M., and Moore, B.A.: A dose-duration trial with propanidid. Br. J. Anaesth., 39:573, 1967.
29. Howells, T.H., Odell, J.R., Hawkins, T.J., and Steane, P.A.: An introduction to FBA 1420: a new non-barbiturate intravenous anaesthetic. Br. J. Anaesth., 36:295, 1964.
30. Swerdlow, M.: A trial of propanidid (FBA 1420) a new ultrashort-acting anaesthetic. Br. J. Anaesth., 37:785, 1965.
31. Goldman, V., and Kennedy, P.: A non-barbiturate intravenous anaesthetic: report of a pilot trial. Anaesthesia, 19:424, 1964.
32. Dundee, J.W., and Clarke, R.S.J.: Alterations in response to somatic pain associated with anaesthesia. XVII: Propanidid (FBA 1420). Br. J. Anaesth., 37:121, 1965.
33. Doenicke, A., and Kugler, J.: Electrical brain function during emergence time after methohexital and propanidid anaesthesia. Acta Anaesthesiol. Scand. [Suppl.], 17:99, 1965.
34. Doenicke, A., Kugler, J., and Laub, M.: Evaluation of recovery and "street fitness" by E.E.G. and psychodiagnostic tests after anaesthesia. Can. Anaesth. Soc. J., 14:567, 1967.
35. Kreuscher, H.: Zur Strassenverkehrstuechtigkeit nach Anwendung von Propanidid. *In* Die intravenoese Kurznarkose mit dem neuen Phenoxyessigsaeurederivat Propanidid (Epontol). Edited by K. Horatz, R. Frey, and M. Zindler. Berlin, Springer, 1965.
36. Korttila, K., Linnoila, M., Ertama, P., and Haekkinen, S.: Recovery and simulated driving after intravenous anesthesia with thiopental, methohexital, propanidid or alphaprodine. Anesthesiology, 43:291, 1975.
37. Langrehr, D.: Endoanaesthetische Wirkungen von Propanid und ihre Bedeutung fuer das Verhalten von Kreislauf und Atmung. *In* Die intravenoese Kurznarkose mit dem neuen Phenoxyessigsaeurederivat Propanidid (Epontol). Edited by K. Horatz, R. Frey, and M. Zindler. Berlin, Springer, 1965.
38. Bernhoff, A.: The cardiovascular effect of propanidid (Epontol). Acta Anaesthesiol. Scand., 12:45, 1968.
39. Conway, C.M., Ellis, D.B., and King, N.W.: A comparison of the acute haemodynamic effects of thiopentone, methohexitone and propanidid in the dog. Br. J. Anaesth., 40:736, 1968.
40. Sankawa, H.: Cardiovascular effects of propanidid and methohexital sodium in dogs. Acta Anaesthesiol. Scand. [Suppl.], 17:55, 1965.
41. Soga, D., Beer, R., Andrae, J., and Bader, R.: Die Beeinflussung der linksventrikulaeren Myokardkontraktilitaet und Haemodynamik durch Propanidid beim Hund. *In* Anaesthesiolgie und Wiederbelebung. Edited by R. Frey, F. Kern, and O. Mayrhofer. Berlin, Springer, 1973.
42. Dundee, J.W., and Clarke, R.S.J.: Clinical studies of induction agents. IX: a comparative study of a new eugenol derivative, FBA 1420, with G 29.505 and standard barbiturates. Br. J. Anaesth., 36:100, 1964.
43. Clarke, R.S.J., and Dundee, J.W.: Toxic effects of intravenous anaesthesia: a comparison of propanidid with thiopentone. *In* Progress in Anaesthesiology. Proceedings of the 4th World Congress of Anesthesiology. Edited by T.B. Boulton, R. Bryce-Smith, M.K. Sykes, G.B. Gillett, and A.L. Revell. Amsterdam, Excerpta Medica, 1970.
44. Illes, I.: Cardiovascular effects of propanidid. Acta Anaesthesiol. Scand. [Suppl.], 17:45, 1965.
45. Van Wyk, A.P., and Kok, O.V.S.: Fabantol (Epontol, propanidid, FBA 1420): preliminary report of 200 cases. Med. Proc., 12:230, 1966.
46. De Oliviera, R.: Repercussoes cardiaces do FBA 1420. Rev. Bras. Anest., 18:59, 1968.
47. Johnstone, M., and Barron, P.T.: The cardiovascular effects of propanidid. A study of radiotelemetry. Anaesthesia, 23:180, 1968.
48. List, W.F.: Endoskopie in Allgemeinnarkose, Erfahrungen mit Propanidid. Anaesthesist, 16:163, 1967.
49. Radnay, P.A.: Allergic and anaphylactic reactions, decrease in blood pressure. Acta Anaesthesiol. Scand. [Suppl.], 17:80, 1965.
50. Zindler, M.: Allergic and anaphylactic reactions, decrease in blood pressure. *In* Intravenous Anaesthesia for Outpatients. Edited by M. Zindler. Acta Anaesthesiol. Scand. [Suppl.], 17:79, 1965.
51. Gjessing, J.: Hypotension, hypoventilation and delayed recovery after propanidid (correspondence). Br. J. Anaesth., 41:1012, 1969.
52. Kay, B.: Hypotensive reaction after propanidid and atropine. Br. Med. J., 3:413, 1969.
53. Johns, G.: Hypotensive reaction after propanidid and atropine. Br. Med. J., 4:52, 1969.
54. Mark, L.C., Cooper, J.R., and Brody, B.B.: Studies on Diethylaminoethanol. II. Antiarrhythmic activity in two homologous alcohol series. J. Pharmacol. Exp. Ther., 98:405, 1950.

55. Harnik, E.: A study of the biphasic ventilatory effects of propanidid. Br. J. Anaesth., *36*:655, 1964.
56. Gordh, T.: Analysis of hyperventilation in propanidid anaesthesia. *In* Anaesthesiology und Wiederbelebung. Edited by R. Frey, F. Kern, and O. Mayrhofer. Berlin, Springer, 1973.
57. Brassfield, C.R., and Corssen, G.: Respiratory and circulatory effects of 2 methoxy-4-allyl-phenoxyacetic acid G 29505) in dogs. Arch. Int. Pharmacodyn. Ther., *147*:311, 1964.
58. Reichel, G., Podlesch, T., Ulmer, W.T., and Zindler, M.: Untersuchugen ueber die Wirkung des Kurznarkotikums Propanidid auf die Ventilation und den Gasstoffwechsel. Anaesthesist, *14*:184, 1965.
59. Davis, J.A.: Blind nasal intubation with propanidid. Br. J. Anaesth., *44*:528, 1972.
60. Torda, T.A., Burkhart, J., and Toh, W.: The interaction of propanidid with suxamethonium and decamethonium. Anaesthesia, 27:159, 1972.
61. Gross, E.G., and Cullen, S.C.: The effects of anesthetic agents on muscular contraction. J. Pharmacol. Exp. Ther., 78:358, 1943.
62. Clarke, R.S.J.: Clinical studies of induction agents. XXIV: The influence of anaesthesia with thiopentone and propanidid on the blood sugar level. Br. J. Anaesth., *40*:46, 1968.
63. Podlesch, I., and Zindler, M.: Klinische Erfahrungen mit Propanidid. *In* Die intravenoese Kurz-narkose mit dem neuen Phenoxyessigsaeurederivat Propanidid (Epontol). Edited by K. Horatz, R. Frey, and M. Zindler. Berlin, Springer, 1965.
64. Clarke, R.S.J., Kirwan, M.J., Dundee, J.W., Neill, D.W., and Mitchell, E.S.: Clinical studies of induction agents. XIII: Liver function after propanidid and thiopentone anaesthesia. Br. J. Anaesth., *37*:415, 1965.
65. Van De Walle, J.: Nierenfunktionspruefung bei Anwendung von Propanidid. *In* Die intravenose Kurznarkose mit dem neuen Phenoxyessigsaeurederivat Propanidid (Epontol). Edited by K. Horatz, R. Frey, and M. Zindler. Berlin, Springer, 1965.
66. Guertner, Th., Kreutzberg, G., and Schellenberger, A.: Tierexperimentelle Untersuchungen zur Leberbelastung nach Propanidid-Narkosen. Ther. Berichte, *39*:62, 1967.
67. Hoffmeister, F., Grunvogel, E., and Wirth, W.: Tierexperimentelle Untersuchungen zur in-traarteriellen Vertraeglichkeit von Narkotika. *In* Die intravenoese Kurznarkose mit dem neuen Phenoxyessigsaeurederivat Propanidid (Epontol). Edited by K. Horatz, R. Frey, and M. Zindler. Berlin, Springer, 1965.
68. Liebegott, G.: Pathologisch-anatomische Befunde nach Anwendung von Kurznarkotika. *In* Die intravenoese Kurznarkose mit dem neuen Phenoxyessigsaeurederivat Propanidid (Epontol). Edited by K. Horatz, R. Frey, and M. Zindler. Berlin, Springer, 1965.
69. Harrfeldt, H.P.: Technik and Erfahrung bei 2700 Kurznarkosen mit Propanidid. *In* Die intra-venoese Kurznarkose mit dem neuen Phenoxyessigsaeurederivat Propandid (Epontol). Edited by K. Horatz, R. Frey, and M. Zindler. Berlin, Springer, 1965.
70. Radnay, P.A.: Venous irritation. Acta Anaesthesiol. Scand. [Suppl.], *17*:83, 1965.
71. Hewitt, J.C., Hamilton, R.C., O'Donnell, J.F., and Dundee, J.W.: Clinical studies of induction agents. XIV: A comparative study of venous complications following thiopentone, methohexitone and propanidid. Br. J. Anaesth., *38*:115, 1966.
72. O'Donnell, J.F., Hewitt, J.C., and Dundee, J.W.: Clinical studies of induction agents. XXVIII: A further comparison of venous complications following thiopentone, methohexitone and pro-panidid. Br. J. Anaesth., *41*:681, 1969.
73. Lind, B., and Roland, P.: Methohexitone and propanidid: a comparative investigation of the side effects. Br. J. Anaesth., *41*:150, 1969.
74. Clarke, R.S.J., and Dundee, J.W.: Clinical studies of induction agents. XXI: The influence of some premedicants on the course and sequelae of propanidid anesthesia. Br. J. Anaesth., *37*:51, 1965.
75. Schneider, W., and Koster, H.J.: Propanidid-Narkose: Erfahrungsbericht ueber 500 Kurznar-kosen. Muench. Med. Wschr., 52:2607, 1965.
76. Dundee, J.W.: Comparison of side effects of methohexital and thiopentone with propanidid. Acta Anaesthesiol. Scand [Suppl.], *17*:55, 1965.
77. Dundee, J.W., Kirwan, M.J., and Clark, R.S.J.: Anaesthesia and premedication as factors in postoperative vomiting. Acta Anesthesiol. Scand., *9*:223, 1965.
78. Whitwam, J.G.: Adverse reactions to i.v. induction agents. Br. J. Anaesth., *50*:677, 1978.
79. Lorenz, W., and Doenicke, A.: Anaphylactoid reactions and histamine release by intravenous drugs used in surgery and anaesthesia. *In* Adverse Response to Intravenous Drugs. Edited by J. Watkins and A.M. Ward. Edinburgh, Academic Press, 1978.
80. Beck, L.: Podiumgespraech ueber das Kurnarkotikum Propanidid. *In* Die intravenoese Kurz-narkose mit dem meuen Phenoxyessigsaeurederivat Propanidid (Epontol). Edited by K. Horatz, R. Frey, and M. Zindler. Berlin, Springer, 1965.
81. Manz, R., and Frank, G.: Zur Frage allergischer Reaktionen nach Epontol. Anaesthesist, *18*:223, 1969.
82. Larard, D.G.: Caridac arrest following induction with propanidid. Br. J. Anaesth., *42*:652, 1970.

83. Bradburn, C.C.: Severe hypotension following induction with propanidid. Br. J. Anaesth., *42*:362, 1970.
84. Miloschewsky, D., and Cervenkova, M.: Cardiovascular collapse following induction with propanidid. Br. J. Anaesth., *42*:833, 1970.
85. Speadbury, T.H., and Marrett, H.R.: Cardiovascular collapse after propanidid. Br. J. Anaesth., *43*:925, 1971.
86. Stovner, J., and Endresen, R.: Repeated propanidid in cancer. Br. J. Anaesth., *43*:207, 1971.
87. Thornton, M.L.: Apparent anaphylactic reaction to propanidid. Anaesthesia, *26*:490, 1971.
88. Lorenz, W., Doenicke, A., Meyer, R., Reimann, H.J., Kusche, J., Barth, H., Geesing, H., Hutzel, M., and Weissenbacher, B.: Histamine release in man by propanidid and thiopentone: pharmacological effects and clinical consequences. Br. J. Anaesth., *44*:355, 1972.
89. Russell, J.T.: Cyclizine anaphylaxis, when administered with propanidid. Anaesthesia, *24*:76, 1969.
90. Doenicke, A., and Lorenz, W.: Nachweis von Histaminfreisetzung bei hypotensiven Reaktionene nach Propanidid und ihre Propylaxe und Therapie mit Corticosteroiden. *In* Intravenose Narkose mit Propanidid. Edited by M. Zindler, H. Yamamura, and W. Wirth. Berlin, Springer, 1973.
91. Wyands, J.E., and Burfoot, M.F.: A clinical study of propanidid (FBA 1420). Can. Anaesth. Soc. J., *12*:587, 1965.
92. Clark, M.M., and Swerdlow, M.: The use of propanidid for minor surgery. Br. J. Anaesth., *38*:823, 1965.
93. Goldman, V., and Kennedy, P.: A non-barbiturate intravenous anaestheic: report of a pilot trial. Anaesthesia, *19*:424, 1964.
94. Reference deleted.
95. Wolfson, R.: A comparison of the induction agents propanidid and methohexitone in dental anaesthesia. Dent. Practitioner, *19*:269, 1959.
96. Cadle, D.R., Boulton, T.B., and Spencer-Swaine, M.: Intermittent intravenous anaesthesia for outpatient dentistry. Anaesthesia, *23*:65, 1968.
97. Boulton, T.B., and Rushman, G.B.: The intermittent administration of propanidid for dental outpatients. *In* Intravenoese Narkose mit Propanidid. Edited by M. Zindler, H. Yamamura, and W. Wirth. Berlin, Springer, 1973.
98. Rothbauer, G.: Propanidid-Narkose in der Zahnheilkunde. *In* Intravenoese Narkose mit Propanidid. Edited by M. Zindler, H. Yamamura, and W. Wirth. Berlin, Springer, 1973.
99. Schellenberger, A.: Propanidid in der Zahnheilkunde. *In* Intravenoese Narkose mit Propanidid. Edited by M. Zindler, H. Yamamura, and W. Wirth. Berlin, Springer, 1973.
100. Howells, T.H.: Intravenous anaesthetic agents in dental anaesthesia. Br. J. Anaesth., *40*:182, 1968.
101. Crossham, P.S., and Dixon, R.A.: Subanaesthetic dosage of propanidid as a sedative for dentistry: a controlled clinical trial. Br. J. Anaesth., *45*:369, 1973.
102. Grimm H., and Bochmann, K.: Epontol-Narkose zur Kardioversion. *In* Intravenoese Narkose mit Propanidid. Edited by M. Zindler, H. Yamamura, and W. Wirth. Berlin, Springer, 1973.
103. Soeder, G.: The use of propanidid in obstetrical analgesia-anaesthesia. *In* Intravenoese Narkose mit Propanidid. Edited by M. Zindler, H. Yamamura, and W. Wirth. Berlin, Springer, 1973.
104. Hennis, H.H.: Propanidid-Narkosen fuer Schnittentbindungen. *In* Intravenoese Narkose mit Propanidid. Edited by M. Zindler, H. Yamamura, and W. Wirth. Berlin, Springer, 1973.
105. Downing, J.W., Coleman, A.J., and Meer, F.M.: An intravenous method of anesthesia for cesarean section. Part I: Propanidid. Br. J. Anaesth., *44*:1069, 1972.
106. Picinelli, G., and Angioloillo, M.: Propanidid-infusion for anaesthesia of long duration in obstetrics. *In* Intravenoese Narkose mit Propanidid. Edited by M. Zindler, H. Yamamura, and W. Wirth. Berlin, Springer, 1973.
107. Stockhausen, H.: Der Platz der Epontal Langzeitnarkose in der Geburtshilfe. *In* Intravenoese Narkose mit Propanidid. Edited by M. Zindler, H. Yamamura, and W. Wirth. Berlin, Springer, 1973.
108. Maus, H., and Shaban, J.: Anwendung von Propanidid fuer Schnittentbindungen. *In* Intravenoese Narkose mit Propanidid. Edited by M. Zindler, H. Yamamura, and W. Wirth. Berlin, Springer, 1973.
109. Schara, J., Hullmann, R., Adolf, M., Berta, J., Gude, G., Harrfeldt, H.P., Heinze, W., Kirschbaum, M., Kuepper, D., Langrehr, D., Linneweber, G., Oehmig, H., and Stockhausen, H.: Langzeitnarkosen mit Propanidid. *In* Intravenoese Narkose mit Propanidid. Edited by M. Zindler, H. Yamamura, and W. Wirth. Berlin, Springer, 1973.
110. Stoffregen, J., and Meyer, E.: Narkose mit Infusion von Propanidid. *In* Intravenoese Narkose mit Propanidid. Edited by M. Zindler, H. Yamamura, and W. Wirth. Berlin, Springer, 1973.
111. Bergmann, H.: Die Verwendung von Propanidid bei der Adenotonsillectomy. *In* Intravenoese Narkose mit Propanidid. Edited by M. Zindler, H. Yamamura, and W. Wirth. Berlin, Springer, 1973.

112. Podlesch, I.: Propanidid-Narkose bei Myasthenie. *In* Intravenoese Narkose mit Propanidid. Edited by M. Zindler, H. Yamamura, and W. Wirth. Berlin, Springer, 1973.

113. DeRenzo, A., Rochat, D., Paderni, E., and Baglione, L.: Epontol (Bayer 1420) as the anesthetic of choice in bronchological practice. Ann. Laryngol. (Torino), 67:477, 1968.

114. Maini, O.P.: Anesthetic technique for cerebral angiography. East Afr. Med. J., 46:382, 1969.

115. Guerrieri, S., Azzea, G.F., Malagu, I., and Guberti, A.: Anesthesia with propanidid in diagnostic angiograpy. Minerva Anesthesiol., 35:17, 1969.

116. Bona, G.: Propanidid-Narkose bei Porphyrie. *In* Intravenoese Narkose mit Propanidid. Edited by M. Zindler, H. Yamamura, and W. Wirth. Berlin, Springer, 1973.

117. Smalhout, B.: Die Einfuehrung von Epontol in die allgemeine und spezielle Anesthesie. *In* Intravenoese Narkose mit Propanidid. Edited by M. Zindler, H. Yamamura, and W. Wirth. Berlin, Springer, 1973.

118. Heifetz, M.J., Birkhan, H.J., and Davidson, L.J.: Clinical evaluation of propanidid in electroconvulsion therapy. Anaesth. Analg., 48:293, 1969.

119. Van de Walle, J., and Baro, F.: Propanidid for electroconvulsive therapy. *In* Intravenoese Narkose mit Propanidid. Edited by M. Zindler, H. Yamamura, and W. Wirth. Berlin, Springer, 1973.

Chapter 11

ALTHESIN

HISTORY

In 1941, Selye, first observed anesthetic properties of several steroid hormones in rats.[1] In subsequent screening of 75 different steroids, this researcher found that, for a steroid compound to possess anesthetic properties, an oxygen atom at either end of the steroid molecule was necessary. Such molecular construction was exemplified by pregnanedione, which proved to be the most potent of the various steroids tested.[2] From results of these early studies, steroids were assumed to be superior to barbiturates in the induction and maintenance of anesthesia by offering a greater margin of safety and facilitating recovery through rapid elimination of the steroid from the blood by the liver and not relying on redistribution. Insolubility in water, however, was a major drawback of such steroid use.

After a delay of more than a decade, findings from laboratory studies of the steroid hydroxidione were reported.[3] Initial clinical experience with this steroid in the United States and in England revealed that pain on injection and, particularly, post-anesthetic thrombophlebitis were frequently observed, as were delayed onset of asthma and prolonged recovery.[4,5] In spite of some positive features with its use, including less respiratory and cardiovascular depression than is observed with barbiturates, and good muscle relaxation, including adequate relaxation of the jaw, thereby facilitating endotracheal intubation, it became increasingly evident that hydroxydione was unsuitable for general clinical use.

Continued screening of other steroids led to the observation that rapid induction and high potency were associated with the presence of a free 3d-hydroxy group in the steroid molecule.[6] GR2/234, alphaxalone, evolved as the most potent steroid of the many compounds tested. Because of its insolubility in water, the steroid was dissolved in a biologically acceptable medium, of which the polyoxylated castor oil, Cremophor EL, proved most successful. The addition of a small amount of another steroid related to alphaxalone, alphadolone acetate (GR2/1574), increased the solubility of alphaxalone in Cremophor more than threefold.[6] By combining alphaxalone and alphadolone acetate in a 3:1 ratio and dissolving them in Cremophor EL, althesin was formed.

GENERAL CHARACTERISTICS

Althesin is the first rapid-acting steroid anesthetic; the onset of CNS depressant action occurs within one arm-brain circulation time. The duration of anesthesia is dose dependent. A clinically useful dose of althesin, ranging from 0.05 to 0.075 ml/kg, produces unconsciousness for 5 to 10 minutes; anesthesia that is suitable for surgical procedures is present for about one half of that amount of time.

Recovery occurs about as promptly as is noted after methohexital anesthesia, but it is slower than after propanidid anesthesia. Unlike the ultra-short-acting barbiturates and similar to propanidid, no relapse into sleep occurs after recovery from althesin. Although althesin has a wide margin of safety, marked cardiovascular depression occurs in some patients, associated with a sharp reduction in peripheral resistance. Althesin reduces the cerebral metabolic rate and cerebral flow, resulting in a decrease in intracranial pressure. A relatively high incidence of severe hypersensitivity reactions to althesin, associated with bronchospasm, cardiovascular collapse, and cardiac arrest, has dampened the initial enthusiasm for the use of althesin as an induction agent and as the sole anesthetic for diagnostic and minor, brief surgical procedures. Widespread clinical acceptance of the drug may also be limited.

CHEMISTRY AND PHYSICAL PROPERTIES

Alphaxalone (GR2/234) is 3 α-hydroxy-5 alpha-pregnane-11-20 dione. Alphadolone acetate (GR2/1574) is 21-acetoxy-3 alpha-hydroxy-5 alpha-pregnane-11, 20 dione.[6-8] The structural formulae of these two compounds are shown in Figure 11–1.

For clinical use, the steroid mixture is formulated such that it is isotonic with blood: alphaxalone, 0.9 g; alphadolone acetate, 0.3 g; polyoxethylated castor oil, 20.0 ml; sodium chloride, 0.25 g; and water, to 100 ml. Althesin should be stored at room temperature; if refrigerated, the steroids may crystallize, and the solution difficult to resolubilize. The preparation should be protected from light.

Alphadolone acetate is approximately 50% as potent as alphaxalone. The main reason for combining the drug with alphaxalone is its solubilizing effect. The pH of the solution is about 7. The polyoxyethylated castor oil, Cremophor El, is the same agent that is used to solubilize propanidid, but the amount contained in althesin is considerably less than that in propanidid. The commercially available preparation of althesin contains 9 mg of alphaxalone and 3 mg of alphadolone acetate, and it is referred to in volume (ml, ml/kg, or μl/kg) rather than in milligrams of total steroid.

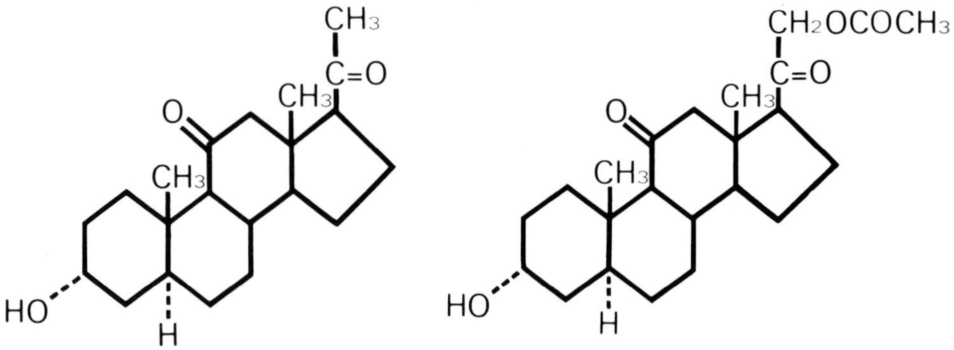

Alphaxalone   Alphadolone acetate

Fig. 11–1. Structural formulae of alphaxalone and alphadolone acetate.

PHARMACOLOGY

Potency, Onset, and Duration of Action

A dose of 50 to 60 μl/kg of althesin given intravenously is the ideal dose—that which consistently induces unconsciousness—but the range of 40 to 100 μl/kg is acceptable in most patients.[9]

The duration of surgical anesthesia induced by althesin is dose dependent. After a dose of 60 to 80 μl/kg intravenously, the mean duration of analgesia (time from beginning of injection of the drug until the patient starts to respond to the surgical stimulus) ranges from 2.4 to 5.0 minutes.[10] The duration of anesthetic action after any intravenous dose of althesin appears to be longer in patients over 40 years of age than in younger patients, but there is no difference in the duration of response between male and female recipients. When minimal induction doses of althesin (35 to 40 μl/kg) were compared with those of methohexital (0.8 to 1.0 mg/kg), althesin was slightly longer-acting than methohexital. With respect to cumulative effects, althesin occupies a position between the ultra-short-acting barbiturates, thiopental and thiamylal, and propanidid, the latter being less cumulative than either of the barbiturates.[7]

Recovery

Immediate clinical recovery after althesin anesthesia is about as rapid as occurs after thiopental anesthesia, but it is not as prompt as that which occurs after methohexital or propanidid anesthesia.[11–13] A simulated driving performance test conducted in healthy volunteers 6 hours after recovery from 85 μl/kg of althesin revealed late impairment of driving skills. Driving performance was better after althesin, however, than after thiopental and methohexital anesthesia, and is similar to unanesthetized control subjects monitored 2 and 4 hours after drug injection.[14]

Distribution, Metabolism, and Excretion

The plasma half-life of alphaxalone is about 7 minutes. When alphaxalone is labeled with a radioactive tracer, the drug persists in the blood for a longer period.[15] The prolonged radioactivity appears to indicate the presence of metabolites rather than the persistence of the active drug circulating in the plasma. Whether the metabolites have some pharmacologic activity is not clear.

Alphaxalone and alphadolone are initially widely distributed in body tissues. Localization in the central nervous system (CNS) is apparent after 1 minute. No selective uptake by specific regions of the cortex or cerebellum is evident.

The highest concentration of the 2 steroids occurs in the liver 3 minutes after injection of the compound, and radioactive althesin appears rapidly in the bile as glucuronide. By 1 hour, the drug almost completely disappears from body tissues, and the bulk is present in the lumen of the gut and bladder. The main route of excretion of alphaxalone and alphadolone is in the bile. Approximately 60 to 70% of a radioactive dose is excreted as metabolic products in the feces for 5 days; the remaining 20 to 30% appears in the urine during the same period. The major biliary metabolite of alphaxalone was identified as a glucuronide of hydroalphaxalone.

In pregnant laboratory animals, small amounts of radioactive althesin are found in the fetus 3 to 10 minutes after drug delivery. The intestine is the only site in which the concentration of althesin exceeds the concentration present in maternal blood.

Only about 40% of the quantity of alphaxalone and alphadolone is bound to plasma protein in humans. Therefore, variations in concentrations in serum proteins or the presence of protein-displacing drugs probably have little influence on the pharmacologic activity of althesin.[16]

Both alphaxalone and alphadolone are biotransformed in rats by hydroxylation.[17] With alphadolone, the acetate group may be hydrolyzed to alcohol. In humans, plasma alphaxalone levels rapidly decline after the administration of 50 to 200 mg/kg, reflecting a short half-life (6 to 9.4 minutes).[7] Two metabolites, representing approximately 20% of the total quantity of steroid administered, can be identified in the urine. They are excreted in a conjugated form within 8 hours of the administration of the drug.[7]

Althesin is devoid of hormonal effects, as documented in various animals species, and does not affect urinary electrolyte excretion when administered to adrenalectomized rats.[18]

Central Nervous System (CNS)

Sleep is produced in one arm-brain circulation time. The pupils tend to dilate, and the eyelash reflex disappears within about 30 seconds of the loss of consciousness.[9,10] Muscle tone is usually decreased. With very slow intravenous injection of althesin (over a period of 60 seconds), onset of anesthesia is delayed.

Electroencephalographic (EEG) Changes

Althesin-induced alterations in the EEG resemble those observed with other intravenous anesthetics: initial mixed theta and delta wave activity with subsequent fast, high-voltage, delta wave patterns. As anesthesia deepens, burst suppression patterns become prevalent.[19,20] After a single dose of althesin, EEG changes are mainly characterized by increased slow-wave activity. The althesin-induced EEG alterations are not restricted to one area of the cortex.[21]

Cardiovascular System

In laboratory animals, the cardiovascular effects of althesin are similar to those of equivalent doses of thiopental and methohexital, with the exception that in the cat heart in situ, althesin exerts a smaller negative inotropic effect.[22–24] At an intravenous dose of 50 μl/kg, the cardiovascular effects of althesin do not differ from those of equipotent doses of methohexital and thiopental. All 3 drugs produce similar falls in blood pressure, central venous pressure, and stroke volume. When althesin use (at intravenous doses of 60 and 150 μl/kg) was compared with thiopental use (at an intravenous dose of 4 mg/kg) in man, a decrease in arterial blood pressure and a compensatory increase in heart rate were observed; cardiac output either was slightly increased or remained unchanged.[25] The decrease in peripheral resistance was significantly greater with both doses of althesin as compared to thiopental. Other investigators reported similar observations regarding the cardiovascular effects of althesin in umpremedicated and premedicated patients.[26–28] With a 75-μl/kg intravenous dose of althesin, a fall in arterial blood pressure was recorded in association with a decrease in peripheral resistance and stroke volume and compensatory tachycardia, resulting in an increase in cardiac output.[29] Preload remained unchanged, whereas afterload decreased. A fall in dp/

dt (rate of pressure change versus time) by 20% seemed to indicate a moderate reduction in myocardial inotropism. The energy demand of the heart decreased initially by only 15%.

In heavily premedicated cardiac patients undergoing heart surgery, the blood pressure depressant action of althesin at a dose of 50 μl/kg is similar to the action of 4 mg/kg of thiopental or 1.5 mg/kg of methohexital. A more marked increase in heart rate occurs with the use of althesin than with the use of barbiturates.[30] When similar studies were conducted in hypertensive patients, no significant difference was noted between the cardiovascular effects of althesin and those of the ultra-short-acting barbiturates, although cardiac output was more adequately maintained with althesin.[31]

Althesin does not cause any significant changes in pulmonary artery pressure.[32] The solubilizing agent Cremophor EL causes a small, statistically significant drop in blood pressure and an elevation in pulse rate in humans.[33]

Respiratory System

Althesin has clinically insignificant effects on respiratory function.[34,35] After completion of the injection of althesin, a short phase of hyperventilation is usually followed by apnea, which lasts for no more than 1 minute. Spontaneous, regular breathing is re-established after a short period of tachypnea. These brief changes in respiratory function may be accompanied by a small increase in arterial CO_2 tension and moderate decrease in arterial oxygen tension.[26]

Respiratory upset, including cough, hiccoughs, and laryngospasm, is rarely encountered with the use of althesin when it is administered in clinically useful doses.[28] Large doses that exceed clinically recommended dose ranges, however, may result in respiratory depression. Laryngeal reflexes are depressed with clinical doses of althesin, which may facilitate aspiration of foreign material.[36]

Cerebral Perfusion, Metabolism, and Intracranial Pressure

Pickerodt, et al., found that, in the baboon, althesin reduces cerebral oxygen consumption, thus resulting in a secondary reduction in cerebral blood flow and cerebrospinal fluid (CSF) pressure.[37,38] Similar observations were made in the dog, although in subsequent studies also performed in dogs, other researchers recorded no increase in cerebral blood flow or CSF pressure.[39–41] In human volunteers, althesin caused a significant decrease in CSF pressure.[42] In a later study, althesin caused cerebral metabolic depression, which was accompanied by a decrease in CSF pressure and an increase in cerebrovascular resistance.[43] The reactivity of cerebral vessels to alterations in $Paco_2$ is maintained under the effect of althesin.

In patients undergoing neurosurgical procedures, a reduction in intracranial pressure occurred after 50 μl/kg of althesin was given, with a return of the preinjection pressure within 10 minutes.[44] In a more recent study, which involved patients about to undergo a neurosurgical procedure who were induced with althesin or thiopental, both drugs produced similar effects on intracranial pressure in connection with the placement of the endotracheal tube (including patients with an elevated level).[45]

Miscellaneous Effects

Althesin has antanalgesic properties; when the drug is administered at sub-anesthetic doses, a transient increase occurs in the appreciation of somatic pain.[46]

After large doses of althesin, antanalgesia is of shorter duration than after comparable doses of thiopental. The antanalgesic property of althesin may be of no great clinical significance.

Althesin does not modify the neuromuscular blocking effects of succinylcholine in cats.[47] No prolongation of succinylcholine-induced apnea was observed in ambulatory patients who were anesthetized for electroconvulsive therapy.[48] A slight potentiation by althesin of the neuromuscular blocking action of d-tubocurare and pancuronium in man was documented.[49]

The incidence of venous complication, including phlebothrombosis, after the use of althesin is about the same as is seen after the administration of thiopental (2.5%) and methohexital (1%). The rate of occurrence is considerably less, however, than that associated with propanidid or after the use of more concentrated barbiturate solutions.[50,51]

At recommended doses, althesin does not cause any detectable depression of liver function.[7] Large doses of althesin may result in a significant elevation of the serum bilirubin level, similar to increases in bilirubin that are recorded with the use of other anesthetics.[52] Liver function tests performed in patients with chronic liver diseases did not reveal any drug-induced changes in the tests conducted 24 hours and 5 days after induction of anesthesia with althesin. Although althesin is metabolized in the liver, impaired liver function does not result in prolonged action of the drug, because patients with chronic liver disease seem to be capable of clearing ^{14}C-labeled althesin at the same rate as do patients with normal liver function.[53,54] Prolonged recovery after the use of althesin may be observed, however, in patients with severe hepatic insufficiency.[55]

Information regarding the transfer of althesin across the placental barrier is incomplete. Some degree of fetal depression was observed when althesin was used for induction and maintenance of anesthesia along with nitrous oxide-oxygen in patients undergoing cesarean section.[56] No depressant effects of the fetus were observed when 50 μl/kg of althesin was employed for induction of anesthesia for cesarean section.[7]

There is no evidence of interaction of althesin with other intravenous or inhalational anesthetics resulting in adverse reactions, with the possible exception of methoxyflurane. This interaction resulted in the development of tachycardia after anesthesia with althesin.[57] Althesin blocked the initiation of malignant hyperpyrexia by halothane in susceptible swine.[58,59]

TOXICITY AND SIDE-EFFECTS

The LD_{50} of althesin in mice is 54.7 mg/kg, as compared to 90.5 mg/kg for thiopental or 39.4 mg/kg for methohexital. The safety margin as expressed as the therapeutic index, LD_{50}/AD_{50}, was narrow with thiopentone (6.9) and methohexital (7.4) as compared with althesin (30.6).[6,8] When testing the cumulative effect of repeated doses in mice, thiopental (40 mg/kg intravenously) proved to have the most rapid rate of accumulation, with only 5 consecutive doses given to produce a sleep time in excess of 300 minutes. Methohexital (28 mg/kg intravenously) was only moderately cumulative, and althesin (12 mg/kg), apart from a slight increase in sleep time between the first and second dose, had a minimal cumulative effect.[6] Recovering animals showed no adverse effects, and tissues examined histologically showed no lesions that could be attributed to the treatment with althesin. Intra-arterial injection of althesin into the rabbit ear did not cause an adverse response in contrast to thiopental (5%), which resulted in thrombophlebitis. When administered to rats in daily doses of 0.2 to 1.8 ml/kg, no evidence of immediate or delayed toxicity of althesin was found when all major organs were examined microscopically. Althesin proved to be acceptable in pregnant mice and rats; no toxic effects were seen in the mother or in the offspring after the administration of 0.5 ml/kg daily for a total of 20 consecutive days. There was no evidence of teratogenic effects in these animals.

Hypersensitivity Reactions

Sensitivity reactions in response to althesin have occurred.[60–65] The incidence of histaminoid-type reactions is estimated at 4.3 per 100,000 administrations, and reaction associated with bronchospasm is estimated at 1.3 per 100,000.[66] In a more recent survey based on 100 reports involving adverse reactions to intravenous anesthetics, the incidence of reactions to althesin was estimated at 1 in 11,000. Discounting all cases in which a muscle relaxant was used, the incidence is 1 in 19,000.[67]

The clinical picture of althesin-induced hypersensitivity responses may vary from an erythematous rash and urticaria, usually confined to the neck and upper chest, to bronchospasm, severe involuntary muscle movements, cardiovascular collapse, and cardiac arrest, usually associated with intense peripheral vasodilation. These potentially disastrous reactions to althesin may be the result of an allergic response, or they may represent a true sensitivity to the drug, causing an exaggerated response to its pharmacologic action. Clearly, histamine release is involved in some of the troublesome complications associated with the use of althesin, as characterized by typical extensive flushing and other skin reactions.[68–70] The possibility that the reactions could be caused by the solubilizing agent, Cremophor EL, has been proposed.[26]

With regard to the mechanisms and mediators of hypersensitivity reactions, it is difficult to distinguish between pharmacologic effects, direct complement activation, and true immune-mediated hypersensitivity reactions solely on the basis of clinical manifestations.[71] Measuring C3 concentrations for 24 hours after a reaction to althesin may determine whether an immune-based response has occurred. In a study, venous blood samples were obtained in 8 patients who had experienced adverse reactions to althesin.[72] In 7 of these patients, there was clear evidence of alternate pathway activation of C3, a process that is known to result in histamine release.[71] One patient of this group showed activation of the classic pathway for complement conversion, with evidence of a true immune-mediated response.

Drug sensitivity is not limited to intravenous anesthetics, but may also occur in response to any of the neuromuscular blocking agents, especially succinylcholine and pancuronium.[73]

Excitatory Phenomena

The incidence of excitatory phenomena during induction with althesin, including muscle twitching, jerking of extremities, coughing, and hiccoughs, is approximately 20%; this value is lower than that associated with methohexital.[74] In pediatric patients, however, greater frequency and severity of undesirable excitatory phenomena were observed with althesin than with methohexital. The occurrence of excitatory phenomena is dose related; in one study, the incidence of these side-effects increased to as much as 60% with a dose of 150 μl/kg.[70,74] A fast rate of injection of althesin also predisposes to a higher incidence of excitatory phenomena, as does the use of hyoscine as a premedicant. The administration of opiates, on the other hand, reduces the incidence of excitatory phenomena.[9]

Nausea and Vomiting

Althesin is associated with a relatively low incidence of postoperative nausea and vomiting (15%).[9]

Miscellaneous Side-Effects

When premedication involves the use of atropine, slight muscle movements and tremor may occur in approximately 20% of patients, a lesser frequency than is seen after an equivalent dose of methohexital.[75] Transient disorientation and emotional upset, as well as restlessness, have been observed during emergence from althesin anesthesia.[76–78]

CLINICAL APPLICATIONS

Its short duration of action with rapid recovery and broad margin of safety, along with other favorable qualities, including the small volume required for anesthesia induction (especially appreciated in pediatric anesthesia), good tissue compatibility, and excellent rate of patient acceptance, make althesin a valuable alternative to thiopental and methohexital as an anesthesia induction agent and as the sole anesthetic in diagnostic and brief surgical manipulations. Whether it is advantageous to employ althesin by continuous infusion (11 ml/kg/hour) in combination with analgesics and neuromuscular blocking for use in neuroradiologic examinations, in orthopedic surgery, or as a sedative remains unclear.[55,79]

When althesin is used as the sole anesthetic for minor surgery, premedication is not required, with the possible exception of atropine sulfate as an antisialogogue. Substitution of hyoscine for atropine increases the incidence of althesin-induced excitatory effects to an unacceptable level.[80] Apparently, the use of a sedative premedication, particularly opiates, holds no advantage. Although opiates decrease the occurrence of excitatory phenomena, they not only prolong recovery from althesin anesthesia, but also increase the incidence of postoperative nausea and vomiting.[81,82]

Induction of Anesthesia

Relatively rapid onset and short duration of action are the main reasons for the use of althesin predominantly as an induction agent. Althesin can safely and effectively be used in a large dose range to induce anesthesia (40 to 150 μl/kg).[7,32] With doses that exceed 150 μl/kg, marked respiratory depression frequently occurs, and the incidence of excitatory phenomena may increase, including muscle movements and respiratory upset. For the induction of balanced anesthesia, no distinct clinical advantages were noted relative to the use of thiopental, but the drug may be a useful alternative to use of barbiturates.[83]

In cardiovascular surgical patients, althesin can be used satisfactorily to induce anesthesia in persons with poorly compensated myocardial and valvular disease, when small increments are administered slowly.[84] Cardiac output decreases, similar to the decrease observed after delivery of thiopental, and althesin offers no advantage over thiopental in this respect. No statistically different cardiovascular effects have been found between althesin and thiopental or methohexital when employed for the induction of anesthesia in patients about to undergo open or closed cardiac surgical procedures.[30]

Althesin may be a suitable anesthesia induction agent for use in patients undergoing intraocular surgery. The administration of this drug is accompanied by a marked decrease in intraocular tension.[85]

Minor Operative Procedures

Althesin is suitable and safe when used for the induction and maintenance of anesthesia for brief surgical and diagnostic manipulations at intravenous doses ranging from 40 to 120 μl/kg. If the procedure outlasts the anesthetic effect, one half of the initial dose is administered to prolong anesthesia.[9,86]

Dentistry

Satisfactory results were reported when althesin (50 μl/kg) was employed in 100 patients undergoing single and multiple dental extractions.[77] In two thirds of this patient group, althesin anesthesia was supplemented by nitrous oxide-oxygen mixtures and halothane. In most patients, the procedure lasted less than 3 minutes. Induction was smooth, pain free, and took one arm-brain circulation time in all patients. Operating conditions were very satisfactory in almost 75% of the group of patients. Of the 100 patients, 6 were considerably restless, making extraction difficult; 4 of these 6 patients had received only 40 μl/kg of althesin, a dose that the author of this study no longer recommends. In spite of some emotional reactions that occurred in about one third of the subjects during awakening from anesthesia, the rate of patient acceptance was excellent.

Althesin has been used in subanesthetic doses as a sedative for conservative dentistry.[87] An initial dose of 25 μl/kg was administered, and its effect on sleepiness, slowing of speech, and response to commands was observed. Further incremental subanesthetic doses were administered to maintain drowsiness while keeping the patient cooperative. Satisfactory analgesia was provided with local anesthetic injections. Initial shivering, jaw tremor, and transient loss of verbal contact after the first administration of althesin sometimes delayed the beginning of the procedure until consciousness returned and the patient was able to co-operate. There was no clear-cut advantage with the use of althesin over diazepam as a sedative in dentistry. The anxiolytic action of althesin was at least as marked as that of diazepam.

Cardioversion

Althesin administration was compared with thiopental use for anesthesia in patients undergoing cardioversion.[88] Patients preferred the althesin as compared to thiopental because it caused less postoperative drowsiness. Also, the success rate of conversion of arrhythmias was slightly higher with althesin anesthesia; excitatory effects were noted more often, however. Although althesin is safe to use as an anesthetic for cardioversion, it is probably not superior to thiopental.

Electroconvulsive Therapy

Althesin is a suitable anesthetic to administer to patients undergoing electroconvulsive therapy. The effectiveness of 36 μl/kg of althesin was compared to that of 50 mg of methohexital, followed by 25 mg of succinylcholine administered intravenously; no distinct difference was noted in the response of these agents in their respective interactions with succinylcholine.[11] The duration of apnea was similar with both agents, as was the incidence of hiccoughs and the occurrence of facial flushing. The mean recovery time after induction, however, was significantly longer with althesin (309 seconds) than with methohexital (251 seconds) use.

Cesarean Section

For patients undergoing cesarean section, the effectiveness of two different doses of althesin, 100 and 150 μl/kg, was explored.[56] The lower dose was well tolerated by the infants. The 150-μl/kg dose of althesin was associated with an unacceptable degree of neonatal depression. Althesin was well accepted by the mothers, because none experienced awareness during anesthesia or had unpleasant dreams. Obviously, more clinical experience with althesin used as an anesthetic for cesarean section is needed, especially in regard to establishing an optimal dose level that provides satisfactory anesthesia for the mother without causing undue fetal depression.

Pediatric Surgery

Minimal doses of althesin have been established for the induction of sleep in 2 age groups of children.[89] Children between the ages of 2 and 10 years received 70 μl/kg of althesin intravenously, and children between the ages of 10 and 16 years received a dose of 50 μl/kg by this same route. Effects of these doses of althesin were compared to those noted after 1.2 mg/kg of methohexital was delivered intravenously. Both anesthetic agents provided smooth and pleasant induction in all patients. Painless injection and small injection volume proved to be a significant advantage with the use of althesin over methohexital. Involuntary muscle movements occurred more frequently, however, and were also more marked with althesin than with methohexital. When used for the induction of anesthesia in children undergoing minor otolaryngologic operations, including adenotonsillectomy, althesin did not offer any special advantages over thiopental or ketamine.[90] A need for analgesics during the early postoperative period was greater after althesin anesthesia than after thiopental or ketamine anesthesia.

Neurosurgery

Documentation that althesin causes cerebral metabolic depression associated with a reduction in CSF pressure and intracranial pressure suggests that the drug may be valuable in neurodiagnostic and neurosurgical procedures. In particular, the suitability of althesin in the anesthetic management of patients with an elevated level of intracranial pressure needs to be further explored.

Malignant Hyperthermia

In three patients identified as susceptible to malignant hyperthermia and who received althesin for induction of anesthesia, the administration of halothane did not result in any increase in temperature, degree of muscle rigor, or serum CPK levels.[91,92] Therefore, althesin may be the preferred anesthetic induction agent in patients who have survived episodes of malignant hyperpyrexia or who are known from family history and raised CPK levels to be at risk for developing malignant hyperthermia in response to anesthesia. The use of althesin under these conditions, however, would not justify the subsequent use of halothane in a patient at risk.

Porphyria

Althesin may be a safe agent to induce anesthesia in patients suffering from porphyria. The drug does not precipitate an acute porphyric attack, as may be encountered with the use of barbiturates in this setting.

REFERENCES

1. Selye, H.: Anesthetic effect of steroid hormones. Proc. Soc. Exp. Biol. Med., *46*:116, 1941.
2. Selye, H.: Studies concerning the correlation between anesthetic potency, hormonal activity and clinical structure among steroid compounds. Anesth. Analg., *21*:41, 1942.
3. P'An, S.Y., Gardocki, J.E., Hutcheon, D.E., Rudel, H., Kodet, M.J., and Laubach, G.D.: General anesthetic and other pharmacological properties of a soluble steroid, 21-hydroxypregomedione sodium succinate. J. Pharmacol. Exp. Ther., *115*:432, 1955.
4. Murphy, F.J., Guadagui, N.P., and DeBon, F.: Use of steroid anesthesia in surgery. JAMA, *158*:1412, 1955.
5. Lerman, L.H.: Viadril: a new steroid anaesthetic. Preliminary communication. Br. Med. J., 2:129, 1956.
6. Davis, B., and Pearce, D.R.: An introduction to althesin (CT 1341). *In* Steroid Anesthesia. Proceeding of the Conference of the Royal College of Physicians, London, 1972.
7. Dundee, J.W., and Wyant, G.M.: Steroids. *In* Intravenous Anaesthesia. Edited by J.W. Dundee and G.M. Wyant. Edinburgh, Churchill Livingstone, 1974.
8. Child, K.J., Currie, J.P., Davis, B., Dodds, M.G., Pearce, D.R., and Twissell, D.J.: The pharmacological properties in animals of CT 1341. A new steroid anaesthetic agent. Br. J. Anaesth., *43*:2, 1971.
9. Clarke, R.S.J., Montgomery, S.J., Dundee, J.W., and Bovill, J.G.: CT 1341: a new steroid anaesthetic. Br. J. Anaesth., *43*:947, 1971.
10. Swerdlow, M., Chakraborty, S.K., and Zahangir, M.A.H.M.: A trial of CT 1341. Br. J. Anaesth., *43*:1075, 1971.
11. Foley, E.T., Walton, B., Savege, T.M., and Strunin, L.: A comparison of recovery times between althesin and methohexitone following anaesthesia for electroconvulsive therapy. Postgrad. Med. J., *48*:112, 1972.
12. Hannington-Kiff, J.G.: Comparative recovery rates following induction of anaesthesia with althesin and methohexitone. Postgrad. Med. J., *48*:116, 1972.
13. Korttilla, K.: Propanidid and Althesin. *In* Trends in Intravenous Anesthesia. Edited by J.A. Aldrete and T.H. Stanley. Miami, Symposia Specialists, 1980.
14. Korttilla, K., Linnoila, M., Ertama, P., and Haekkinen, S.: Recovery and simulated driving after intravenous anaesthesia with thiopental, methohexital, propanidid or alphadione. Anesthesiology, *43*:291, 1975.
15. Child, K.J., Gibson, W., Harney, G., and Hart, J.W.: Metabolism and excretion of althesin (CT 1341) in the rat. Postgrad. Med. J., *48*:37, 1972.
16. Ghoneim, M.M., and Korttilla, K.: Pharmacokinetics of intravenous anaesthetics: implications for clinical use. Clin. Pharmacokinet., 2:344, 1977.
17. Card, B., McCullough, R.J., and Pratt, D.A.H.: Tissue distribution of CT 1341 in the rat. Postgrad. Med. J., June, 34, 1972.
18. Child, K.J., English, A.F., Gilbert, H.G., and Woollett, W.A.: An endocrinological evaluation of CT 1341 (althesin) with special reference to reproduction. Postgrad. Med. J., June, 51, 1972.
19. Scott, D.F., and Sully, M.: Testing a new anaesthetic drug. Proceedings of the Electro-Physiological Technologists' Association, 1972.
20. Scott, D.F., and Virden, S.: Comparison of the effect of Althesin with other induction agents on electroencephalographic patterns. Postgrad. Med. J., *48*:93, 1972.
21. Takahashi, T.: Wave-band analysis of EEG patterns during anaesthesia produced by althesin. Postgrad. Med. J., *48*:96, 1972.
22. Child, K.J., Davis, B., Dodds, M.G., and Twissel, D.J.: Anaesthetic cardiovascular and respiratory effects of a new steroidal anaesthetic CT 1341: a comparison with other intravenous anesthetic drugs in the unrestrained cat. Br. J. Pharmacol., *46*:189, 1972.
23. Foex, P., and Prys-Roberts, C.: Pulmonary haemodynamics and myocardial effects of althesin (CT 1341) in the goat. Postgrad. Med. J., *48*:24, 1972.
24. Gordh, T.: The effect of althesin on the heart in situ in the cat. Postgrad. Med. J., *48*:31, 1972.
25. Coleman, A.J., Downing, J.W., Leary, W.P., Moyes, D.G., and Styles, M.: The immediate cardi-

ovascular effects of althesin (Glaxo CT 1341), a steroid induction agent, and thiopentone in man. Anaesthesia, 27:373, 1972.

26. Savege, T.M., Foley, E.I., Coultas, R.J., Walton, B., Strunin, L., Simpson, B.R., and Scott, D.F.: CT 1341: some effects in man. Anaesthesia, 26:402, 1971.

27. Savege, T.M., Foley, E.I., Ross, L., and Maxwell, M.P.: A comparison of the cardiorespiratory effects during induction of anaesthesia with althesin, thiopentone and methohexitone. Postgrad. Med. J., 48:66, 1972.

28. Clarke, R.S.J., Dundee, J.W., and Carson, I.W.: A new steroid anaesthetic: althesin. Proc. R. Soc. Lond. [Biol.], 66:1027, 1973.

29. Patschke, D., Hess, W., Tarnow, J., and Weymar, A.: Die Wirkung von Fentanyl und Althesin auf die Haemodynamik, die Herzinotropie und den myokardialen Sauerstoffverbrauch des Menschen. Anaesthesist, 25:10, 1976.

30. Lyons, S.M., and Clarke, R.S.J.: A comparison of different drugs for anaesthesia in cardiac surgical patients. Br. J. Anaesth., 44:575, 1972.

31. Prys-Roberts, C., Foex, P., and Biro, B.P.: Cardiovascular responses of hypertensive patients to induction of anaesthesia with Althesin. Postgrad. Med. J., 48:80, 1972.

32. Campbell, D., Forrester, A.C., Miller, D.C., Hutton, J., Kennedy, J.A., Lawrie, D.V., Lorimer, A.R., and McCall, D.: A preliminary clinical study of CT 1341—a steroid anaesthetic. Br. J. Anaesth., 43:14, 1971.

33. Savege, T.M., Foley, E.I., and Simpson, B.R.: Some cardiorespiratory effects of Cremophor EL. Br. J. Anaesth., 45:515, 1973.

34. Hall, G.M., Whitman, J.G., and Morgan, M.: Some respiratory effects of althesin. Br. J. Anaesth., 45:629, 1973.

35. Tomlin, P.J.: The respiratory effects of althesin. Postgrad. Med. J., 48:85, 1972.

36. Carson, I.W., Moore, J., Balmer, J.P., Dundee, J.W., and McNabb, G.: Laryngeal competence with ketamine and other drugs. Anesthesiology, 38:128, 1973.

37. Pickerodt, V.W.A., McDowall, D.G., Coroneos, N.J., and Kearney, N.P.: Effect of althesin on cerebral metabolism and intracranial pressure in the anaesthetised baboon. Br. J. Anaesth., 44:751, 1972.

38. Pickerodt, V.W.A., McDowall, D.G., Coroneos, N.J., and Kearney, N.P.: Effect of althesin on carotid blood flow and intracranial pressure in the anaesthetised baboon: a preliminary communication. Postgrad. Med. J., 48:58, 1972.

39. Steward, D.J.: The effects of CT 1341 on cerebral blood flow and intracranial pressure. In Proceedings of the Fifth World Congress of Anaesthesiologists. Amsterdam, Excerpta Medica, 1972.

40. Cohen, R.S., Creighton, R.E., Nisbet, H.I.A., McDonald, P., and Steward, D.J.: The effects of althesin on cerebral blood flow and intracranial pressure. Can. Anaesth. Soc. J., 20:754, 1973.

41. Cohen, R.S., Nisbet, H.I.A., Creighton, R.E., and McDonald, P.: The effects of hypoxemia on cerebral blood flow and cerebrospinal fluid pressure in dogs anaesthetized with althesin, pentobarbitone and methoxyflurane. Can. Anaesth. Soc. J., 20:757, 1973.

42. Takahashi, T., Takasaki, M., Naniki, A., and Dohi, S.: Effects of althesin on cerebrospinal fluid pressure. Br. J. Anaesth., 45:179, 1973.

43. Sari, S., Mazkawa, T., Tohjo, M., Okuda, Y., and Takeshita, H.: Effects of althesin on cerebral blood flow and oxygen consumption in man. Br. J. Anaesth., 48:545, 1976.

44. Turner, J.M., Coroneos, N.J., Gibson, R.M., Powell, D., Ness, M.A., and McDowall, D.G.: The effect of althesin on intracranial pressure in man. Br. J. Anaesth., 45:168, 1973.

45. Moss, E., Powell, D., Gibson, R.M., and McDowall, D.G.: Effects of tracheal intubation on intracranial pressure following induction of anaesthesia with thiopentone or althesin in patients undergoing neurosurgery. Br. J. Anaesth., 50:353, 1978.

46. Arera, M.V., Carson, I.W., and Dundee, J.W.: Alterations in response to somatic-pain associated with anaesthesia. XXI: Althesin (CT 1341). Br. J. Anaesth., 44:590, 1972.

47. Child, K.J., Currie, J.P., Davis, B., Dodds, M.G., Pearce, D.R., and Twissel, D.J.: The pharmacological properties in animals of CT 1341—a new steroid anaesthetic. Br. J. Anaesth., 43:2, 1971.

48. Cooper, J.: Althesin in outpatient psychiatric practice. Postgrad. Med. J., 48:115, 1972.

49. Bradford, E.M.W., Campbell, D., Forrester, A.C., and Miller, D.C.: CT 1341—further studies in man. Br. J. Anaesth., 43:722, 1971.

50. Carson, I.W.: Group trial of althesin as an intravenous anaesthetic. Postgrad. Med. J., 48:108, 1972.

51. Carson, I.W., Alexander, J.P., Hewitt, J.C., and Dundee, J.W.: Clinical studies of induction agents. XLI: Venous sequelae following the use of the steroid anaesthetic agent, althesin. Br. J. Anaesth., 44:1311, 1972.

52. Clarke, R.S.J., Dundee, J.W., Doggart, J.R., and Lavery, T.: The effect of single and intermittent administrations of althesin and other intravenous anaesthetics on liver function. Anaesth. Analg., 53:461, 1974.

53. Strunin, L., Strunin, J.M., Knights, K., and Ward, M.P.: Metabolism of ^{14}C-labeled alphaxalone in man. *In* Recent Progress in Anaesthesiology and Resuscitation. Edited by A. Arias, R. Llaurado, M. Nalda, and J. Lunn. Amsterdam, Exerpta Medica, 1974.

54. Ward, M.E., Adu-Gyamfi, V., and Strunin, L.: Althesin and pancuronium in chronic liver disease. Br. J. Anaesth., 47:1199, 1975.

55. Du Cailar, J.: The effects in man of infusions of althesin with particular regard to the cardio-vascular system. Postgrad. Med. J., 48:72, 1972.

56. Downing, J.W., Coleman, A.J., and Meer, F.M.: An intravenous method of anaesthesia for cesarian section. Br. J. Anaesth., 45:381, 1973.

57. Hunter, A.R.: New drugs. Althesin. *In* Recent Advances in Anaesthesia and Analgesia. Int. Anaesthesiol. Clin., 16:8, 1978.

58. Harrison, G.G.: Althesin and malignant hyperpyrexia. Br. J. Anaesth., 45:1019, 1973.

59. Hall, L.W., Trim, C.M., and Woolf, N.: Further studies of porcine malignant hyperthermia. Br. Med. J., April:145, 1972.

60. Austin, T.R., Anderson, J., and Richardson, J.: Bronchospasm following althesin anaesthesia. Br. J. Anaesth., 11:661, 1973.

61. Avery, A.F., and Evans, A.: Reactions to althesin. Br. J. Anaesth., 45:301, 1973.

62. Horton, J.N.: Adverse reaction to althesin. Anaesthesia, 28:182, 1973.

63. Hester, J.B.: Reactions to althesin. Br. J. Anaesth., 45:303, 1973.

64. Evans, J.M., and Keogh, J.A.M.: Adverse reactions to intravenous anaesthetic induction agents. Br. Med. J., 2:735, 1977.

65. Clarke, R.S.J., Fee, J.H., and Dundee, J.W.: Hypersensitivity reactions to intravenous anaes-thetics. *In* Adverse Response to Intravenous Drugs. Edited by J. Watkins and A.M. Ward. London, Academic Press, 1978.

66. Dundee, J.W., Assem, E.S.K., Gaston, J.M., Keilty, S.R., Sutton, J.A., Clarke, R.S.J., and Grainger, D.: Sensitivity to intravenous anaesthetics: report of three cases. Br. Med. J., 1:63, 1974.

67. Clarke, R.S.J., Dundee, J.W., Garrett, R.T., McArdle, G.K., and Sutton, J.A.: Adverse reactions to intravenous anaesthetics, a survey of 100 reports. Br. J. Anaesth., 47:575, 1975.

68. Lorenz, W., Doenicke, A., Meyer, R., Reimann, J., Kusche, J., Barth, H., Gessing, H., Hutzel, M., and Weissenbacher, B.: Histamine release in man by propanidid and thiopentone: phar-macological effects and clinical consequeneces. Br. J. Anaesth., 44:355, 1972.

69. Doenicke, A., Lorenz, W., Beigl, R., Bezecny, H., Uhlig, G., Kalmar, L., Praetorius, B., and Mann, B.: Histamine release after intravenous application of short-acting hypnotics: a comparison of etomidate, althesin (CT 1341) and propanidid. Br. J. Anaesth., 45:1097, 1973.

70. Thorton, H.L.: Apparent anaphylactic reactions to propanidid. Anaesthesia, 26:490, 1971.

71. Watkins, J., Udnoon, S., and Taussig, P.E.: Mechanisms of adverse response to intravenous agents in man. *In* Adverse response to intravenous drugs. Edited by J. Watkins and A.M. Ward. London, Academic Press, 1978.

72. Beamish, D., and Brown, D.T.: Adverse responses to I.V. anaesthetics. Br. J. Anaesth., 53:55, 1981.

73. Dundee, J.W.: Editorial. Hypersensitivity to intravenous anaesthetic agents. Br. J. Anaesth., 48:57, 1976.

74. Clarke, R.S.J., Dundee, J.W., and Carson, I.: Some aspects of the clinical pharmacology of althesin. Postgrad. Med. J., 48:62, 1972.

75. Dundee, J.W., Carson, I.W., and Clarke, R.S.J.: A comparison of althesin (CT 1341) with methohexitone and propanidid as induction agents. *In* Proceedings of the Fifth World Congress of Anaesthesiologists. Amsterdam, Excerpta Medica, 1972.

76. Kauste, A.: Intravenous anaesthetic althesin. Comparative clinical studies with thiopentone, propanidid and methohexitone. Dissertation. University of Helsinki, Helsinki, Finland, 1976.

77. Warren, J.B.: Althesin in the dental chair. Postgrad. Med. J., 48:130, 1972.

78. Carson, I.W., Graham, J., and Dundee, J.W.: Clinical studies of induction agents. XLII. Recovery from althesin—a comparative study with thiopentone and methohexitone. Br. J. Anaesth., 47:358, 1975.

79. Savege, T.M.: A new steroid anaesthetic—althesin. Proc. R. Soc. Lond. [Biol.], 66:1029, 1973.

80. Clarke, R.S.J., Dundee, J.W., Carson, M.V., and McCaughey, W.: Clinical studies of induction agents. XL: Althesin with various premedicants. Br. J. Anaesth., 44:485, 1972.

81. Dundee, J.W., Moore, J., and Clarke, R.S.J.: Studies of drugs given before anaesthesia. V: Peth-idine 100 mg alone and with atropine or hyoscine. Br. J. Anaesth., 36:703, 1964.

82. Clarke, R.S.J., Dundee, J.W., Carson, I.V., Arora, M.V., and McCaughey, W.: Clinical studies of induction agents. XL: Althesin with various premedicants. Br. J. Anaesth., 43:845, 1971.

83. Tammisto, T., Takki, S., Tigerstedt, I., and Kauste, A.: A comparison of althesin and thiopentone in induction of anaesthesia. Br. J. Anaesth., 45:100, 1973.

84. Broadley, J.M., and Taylor, P.A.: An assessment of althesin for the induction of anaesthesia in cardiac surgical patients: a comparison with thiopentone. Br. J. Anaesth., 46:687, 1974.

85. Fordham, R.M.M., Awdry, P.M., and Paterson, G.M.: The suitability of althesin for use as an induction agent in intra-ocular surgery. Postgrad. Med. J., *48*:129, 1972.
86. Swerdlow, M.: Althesin—a new intravenous anaesthetic. Can. Anaesth. Soc. J., *20*:186, 1973.
87. Dixon, R.A.: Subanaesthetic dosage of althesin as a sedative for conservative dentistry. Br. J. Anaesth., *48*:431, 1976.
88. Heinonen, J., Orko, R., and Louhija, A.: Anaesthesia for cardioversion: a comparison of althesin and thiopentone. Br. J. Anaesth., *45*:49, 1973.
89. Keep, P.J., and Manford, M.L.M.: A comparison of althesin and methohexitone in paediatric anaesthesia. Br. J. Anaesth., *46*:685, 1974.
90. Saarnivaara, L.: Comparison of thiopentone, althesin and ketamine in anaesthesia for otolaryngological surgery in children. Br. J. Anaesth., *49*:363, 1977.
91. Honda, N., Konno, K., Itohda, Y., Nishino, M., Matsushima, S., Haseba, S., Honda, Y., and Gotoh, Y.: Malignant hyperthermia and althesin. Can. Anaesth. Soc. J., *24*:514, 1977.
92. Judelman, H., and Pirie, D.H.: Anaesthesia in a patient with previous malignant hyperpyrexia. Br. J. Anaesth., *46*:519, 1974.

Chapter 12

MINAXOLONE

CHEMISTRY, PHYSICAL PROPERTIES, AND AVAILABILITY FOR INVESTIGATIONAL USE

Minaxolone is 28-ethoxy-3a-hydroxy-11a-dimethylamino-5a-pregnane-20-one (Fig. 12–1). Unlike its forerunner, althesin, this ultra-short-acting steroid anesthetic is soluble in water. The drug is now available in the United Kingdom for investigational use as a 0.5% solution at a pH of 4.

Laboratory Studies and First Clinical Experience

The pharmacologic properties of minaxolone were first studied in laboratory animals, and the drug was found to be effective as an intravenous anesthetic.[1] Initial investigations with minaxolone in human volunteers and surgical patients established its suitability and safety as an intravenous anesthetic induction agent.[2,3] These reports were confirmed by findings from studies in which minaxolone was used in doses of either 0.25 or 0.5 mg/kg intravenously to induce anesthesia in 62 patients undergoing minor urologic and gynecologic procedures.[4] The drug was effective in inducing anesthesia in 92% of 36 patients receiving the 0.5-mg/kg dose; loss of consciousness occurred within 1 arm-brain circulation time. In most of the 62 patients, excitatory effects were recorded, including hypertension, involuntary muscle movements, and tremor. These side-effects were mainly observed in patients who appeared inadequately anesthetized and, therefore, received more frequent administrations of minaxolone in the lower

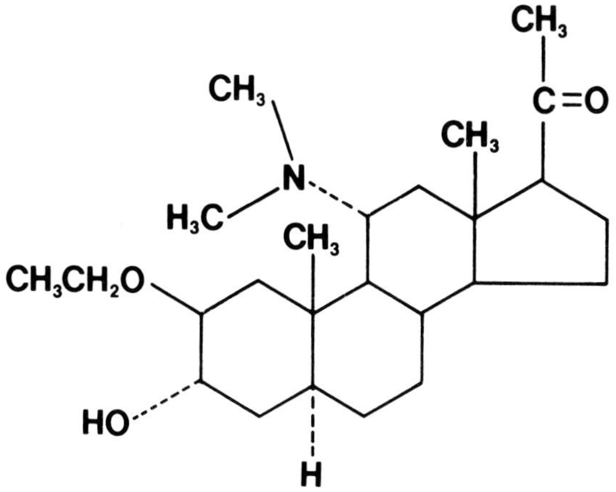

Fig. 12–1. Structural formula of minaxolone.

dose (0.25 mg/kg). This finding suggests that the lower dose failed to produce an adequate depth of anesthesia consistently.

The duration of succinylcholine-induced apnea during minaxolone anesthesia is similar to that observed with thiopental and methohexital, but is shorter than that seen with propanidid, which competes with plasma cholinesterase.

These initial favorable results were further supported by data from a study in which minaxolone was used as the anesthetic induction agent in 100 female patients undergoing minor gynecologic or genitourinary surgery.[5] All patients received atropine (0.6 mg intravenously), followed randomly by fentanyl (75 to 150 μg/kg intravenously, according to body weight) or the corresponding volume of normal saline solution. Anesthesia was then induced with minaxolone (1 mg/ second intravenously) until loss of consciousness occurred. Anesthesia was maintained with nitrous oxide-oxygen mixtures supplemented by incremental doses of minaxolone (5 to 10 mg intravenously) to control spontaneous muscle movements. The time needed for onset of anesthesia was comparable to that of thiopental but was shorter than that of althesin. Apnea occurred less frequently with minaxolone use than with other intravenous anesthetics. A few patients experienced mild pain during injection of the drug.

The incidence of excitatory phenomena, including tremors and involuntary muscle movements, was similar to that observed by Dundee and associates.[4] The period of recovery from minaxolone anesthesia was considerably longer than that reported with the use of methohexital or etomidate.

Fentanyl administration significantly reduces the total dose of minaxolone required for anesthesia. Fentanyl also reduces the incidence of excitatory phenomena during the induction of and emergence from minaxolone-induced anesthesia, thus improving the number of satisfactory anesthetic procedures. The cardiovascular effects of minaxolone appear to be similar to those of other intravenous anesthetic agents, but are somewhat enhanced when fentanyl is administered. Fentanyl tends to increase the incidence of nausea and vomiting during the postoperative period.

In another study, minaxolone was compared with althesin as an anesthesia induction agent, intermittently supplemented by nitrous oxide and oxygen, for short surgical procedures.[6] Short-term recovery after minaxolone use was significantly slower than that noted after althesin anesthesia; 1 hour after the end of the administration of anesthesia, no differences could be detected between patients recovering from minaxolone use compared to those recovering from althesin anesthesia.

When administered at a minimum infusion rate of 11.3 mg/kg/minute in patients premedicated with morphine (10 mg intramuscularly) and spontaneously breathing 66% nitrous oxide in oxygen, the cardiovascular and respiratory effects of minaxolone were similar to those observed with althesin employed under comparable conditions.[7] The prolonged short-term recovery from minaxolone compared to that associated with althesin was suggested by the authors to be due to the solubility of the drug in water and to its greater volume of distribution.

In a study concerned with the effect of premedication on induction, maintenance, and recovery characteristics of minaxolone administered as a supplement to nitrous oxide-oxygen anesthesia, premedication with morphine combined with atropine provided better operative conditions and was associated with fewer side-effects when compared to the use of atropine alone or of diazepam combined with atropine.[8] The ventilatory response to the morphine-atropine premedication resulted in increased respiratory frequency and decreased tidal volume in all patients. This effect was most marked in the diazepam-atropine group of patients. The total dose of minaxolone required for anesthesia was less when the morphine-atropine combination was employed, which may explain the shorter recovery times recorded with this premedication.

Because minaxolone shares most of the advantageous properties of althesin but with a lesser incidence of undesirable side-effects, investigators agree that the overall favorable results obtained during the initial clinical trials with this drug warrant more thorough clinical examination of the usefulness and safety of this drug as an intravenous anesthetic induction agent.

REFERENCES

1. Davis, B., Dodds, M.G., Dolamore, P.G., Gardner, C.J., Sawyer, P.R., Twissel, D.J., and Vallance, D.K.: Minaxolone: a soluble steroid anesthetic. Br. J. Anaesth., 51:564, 1979.
2. Aveling, W., Sear, J.W., Fitch, W., Chang, H., Waters, A., Cooper, G.M., Simpson, P., Savege, T.M., Prys-Roberts, C., and Cooper, D.: Early clinical evaluation of minaxolone: a new intravenous steroid anaesthetic agent. Lancet, 2:71, 1979.
3. McNeill, H.G., Clarke, R.S.J., and Dundee, J.W.: Minaxolone: a new water-soluble steroid anaesthetic. Lancet, 2:73, 1979.
4. Dundee, J.W., Clarke, R.S.J., and McNeill, H.G.: Minaxolone: a preliminary communication. *In* Trends in Intravenous Anesthesia. Edited by J.A. Aldrete and T. Stanley. Miami, Symposia Specialists, 1980.
5. Punchihewa, V.G., Morgan, M., Lumley, J., and Whitwam, J.F.: Initial experience with minaxolone, a water-soluble steroid intravenous anaesthetic agent. Anaesthesia, 35:214, 1980.
6. Sear, J.W., Cooper, G.M., Williams, N.B., Simpson, P.J., and Prys-Roberts, C.: Minaxolone or althesin supplemented by nitrous oxide: a study in anaesthesia for short operative procedures. Anaesthesia, 35:169, 1980.
7. Sear, J.W., Prys-Roberts, C., Gray, A.G.J., Walsh, E.M., Curnow, J.S.H., and Dye, J.: Infusions of minaxolone to supplement nitrous oxide-oxygen anaesthesia: a comparison with althesin. Br. J. Anaesth., 53:339, 1981.
8. Gray, A.J.G., Cooper, G.M., Chapman, J.A., Sear, J.W., Simpson, P.J., and Prys-Roberts, C.: Studies on premedication and ventilatory responses to minaxolone. Acta Anaesthesiol. Belg., 32:121, 1981.

Chapter 13

ETOMIDATE

HISTORY

In the continuing search for the "ideal" intravenous anesthetic induction agent, which provides rapid and short duration of action, pleasant loss of consciousness, minimal cardiovascular alterations, and no significant undesirable side-effects, Godefroi and co-workers synthesized the carboxylated imidazole etomidate in 1965. Janssen, et al., reported its hypnotic properties as noted in laboratory animals in 1971.[1,2]

The first clinical study of the use of etomidate as an anesthetic induction agent was conducted by Doenicke in 1975.[3] Since then, the drug has been extensively evaluated, when used in both laboratory animals and man, as an anesthetic induction agent, continuous hypnotic anesthetic supplement, complete intravenous anesthetic, "brain protective" agent, and a postoperative and intensive care unit sedative-hypnotic.[4] Pain on injection, superficial thrombophlebitis, and myoclonia are the most frequent side-effects associated with the use of etomidate. In addition, nausea and vomiting are troublesome, especially after the use of multiple doses of this drug.

In spite of these annoying side-effects, etomidate may represent an important advance in the present-day practice of anesthesia. Because etomidate produces minimal changes in cardiovascular dynamics and respiratory functions, it is particularly suitable and safe for use in the induction of anesthesia and as a sole anesthetic for short, relatively painless diagnostic and therapeutic procedures in high-risk patients with reduced cardiac reserve, hypovolemia, and severe pulmonary dysfunction.

CHEMISTRY AND PHYSICAL PROPERTIES

Etomidate (R-(+)-ethyl-1-(1-phenylethyl)-1*H*-imidazole-5-carboxylate sulfate) is a potent, short-acting intravenous hypnotic agent (Fig. 13–1).[2] Etomidate has 2 isomers; only the (+) isomer possesses the hypnotic properties. Etomidate (R 16 659, Hypnomidate, and Amidate) is supplied as a sulfate and is dissolved in 1.8 mg Na_2HPO_4 and 2.2 mg of Na_2HPO_4, with a 4.2% glucose solution in a concentration of 1.5 mg of etomidate base per 1 ml. The pH is about 3.4. The molecular weight of etomidate is 342.36.[5]

Potency and Toxicity

In rats, etomidate has an ED_{50} of 0.57 mg/kg. It is 6 times as potent as methohexital and is about 25 times more potent than propanidid.[2,6] The safety margin of etomidate (LD_{50}/ED_{50}) is 26.0, as compared to 9.5 for methohexital, 6.7 for

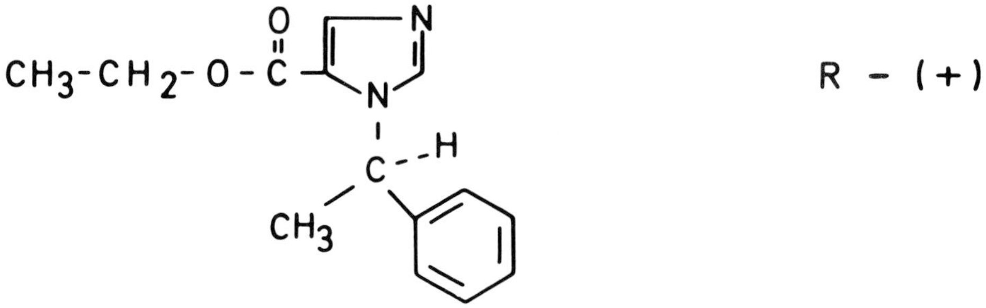

Fig. 13–1. Structural formula of etomidate.

propanidid, and 4.6 for thiopental. No adverse effects with prolonged administration of etomidate have been observed after hematologic and biochemical analyses, urinalysis, and histopathologic and teratogenetic tests.[6] Effective concentrations of etomidate do not affect essential tissue metabolism or uptake of transmitter substances.[7]

Metabolism, Distribution, and Excretion

Etomidate is moderately lipid soluble. It is rapidly metabolized, primarily in the liver by hydrolysis of the ester group to form the main metabolite, the carboxylic acid of etomidate. The metabolite is pharmacologically inactive.[8] Ester hydrolysis does not take place in human blood.[7] Plasma levels of the drug decline according to a triexponential curve with distribution half-lives of 2.6 minutes (initial $t\frac{1}{2}$) and 29 minutes (intermediate $t\frac{1}{2}$) and with an elimination half-life ($t\frac{1}{2}$ β) of 4.6 ± 2.6 hours.[9] Hepatic clearance is approximately 15% of the total drug dosage per hour.[10] The rapid rate and extensive distribution of the drug into peripheral tissues are reflected by its large volume of distribution (4.5 L/kg); these factors are also probably responsible for the very short duration of action. The slow redistribution of etomidate from the deep peripheral compartment explains the relatively long elimination half-life. To maintain pharmacologically effective plasma concentrations for "total" intravenous anesthesia, etomidate is administered by continuous intravenous infusion.[11,12] Plasma levels of etomidate required for hypnosis exceed 0.25 μg/ml in man.[13]

In humans, 75% of an intravenously delivered dose of etomidate is excreted in the urine during the first 24 hours after administration, mainly as an inactive acid metabolite; 10% is noted in bile and 13% of the administered dose is found in the feces.[14]

PROTEIN BINDING

Etomidate readily binds to human plasma proteins. At a pH of 7.4, the drug is 76% bound to human albumin.[15,16] Because only the unbound fraction of etomidate exerts the pharmacologic effect, variations in albumin concentrations may alter the free drug fraction and thus the potency of the drug.

PHARMACOLOGY

Central Nervous System (CNS)

Etomidate is a pure hypnotic and has no analgesic activity. It has a rapid rate of onset of action and induces hypnosis within one arm-brain circulation.[2,17] The duration of hypnosis with etomidate is dose dependent; the hypnotic effect doubles when the dose is doubled. No tolerance develops after repeated administrations. The time of recovery from hypnosis is short and is related to the duration of the hypnosis. At low doses, recovery time is approximately four to five times the duration of hypnosis; at high doses, recovery time is about one to five times the duration of the hypnotic effect.[4]

Results of initial studies in which etomidate was administered to human subjects established that an intravenous dose of 0.15 mg/kg produced hypnosis that in most patients proved too short and shallow to provide a satisfactory state of unconsciousness.[17] By doubling the dose to 0.3 mg/kg, a considerably deeper sleep was produced with hypnosis being prolonged by approximately 2 minutes. A second intravenous injection with the same dose resulted in marked prolongation of sleep, indicating some cumulative effect. An intravenous, 0.15-mg/kg dose of etomidate provides the same degree of hypnotic potency as 5 mg/kg of propanidid given intravenously. Prolonged periods of fatigue were recorded in human volunteers after receiving thiopental and methohexital, but no fatigue was observed 10 minutes after awakening from propanidid or etomidate anesthesia.[17]

ELECTROENCEPHALOGRAPHIC (EEG) EFFECTS

Etomidate-induced EEG changes have been studied in human volunteers.[18] Alterations in the EEG produced by etomidate resemble EEG changes observed with the use of barbiturates. The first noticeable change during a 60-second intravenous injection of the drug occurs after 30 to 40 seconds; a diffuse and irregular rapid-wave activity occurs that is comparable to the induction stage associated with barbiturate use. After a few seconds, transitional mixed activity occurs, with slow waves superimposed by rapid activity corresponding to light anesthesia. Subsequently, increased slow-wave activity develops that corresponds to a medium stage of anesthesia and is sufficient in hypnotic action to allow surgical manipulations.

EEG changes produced by etomidate in humans clearly reflect a hypnotic action that is based mainly on an impairment of neocortical function.[18] Because the drug does not sufficiently block afferent impulses to thalamic regions or has little influence on intrinsic brain stem electric activity, it has no analgesic activity. A comparison of etomidate- and thiopental-induced EEG changes showed a lack of beta activity associated with a considerably longer duration of the "deep stage" of anesthesia with etomidate, which contrasts with the absence of periodic burst suppression pattern observed with thiopental administration.[19] The myoclonic movements that may occur after etomidate administration are not associated with epileptiform discharges in the EEG.[18,19]

Cardiovascular System

ANIMAL STUDIES

The cardiovascular effects of etomidate at intravenously administered doses of 1.25 and 2.5 mg/kg in dogs were minimal.[20] A slight decrease in aortic blood pressure occurred, associated with a moderate increase in heart rate, but no significant effects were observed related to left ventricular pressure dynamics at a constant heart rate or on mean aortic and mean coronary blood flow. At these intravenous doses, etomidate, unlike propanidid, does not induce histamine release, which may contribute to the cardiovascular stability noted during and after anesthetic induction with etomidate.[21,22]

When comparing the acute hemodynamic effects of etomidate in dogs with those of various induction agents (including thiopental, methohexital, propanidid, althesin, ketamine, and piritramide), external cardiac work remained unchanged after propanidid and althesin, but myocardial contractility decreased and myocardial consumption increased, probably because of an increase in heart rate with simultaneous increase in blood flow.[23] Also, with propanidid, coronary dilatation was initially noted, whereas with use of the barbiturates and ketamine, these vessels were constricted. Cardiac efficiency decreased under the influence of barbiturates and ketamine, resulting in an uneconomic use of the heart. In contrast, etomidate and piritramide had no adverse effects on hemodynamics; in particular, coronary blood flow and myocardial oxygen consumption determinations remained constant.

In pigs, the cardiovascular effects of etomidate administered by continuous infusion, at doses ranging from 0.03 to 0.24 mg/kg, were studied with emphasis on regional blood flow, cardiac performance, and metabolism.[24] Etomidate caused moderate, dose-dependent decreases in cardiac output, arterial pressure, and left ventricular pressure determinations, whereas those of heart rate, myocardial blood flow distribution, and myocardial metabolism of lactate, glucose, and free fatty acids remained unchanged.

In heart-lung preparations obtained from cats, a slight, direct negative inotropic effect was noted with etomidate administered at low and medium concentrations.[25] A direct negative chronotropic action with etomidate was detectable only at higher drug concentrations. When compared to hexobarbital, etomidate revealed a significantly larger therapeutic range with regard to both inotropic and chronotropic action. With the exception of a marked reduction in stroke volume, all other parameters related to qualitative and quantitative effects of etomidate remained constant. When testing cardiac adaptability in response to gradual changes in volume and pressure loads caused by doses of etomidate and hexobarbital sufficient to reduce myocardial contractility, ventricular performance was less adversely affected by etomidate than by hexobarbital.[25]

The possible interaction between etomidate and antihypertensive agents (such as propranolol and α-methyl-dopa) was investigated in dogs.[26] There was no indication that antihypertensive agents interfere with the action of etomidate with regard to the effect of the latter drug on heart rate, aortic blood pressure, respiratory function, and duration of sleep.

Marked and long-lasting etomidate-induced depression of sympathetic activity was documented in normal and baroreceptor-denervated cats.[27] Depression of preganglionic cervical sympathetic activity was barely reflected by changes in arterial blood pressure. Because the mild tachycardia observed in normal cats may have only partially counteracted the depression in arterial pressure expected from the severely depressed sympathetic tone, one can assume that etomidate exerts minimal direct cardiovascular depression. Baroreceptor-denervated cats responded to etomidate with bradycardia instead of tachycardia. This response may be explained by the diminished sympathetic tone, but may also be caused in part by a direct negative inotropic effect of the drug. In addition, a possible vagolytic action of etomidate cannot be excluded.[27]

HUMAN STUDIES

Results of studies concerned with the effect of etomidate on cardiovascular parameters in humans generally confirm the remarkable hemodynamic stability that was documented in animals. After initial investigations into the value and efficiency of the drug as an anesthetic induction agent in humans, the importance of its minimal effects on cardiovascular function was documented.[28] The remarkable hemodynamic stability afforded by etomidate was confirmed in a subsequent study concerned with cardiovascular and pulmonary responses to etomidate (0.3 mg/kg intravenously) in human volunteers.[29] From all parameters studied, including heart rate, mean systemic arterial pressure, pulmonary artery pressure, central venous pressure, pulmonary capillary wedge pressure, cardiac output, stroke volume, cardiac index, systemic vascular resistance, and pulmonary vascular resistance, a 10% increase in heart rate was the only significant hemodynamic change observed. In another study with etomidate (0.2 mg/kg intravenously), an increase in heart rate of only 2.8% was observed.[30] Similar observations were made in healthy human volunteers and in patients with valvular disease after etomidate was administered in doses of 0.12 mg/kg/minute and 0.3 mg/kg intravenously, respectively.[31] With the exception of a moderate (9%) increase in heart rate, only slight changes in general and coronary hemodynamics were observed in both the healthy subjects and the patients with heart disease.

Another study involving patient volunteers without heart disease also documented minimal effects of etomidate (0.3 mg/kg intravenously) on the cardiovascular system.[32] A slight increase in cardiac index was observed immediately after completion of the injection; mean arterial pressure, left ventricular pressure, and heart rate decreased slightly, with the maximum effect observed 3 minutes after etomidate administration. All cardiovascular parameters returned to control levels 10 minutes after drug delivery.

Healthy volunteers, who were lightly anesthetized with halothane-nitrous oxide or isoflurane-fentanyl, exhibited no significant effect of etomidate (0.3 mg/kg intravenously) on myocardial contractility.[33] With this dose of etomidate, myocardial oxygen consumption was reduced by 14%.

An 18% reduction in myocardial oxygen consumption was observed in patients with congenital and acquired heart disease after receiving etomidate (0.3 mg/kg) combined with fentanyl (0.1 mg).[34] The decrease in myocardial energy demand was considered to be related to the slight etomidate-induced decrease in systolic pressure. Such reduction in myocardial oxygen consumption was not recorded in patients who were free from cardiovascular disease.

In a similar study involving patients with myocardial disease, only minor changes in hemodynamics, including arterial pressure, heart rate, left ventricular pressure, left ventricular end-diastolic pressure, dp/dt_{max}, cardiac index, and stroke index, were recorded.[35] The investigators concluded that, although etomidate exerts a small negative inotropic effect in patients with myocardial insufficiency, the drug is very effective and safe for induction of anesthesia in patients with myocardial disease.

Patients with demonstrated cardiac disease have good tolerance of etomidate-induced anesthesia. In one study, the only significant change in cardiopulmonary dynamics was a slight elevation in arterial CO_2 tension.[36] Slight increases in arterial CO_2 tension have also been recorded in patients with aortic or mitral valve disease, despite a modest increase in respiratory frequency.[37] Interestingly, an increase in heart rate observed after etomidate delivery in subjects without cardiac disease did not occur in these high-risk patients.

Various additional reports from investigators in Europe, and also from the United States and Canada, outline results that generally confirm the minimal amount of cardiovascular impairment associated with clinically effective doses of etomidate.[38,39] Most researchers agree that etomidate comes close to the "ideal" induction agent in both healthy subjects and patients with heart disease. In addition, the use of fentanyl and diazepam as premedicants minimizes pain from etomidate injection and reduces the incidence of involuntary muscle movements; before the use of these agents, these movements were considered a significant and clinically unacceptable disadvantage of the drug.[40]

CEREBRAL BLOOD FLOW (CBF) AND INTRACRANIAL PRESSURE (ICP)

Etomidate decreases CBF and cerebral oxygen consumption.[41–47] In contrast to thiopental, etomidate causes these changes without decreasing arterial blood pressure or the rate of cerebral perfusion. In one study, cerebral blood flow was measured by injecting [133]xenon into the internal carotid artery of patients undergoing carotid angiography.[47] Isotope clearance over a 10-minute period was monitored with the use of scintillation counters and a 10-channel cerebrograph. A significant decrease in CBF was recorded after the administration of etomidate (0.3 mg/kg intravenously). With the exception of significant decrease in heart rate, all other cardiovascular parameters studied, including arterial blood pressure, stroke volume, cardiac output, central venous pressure, and arterial and venous blood gases, remained constant. A substantial decrease in CBF in response to continuous intravenous infusion of etomidate was reported by other investigators.[24]

Intracranial pressure was measured in patients with intracranial space-occupying lesions.[45] The administration of etomidate (0.2 mg/kg) produced a significant decrease in ICP. Mean arterial pressure also decreased in most patients, but the change was statistically significant only at 3 and 4 minutes after the injection of etomidate. Changes in cerebral perfusion pressure and heart rate were minor and were not clinically significant. Increases in ICP after ketamine administration have been successfully treated by etomidate or have been minimized by pretreatment with the drug.

Respiratory System

Respiratory function is minimally affected by etomidate use at an intravenous dose of 0.15 mg/kg. Transient apnea of 20 to 25 seconds' duration was reported, however, after etomidate (0.3 mg/kg) was delivered intravenously to geriatric patients.[48] In patients with myocardial disease (ASA classes III and IV) receiving etomidate by rapid intravenous injection (0.3 mg/kg), a mean decrease in arterial Po_2 (85 to 66 mm Hg) was recorded.[49] When the drug was administered over a period of 60 seconds, a slight increase in arterial CO_2 tension was observed. This change, however, was not considered clinically significant. In patients premedicated with diazepam and atropine, a significant increase in respiratory frequency was noted toward the end of the injection, concomitant with a significant increase in minute volume.[50,51] In patients premedicated with papaveretum and hyoscine, no such increase in respiratory frequency occurred. These patients briefly experienced hyperventilation followed by respiratory depression; some patients experienced apnea that lasted 30 seconds on average. The incidence of apnea was 40% in the diazepam-atropine group and 27% in the opiate group. The brief period of hyperventilation after induction of anesthesia with etomidate was less than that observed with propanidid but was similar to that encountered with althesin.

Respiratory response to etomidate has been investigated in children.[52] From a study of 198 children (age range of 6 to 16 years) who received etomidate (0.2 mg/kg intravenously) for induction of anesthesia, none developed respiratory depression after injection of the drug and none was apneic for more than 10 seconds. Of 37 children who received fentanyl (25 μg/kg intravenously) in addition to the etomidate injection, 12 were apneic for more than 10 seconds. No child required assisted ventilation.

Musculoskeletal System

One undesirable side-effect of etomidate is the occurrence of insufficiently coordinated muscle movements, in the form of myoclonia and dyskinesia, that are probably caused by disinhibition of subcortical structures.[19] These myoclonic muscle movements occur in approximately 30% of lightly premedicated patients.[17] The incidence can be as high as 60% in patients receiving etomidate (0.3 mg/kg intravenously) after atropine premedication. The incidence of involuntary muscle movements is reduced, but not eliminated, by prior administration of diazepam (0.1 mg/kg intravenously). When fentanyl (0.05 to 0.1 mg intravenously) is added to the etomidate-diazepam combination, the myoclonic and dyskinetic activity is further suppressed, whereas the hypnotic activity related to the etomidate is prolonged.[17] Equally good results in reducing the occurrence of etomidate-induced involuntary muscle movements have been observed with the use of meperidine as a premedicant.

Etomidate-induced muscle activity should not be equated with generalized tonic-clonic epileptic seizures. Extensive studies concerned with the possible epileptogenic effects of etomidate in humans have documented neither definite paroxysmal or epileptic discharges nor clinical signs of generalized epileptic seizure activity in the EEG.[18,19] Even in epileptic patients, no activation of paroxysm has been observed during etomidate anesthesia.

Miscellaneous Effects

LOCAL IRRITATION

When injected intra-arterially in rabbits, etomidate displays no serious adverse effects. Although no significant irritant effects are noted when the drug is given intravenously, the administration of etomidate in a buffered solution was accompanied by a burning sensation at the site of injection in 33 to 80% of a group of patients.[28,53,54] The incidence of pain resulting from etomidate injection can be reduced by using large veins and administering the drug more slowly. Gooding, et al., reported a significant reduction in the incidence of localized pain by injecting etomidate that was dissolved in 35% propylene glycol at a pH of 5.0 in place of saline at a pH of 3.4.[55] With this new etomidate preparation, the occurrence of pain at the site of injection is less common.[56]

ELECTROLYTES AND BLOOD GLUCOSE LEVEL

Etomidate does not cause changes in the levels of plasma potassium and blood glucose. In conjunction with succinylcholine, however, etomidate causes a significant rise in plasma potassium and blood glucose values. The hyperglycemic response is greater after etomidate administration than that recorded after the use of thiopental.[57]

OBSTETRICS

No data from adequate and controlled studies of the use of etomidate in pregnant women are available. Therefore, the drug is not recommended for use in obstetric patients, including women who are to undergo cesarean section deliveries. The manufacturer of etomidate suggests that the drug may be used with caution during lactation and pregnancy, but only if the potential benefit justifies a possible increased risk to the fetus.

ADRENOCORTICAL SYSTEM

When etomidate is administered at clinically useful doses to induce anesthesia (0.2 to 0.35 mg/kg intravenously), the levels of serum cortisol and plasma aldosterone decrease during the first 30 to 60 minutes after induction; ACTH levels increase and serum testosterone and catecholamine levels are not influenced.[58,59] The effects of an induction dose of etomidate on the adrenocortical steroidogenesis are clearly reversible, the response to ACTH stimulation is normal 24 hours later, and there seem to be no clinical consequences.[60,61]

CLINICAL APPLICATIONS

Induction of Anesthesia

Because etomidate is a pure hypnotic, the predominant role the drug plays in clinical anesthesia is that of an anesthetic induction agent. Because it has no significant depressant effects on cardiovascular and pulmonary function, the drug is especially valuable for induction of anesthesia and for short surgical procedures in high-risk patients, particularly those with reduced myocardial reserve and compromised pulmonary function for whom alternative induction agents without depressive myocardial actions (e.g., opioids) necessitate postoperative pulmonary support.[62] When rapid induction of anesthesia is essential, as for emergency surgical intervention in a patient in hypovolemic shock for whom time does not allow adequate circulatory volume replacement, etomidate combined with fentanyl may be the anesthetic of choice (with the possible exception of ketamine).[63] Satisfactory results related to the use of etomidate in conjunction with fentanyl and diazepam for brief therapeutic and diagnostic manipulations were reported.[64–67] Etomidate was also found suitable in hastening the induction of fentanyl and neuroleptanesthesia.[68,69] Because etomidate lowers the ICP, it may be the drug of choice for induction of anesthesia in patients with an elevated ICP.[42–47]

Other Clinical Uses

Other areas in which etomidate was found useful include electroconvulsive therapy, cardioversion, bronchoscopy, and tonsillectomy in children.[70–73] Because etomidate significantly lowers intraocular pressure, the drug is effective and safe for use during brief ophthalmic procedures in which a rise in intraocular tension is undesirable.[74]

The value of etomidate when administered by infusion for long-term sedation in intensive care units was confirmed by investigators from the United Kingdom.[75] Preliminary data from European studies suggest the use of etomidate by continuous infusion with the use of an alcohol preparation providing prolonged anesthesia with fewer undesirable effects. Boidin called attention to the possible development of an addisonian crisis resulting from the etomidate-induced blockade of corticosteroid production during prolonged infusion of the drug for long-term sedation in intensive care units.[76] The author suggests the administration of ascorbic acid, thereby increasing the serum cortisol concentration and restoring the relationship between the serum cortisol and serum ACTH concentrations in patients in whom cortisol synthesis was blocked by etomidate infusion.

Etomidate is a promising drug for use when rapid induction of anesthesia and stable hemodynamics are required. Etomidate will probably not replace thiopental, but it represents an alternative with a favorable pharmacokinetic and pharmacodynamic profile.

REFERENCES

1. Godefroi, E., Janssen, P.A.J., Van Der Eycken, C.A.M., Van Heertum, A.H.M.T., and Niemegeers, C.J.E.: DL-1-(1-arylalkyl) imidazole-5-carboxylate esters. A novel type of hypnotic agent. J. Med. Chem., 8:220, 1965.
2. Janssen, P.A.J., Niemegeers, C.J.E., Schellekens, K.H.L., and Lenaerts, F.M.: Etomidate, R-(+)-ethyl-1 (alpha-methyl-benzyl) imidazole-5-carboxylate (R 16 659), a potent, short-acting and relatively atoxic intravenous hypnotic agent in rats. Arzneimittelforschung, 21:1234, 1971.
3. Doenicke, A.: Etomidate, a new intravenous hypnotic. Acta Anaesthesiol. Belg., 25:5, 1975.
4. Giese, J.L., and Stanley, T.H.: Etomidate: a new intravenous anesthetic induction agent. Pharmacotherapy, 3:251, 1983.
5. Reneman, R.S., and Janssen, P.A.J.: The experimental pharmacology of etomidate, a new potent, short-acting intravenous hypnotic. *In* Etomidate. An Intravenous Hypnotic Agent. Edited by A. Doenicke. Berlin, Springer, 1977.
6. Janssen, P.A.J., Niemegeers, C.J.E., and Marsboom, R.P.H.: Etomidate, a potent non-barbiturate hypnotic. Intravenous etomidate in mice, rats, guinea-pigs, rabbits and dogs. Arch. Int. Pharmacodyn. Ther., 214:92, 1975.
7. Xhonneux, R., Canneliet, E., and Reneman, R.S.: The electrophysiological effects of etomidate (R 26 490), a new short-acting hypnotic, in various cardiac tissues. Proceedings of the 4th European Congress of Anaesthesiology, Madrid, September, 1974.
8. Hill, R.G., and Taberner, P.V.: Some neuropharmacological properties of the new non-barbiturate hypnotic etomidate (R(+)-ethyl-1-(alpha-methyl-benzyl) imidazole-5-carboxylate). Br. J. Pharmacol., 54:241p, 1975.
9. Ghoneim, M.M., and Van Hamme, M.J.: Hydrolysis of etomidate. Anesthesiology, 50:227, 1979.
10. Heykants, J.J., Meuldermans, W.E., Michiels, L.J.M., Lewi, P.J., and Janssen, P.A.J.: Distribution, metabolism and excretion of etomidate, a short-acting hypnotic drug in the rat: comparative study of (R)-(+) and (S)-(-)-etomidate. Arch. Int. Pharmacodyn. Ther., 216:113, 1975.
11. Van de Walle, J., Demeyere, R., Vanacker, B., Vermaut, G., and Vandermeersch, E.: Total I.V. anesthesia using a continuous etomidate infusion. Acta Anaesthesiol. Belg., 30:117, 1979.
12. Van Hamme, M.J., Ghoneim, M.M., and Ambre, J.J.: Pharmacokinetics of etomidate, a new intravenous anesthetic. Anesthesiology, 49:274, 1978.
13. Ambre, J.J., Van Hamme, M.J., Ghoneim, M.M., and Gross, E.G.: Pharmacokinetics of etomidate, a new intravenous anesthetic. Fed. Proc., 36:997, 1977.
14. Heykants, J., Brugmans, J., and Doenicke, A.: On the pharmacokinetics of etomidate (R 26 490) in human volunteers: plasma levels, metabolism and excretion. Clinical Research Report R 26 490/1. Beerse, Belgium, Janssen Research Products Information Service, 1973.
15. Mannes, G.A., and Doenicke, A.: Protein binding of etomidate. *In* Etomidate. An Intravenous Hypnotic Agent. Edited by A. Doenicke. Berlin, Springer, 1977.
16. Meuldermans, W.E.G., and Heykants, J.J.P.: The plasma protein binding and distribution of etomidate in dog, rat and human blood. Arch. Int. Pharmacodyn. Ther., 221:150, 1976.
17. Doenicke, A.: Etomidate, a new hypnotic agent for intravenous application. *In* Etomidate. An Intravenous Hypnotic Agent. Edited by A. Doenicke. Berlin, Springer, 1977.

18. Kugler, J., Doenicke, A., and Laub, M.: The EEG after etomidate. *In* Etomidate. An Intravenous Hypnotic Agent. Edited by A. Doenicke. Berlin, Springer, 1977.

19. Ghoneim, M.M., and Yamada, T.: Etomidate: a clinical and electroencephalographic comparison with thiopental. Anesth. Analg., 56:479, 1977.

20. Reneman, R.S., Jageneau, A.H.M., Xhonneux, R., and Laduron, P.: The cardiovascular pharmacology of etomidate (R 26 490), a new, potent and short-acting intravenous hypnotic agent. Proceedings of 4th European Congress of Anaesthesiology, Madrid, September, 1974.

21. Laduron, P., and Janssen, P.A.J.: Histamine release in dogs after intravenous injection of etomidate. Biological Research Report R 26 490/1. Beerse, Belgium, Janssen Research Products Information Service, 1973.

22. Doenicke, A.: Histamine release after intravenous application of short-acting hypnotics. Br. J. Anaesth., 45:1097, 1973.

23. Patschke, D., Brueckner, J.B., Gethmann, J.W., Tarnow, J., and Weymar, A.: A comparison of the acute effects of intravenous induction agents (thiopentone, methohexitone, propanidid, althesin, ketamine, piritramide and etomidate) on haemodynamics and myocardial oxygen consumption in dogs. *In* Etomidate. An Intravenous Hypnotic. Edited by A. Doenicke. Berlin, Springer, 1977.

24. Prakash, O., Dhasmana, M., Verdouw, P.D., and Saxena, P.R.: Cardiovascular effects of etomidate with emphasis on regional myocardial blood flow and performance. Br. J. Anaesth., 53:591, 1981.

25. Fischer, K.J., and Marquart, H.: Experimental investigations on the direct effect of etomidate on myocardial contractility. *In* Etomidate. An Intravenous Hypnotic. Edited by A. Doenicke. Berlin, Springer, 1977.

26. Reneman, R.S., Van Gerven, W., and Kruger, R.: Interaction between etomidate and the antihypertensive agents propranolol and alpha-methyl-dopa. *In* Etomidate. An Intravenous Hypnotic. Edited by A. Doenicke. Berlin, Springer, 1977.

27. Skovsted, P., and Sapthavichaikul, S.: The effects of etomidate on arterial pressure, pulse rate and preganglionic sympathetic activity in cats. Can. Anaesth. Soc. J., 24:565, 1977.

28. Gooding, J.M., and Corssen, G.: Etomidate: an ultra short-acting nonbarbiturate agent for anesthesia induction. Anesth. Analg., 55:286, 1976.

29. Gooding, J., and Corssen, G.: Effect of etomidate on the cardiovascular system. Anesth. Analg., 56:717, 1977.

30. Rifat, K., Gamulin, Z., and Gemperle, M.: Etomidate: effects cardiovasculaires du nouvel agent anesthesique intraveineux. Can. Anaesth. Soc. J., 23:492, 1976.

31. Kettler, D., Sonntag, H., and Donath, K.: Hemodynamics, myocardial mechanics, oxygen requirements and oxygen consumption of the human heart during etomidate induction into anesthesia. Anaesthesist, 23:116, 1974.

32. Brueckner, J.B., Gethemann, J.W., Patschke, D., Tarnow, J., and Weymar, A.: Untersuchungen zur Wirkung von Etomidate auf den Kreislauf des Menschen. Anaesthesist, 23:322, 1974.

33. Patschke, D., Brueckner, J.B., Eberlein, H.J., Hess, W., Tarnow, J., and Weymar, A.: Effects of althesin, etomidate and fentanyl on haemodynamics and myocardial oxygen consumption in man. Can. Anaesth. Soc. J., 24:57, 1977.

34. Hempelmann, G., Seitz, W., and Piepenbrock, S.: Kombination von Etomidate und Fentanyl. Ein Beitrag zur Haemodynamik, Inotropie, myokardialem Sauerstoffverbrauch und selektiver Gefaesswirkung. Anaesthesist., 26:231, 1977.

35. Hempelmann, G., Oster, W., Piepenbrock, S., and Karliczek, G.: Hemodynamic effects of etomidate—a new hypnotic in patients with myocardial insufficiency. *In* Etomidate. An Intravenous Induction Agent. Edited by A. Doenicke. Berlin, Springer, 1977.

36. Gooding, J.M., Weng, J.T., Smith, R.A., Berninger, G.T., and Kirby, R.R.: Cardiovascular and pulmonary responses following etomidate induction of anesthesia in patients with demonstrated cardiac disease. Anesth. Analg., 58:40, 1979.

37. Colvin, M.P., Savege, T.M., Newland, P.E., Weaver, E.J.M., Waters, A.F., Brookes, J.M., and Inniss, R.: Cardiorespiratory changes following induction of anaesthesia with etomidate in patients with cardiac disease. Br. J. Anaesth., 51:551, 1979.

38. Zindler, M.: Etomidate, a new short-acting, intravenous hypnotic. Acta Anaesthesiol. Belg., 27:143, 1976.

39. Karliczek, G.F., Breuken, V., and Schokkenbrock, R.: Etomidate-analgesic combinations for induction of anesthesia in cardiac patients. Anaesthesist, 31:51, 1982.

40. Tarnow, J., Hess, W., and Klein, W.: Etomidate, althesin and thiopentone as induction agents for coronary artery surgery. Can. Anaesth. Soc. J., 27:338, 1980.

41. Renou, A.M., Vernhelt, J., and Macrez, P.: Cerebral blood flow and metabolism during etomidate anesthesia in man. Br. J. Anaesth., 50:1047, 1978.

42. Schulte am Esch, J., Thiemig, I., and Entzian, W.: The influence of etomidate and thiopentone on the intracranial pressure elevated by nitrous oxide. Anaesthesia, 29:525, 1980.

43. Herrschaft, H., Schmidt, H., and Glein, F.: The response of human cerebral blood flow to

anesthesia with thiopentone, methohexitone, propanidid, ketamine and etomidate. Adv. Neurosurg., 3:120, 1975.

44. Cunitz, G., Danhauser, I., and Wickbold, J.: Vergleichende Untersuchungen ueber den Einfluss von Etomidate, Thiopental und Methohexital auf den intracraniellen Druck des Patienten. Anaesthesist, 27:64, 1978.

45. Moss, E., Powell, D., and Gibson, R.M.: The effect of etomidate on intracranial pressure and cerebral perfusion pressure. Br. J. Anaesth., 51:347, 1979.

46. Ekhart, E., and List, W.F.: Die wirkung von Etomidate auf den Liquordruck. Prakt. Anasth. Wiederbel. Intensivther., 13:502, 1978.

47. Van Aken, J.G., and Rolly, G.: Influence of etomidate, a new short-acting anesthetic agent, on cerebral blood flow in man. Acta Anaesthesiol. Belg., 27:175, 1976.

48. Marquardt, B., Waibel, H., and Brueckner, J.B.: The influence of R 26 490 (etomidate sulfate) on ventilation and gas exchange. *In* Etomidate. An Intravenous Hypnotic Agent. Edited by A. Doenicke. Berlin, Springer, 1977.

49. Hempelmann, G., Hemplemann, W., Piepenbrock, S., Oster, W., and Karliczek, G.: Die Beeinflussung der Blutgase und Haemodynamik durch Etomidate bei myokardial vorgeschaedigten Patienten. Anaesthesist, 23:423, 1974.

50. Morgan, M., Lumley, J., and Whitwam, J.: Etomidate, a new water-soluble nonbarbiturate intravenous induction agent. Lancet, 2:955, 1975.

51. Morgan, M., Lumley, J., and Whitwam, J.: Respiratory effects of etomidate. Br. J. Anaesth., 49:233, 1977.

52. Kay, B.: A clinical assessment of the use of etomidate in children. Br. J. Anaesth., 48:207, 1976.

53. Holdcroft, A., Morgan, M., Whitwam, J.G., and Lumley, J.: Effect of dose and premedication on induction, complications with etomidate. Br. J. Anaesth., 48:199, 1976.

54. Fragen, R.J., Caldwell, N., and Brunner, E.A.: Clinical use of etomidate for anesthesia induction: a preliminary report. Anesth. Analg., 55:730, 1976.

55. Gooding, J.M., Smith, R.A., Weng, J.T., Kirby, R.R., and Hanchey, J.A.: Etomidate. Clinical experience with a new solvent. Anaesthesiol. Rev., June 23, 1979.

56. Fragen, R.J., and Caldwell, N.: Comparison of a new formulation of etomidate with pentothal—side effects in awakening times. Anesthesiology, 50:242, 1979.

57. Famewo, C.E., Magbagbeola, J.A.O., and Ogunnaike, I.A.: Plasma potassium, sodium and blood sugar following etomidate and suxamethonium. Anaesthesia, 34:278, 1979.

58. Wagner, R.L., White, P.F., Kan, P.B., Rosenthal, M.H., and Feldman, D.: Inhibition of adrenal steroidogenesis by the anaesthetic etomidate. N. Engl. J. Med., 310:1415, 1984.

59. Duthie, D.J.R., Fraser, R., and Nimmo, W.S.: Effect of induction of anaesthesia with etomidate on corticosteroid synthesis in man. Br. J. Anaesth., 57:156, 1985.

60. Borner, U., Gips, H., Boldt, J., Hose, R., von Borman, B., and Hempelmann, G.: Wirkung einer Einleitungsdosis von Etomidat, Methohexital und Midazolam auf die Funktion der Nebennierenrinde vor und nach ACTH-Stimulation. Dtsch. Med. Wochenschr., 110:750, 1985.

61. Vanden Bossche, H., Willemsens, G., Cools, W., and Bellens, D.: Effects of etomidate on steroid biosynthesis in subcellular fractions of bovine adrenals. Biochem. Pharmacol., 33:386, 1984.

62. Stanley, T.H., Philbin, D.M., and Coggins, C.H.: Fentanyl-oxygen anaesthesia for coronary artery surgery: cardiovascular and anti-diuretic hormone responses. Can. Anaesth. Soc. J., 26:168, 1979.

63. Zindler, M.: Etomidate and fentanyl for emergency anaesthesia in acute bleeding with haemorrhagic shock. *In* Etomidate. An Intravenous Induction Agent. Edited by A. Doenicke. Berlin, Springer, 1977.

64. Lees, N.W., and Hendry, J.G.B.: Etomidate in urological outpatient anaesthesia. A clinical evaluation. Anaesthesia, 32:592, 1977.

65. Schuermans, V., Dom, J., and Dony, J.: Multinational evaluation of etomidate for anesthesia induction. Anaesthesist, 27:52, 1978.

66. Miller, B.M., Hendry, J.G.B., and Lees, N.W.: Etomidate and methohexitone: a comparative clinical study in outpatient anaesthesia. Anaesthesia, 33:450, 1978.

67. Zacharias, M., Clarke, R.S.J., and Dundee, J.W.: Etomidate. *In* Trends in Intravenous Anesthesia. Edited by J.A. Aldrete and T.H. Stanley. Miami, Symposia Specialists, 1980.

68. Kalenda, Z.: The use of etomidate as an induction agent in fentanyl analgesia. *In* Etomidate. An Intravenous Induction Agent. Edited by A. Doenicke. Berlin, Springer, 1977.

69. Doenicke, A., Schellenberger, A., Schmidinger, S., Spiess, W., and Harlass, G.: Etomidate und andere intravenoese Hypnotica in der Einleitungsphase der Neuroleptanalgesie. *In* Probleme der intravenoesen Anaesthesia. Edited by W.F. Henschel. Erlangen, Straube, 1976.

70. Crispin, A., and Crommen, A.M.: A progress in electroconvulsive therapy: the non-barbiturate anesthetic drug etomidate. Acta Psychiatr. Belg., 76:678, 1976.

71. Weymar, A., Patschke, D., Tarnow, J., and Brueckner, J.B.: Etomidate anaesthesia for cardioversion. *In* Etomidate. An Intravenous Hypnotic Agent. Edited by A. Doenicke. Berlin, Springer, 1977.

72. McIntosh, B.M.M., Lumley, J., Morgan, M., and Stradling, P.: Methohexitone and etomidate for bronchoscopy. Anaesthesia, 34:739, 1979.
73. Doom, A., and Mundeleer, P.: Etomidate and tonsillectomy. Acta Anaesthesiol. Belg., 27:181, 1976.
74. Famewo, C.E., Odugbesan, C.O., and Osuntocun, O.O.: Effect of etomidate on intra-ocular pressure. Can. Anaesth. Soc. J., 24:712, 1977.
75. Newby, D.M., and Edbroke, D.L.: Influence of sedation on mortality in trauma patients. Lancet, 2:1381, 1983.
76. Boidin, M.P.: Can etomidate cause an Addisonian crisis? *In* Anaesthesia and Its Interaction with the Components of Critical Care Medicine. Thesis, Erasmus University Rotterdam, 1985.

Chapter 14

ALCOHOL

HISTORY

For centuries, the soporific and pain-relieving properties of alcohol (ethanol, ethyl alcohol, ethyl hydroxide, and spiritus vini rectificatus) have been recognized by members of the medical profession. Its use as an anesthetic during surgical procedures stems back to the early sixteenth century when patients were rendered insensible to pain by inhaling alcohol fumes.[1] Stirius reported the intravenous administration of alcohol in 1668.[2] Few physicians showed an interest in continuing to explore the suitability of alcohol as an intravenous anesthetic until 1921, when Nakagawa conducted experiments with laboratory animals to study the effectiveness of intravenous alcohol combined with either chloroform or diethyl ether for induction of anesthesia.[3] Cardot and colleagues confirmed that the intravenous administration of a mixture of alcohol and chloroform in saline solution produced adequate anesthesia for short surgical interventions in dogs.[4] At about the same time, Behan completed a study of the use of intravenous alcohol as a postoperative sedative in human subjects.[5]

A few years later, Marin presented the first comprehensive study concerned with the use of intravenous alcohol as a general anesthetic in humans. He thus introduced the method into the clinical practice of anesthesia.[6] Marin administered a 25% alcohol solution to several hundred patients. The results varied; some were disappointing. A significant drawback to the intravenous use of alcohol was the frequent occurrence of venous thrombosis. After an exhaustive study of the results of the method of Marin, a committee formed by the Mexican Academy of Medicine condemned the method as unworthy and dangerous.[7]

During the ensuing years, the intravenous application of alcohol for pain relief during surgery continued to meet with little enthusiasm, with the exception of some favorable reports from French, Swiss, German, and British investigators.[8–13] In 1944, various clinical reports concerned with the use of intravenous alcohol for the production of surgical anesthesia were surveyed, leading to the conclusion that the unsatisfactory results and deaths related to the use of this method precluded its use as a safe procedure.[14]

More than 20 years later, interest has been renewed in intravenous alcohol anesthesia as a suitable adjunct to general anesthesia, as an analgesic in the immediate postoperative period, and as a useful and effective method in the pre-, intra-, and postoperative management of the alcoholic patient.[15,16]

CHEMISTRY AND PHYSICAL PROPERTIES

Alcohol is a colorless, volatile, hygroscopic, flammable fluid with a characteristic odor and burning taste. It is obtained by the distillation of fermented saccharine liquids. The specific gravity of alcohol is 0.8337. Ethyl alcohol mixes freely with water and chloroform, is readily volatilized, and boils at 78°C. The structural formula of ethyl alcohol is shown in Figure 14–1.

CLINICAL PHARMACOLOGY

When topically applied, alcohol acts as an astringent. When injected hypodermically, alcohol injures cells by precipitating and dehydrating protoplasm. When alcohol is injected close to or into nerves, neuritis and nerve degeneration may result. Alcohol has germicidal action.

PHARMACOKINETICS

Absorption, Distribution, and Excretion

When ingested, alcohol is rapidly absorbed from the gastrointestinal tract. Vaporized alcohol is absorbed through the lungs and also from subcutaneous sites if its concentration is not excessive. The rate of absorption of alcohol through the stomach is initially rapid and subsequently decreases, with considerable amounts remaining unabsorbed. The rate of gastric emptying is crucial with regard to the time at which absorption from the intestinal tract is complete. In the absence of significant factors delaying the speed of stomach emptying, complete absorption of alcohol may range from 2 to 6 hours. The time of maximum blood levels after ingestion of alcohol also depends on its rate of oxidation and excretion. This determination varies greatly per individual.

With the parenteral use of alcohol, there is also a wide variation in tolerance to the drug, although blood alcohol levels produced by this route of administration are more predictable than those observed when alcohol is ingested.[17,18] When administered by intravenous infusion, complete arteriovenous equilibrium is established within approximately 5 minutes.[19] Total-body alcohol saturation occurs within 1 hour of drug administration, with venous blood alcohol levels rapidly declining during this period at a rate of about 15 mg/100 ml/hour.[18]

After absorption, the alcohol is distributed throughout all body tissues and fluids, cellular as well as extracellular: the concentration in plasma is slightly higher than that found in the erythrocytes. The alcohol content of the brain tends to vary directly with the alcohol content of the blood, with higher concentrations found in the cerebrospinal fluid than in the blood when the blood alcohol level decreases and with lower concentrations noted in the cerebrospinal fluid when the blood alcohol level increases.

Of the total quantity of alcohol that enters the body, as much as 98% is completely oxidized. Oxidation begins immediately upon absorption and continues as long as alcohol remains in the body. The amount of alcohol oxidized per unit

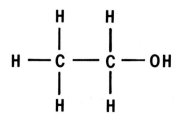

Fig. 14–1.   Structural formula of ethyl alcohol.

of time is proportionate to body weight and amounts to approximately 10 ml/hour. Oxidation is accelerated only slightly with increased blood alcohol concentrations. Maximal daily metabolism of alcohol in humans has been found to be about 380 ml.[20]

Elimination of alcohol from the body is mainly through the kidneys and, to a very small degree, through the lungs. Traces of alcohol can be detected in sweat, tears, saliva, bile, and gastric juice. Approximately 2% of the alcohol that enters the body escapes oxidation and is excreted unchanged in the urine.

After rapid intravenous administration of alcohol (0.8 mg/kg), great variations in peak urinary concentrations of alcohol are observed.[21] These variations generally occur when urinary alcohol levels exceed alcohol levels in venous blood, as a rule within 30 minutes of the end of the alcohol infusion.

PHARMACODYNAMICS

Central Nervous System (CNS)

The CNS is more markedly affected by alcohol than any other system of the body. After an initial stimulatory action, apparently caused by depression of higher inhibitory control mechanisms (resulting in unrestrained activity of lower centers), alcohol causes primary and continuous CNS depression.[22] Inhibition of higher mental processes, especially those related to training and previous experience and those that are responsible for sobriety and self-restraint, results in removal of finer grades of discrimination, memory, and concentration. The personality becomes expansive, and the speech becomes eloquent. Mood swings are often uncontrolled, and emotional outbursts are frequent. Alcohol does not increase mental or physical abilities. It is an irregularly descending depressant, and its effects on the CNS are more marked when blood concentrations are rising than when they are falling, and are more pronounced when the rate of increase is slow.

Alcohol-induced changes in the EEG are characterized by a slowing of brainwave activity similar to the slowing that occurs with hypoxia and hypoglycemia. The mechanisms involved in these EEG changes, however, are not identical to the mechanisms connected with lack of oxygen or lowered blood glucose levels. The parameters of cerebral blood flow, cerebral metabolism, and cerebral vascular resistance are unchanged with moderate increases in alcohol blood concentrations. With severe alcohol intoxication (300 mg/100 ml or more), however, the mean cerebral blood flow determination is increased and cerebral oxygen consumption and cerebral vascular resistance are significantly reduced.[23]

Cardiovascular System

Alcohol exerts only minor effects on the circulation; blood pressure and cardiac output remain essentially unchanged at moderately elevated alcohol blood levels. Very high blood concentrations of alcohol may have a depressant effect on the heart, but cardiac failure does not occur until the alcohol blood concentration is 30% greater than that producing respiratory arrest.[24] Alcohol causes generalized vasodilatation, which especially affects the cutaneous vessels. Warm and flushed skin is produced and results in heat loss, which can be significantly enhanced by sweating and by higher alcohol blood concentrations.

Respiratory System

Alcohol does not markedly affect respiratory function, except in doses that are large enough to cause severe intoxication. In humans, blood concentrations of 400 mg/100 ml or higher are associated with respiratory depression, including apnea. Relatively low blood alcohol levels have a transient respiratory stimulatory effect.[25]

Gastrointestinal System

Alcohol stimulates gastric secretion by a mechanism involving the release of histamine; this process is not inhibited by conventional doses of atropine sulfate.[26] Gastrointestinal motor functions are not influenced by moderate blood alcohol concentrations; high concentrations result in virtual cessation of gastrointestinal activity. Acutely elevated plasma alcohol concentrations do not affect liver function.[27,28]

Genitourinary Tract

Alcohol produces a significant, dose-related diuretic response in humans that results from a decrease in the renal tubular reabsorption of water. Alcohol-induced diuresis occurs when the alcohol blood level is rising, but ceases when the level is stationary or falling. The diuretic response to alcohol can be explained by the action of the drug on the supraopticohypophyseal system, which inhibits the secretion of the posterior pituitary antidiuretic hormone.[29]

CLINICAL APPLICATIONS

Intravenous Analgesia

The effectiveness of intravenously administered alcohol was studied in the control of somatic pain in healthy adult male volunteers by determining their pain threshold before and during infusion of either 0.9% saline solution or 1.5 ml/kg body weight of absolute alcohol in a 10% solution (v/v) in saline over a period of 1 hour.[30] The pain threshold was determined by the application of tibial pressure.[31] During the test, the pain threshold was significantly increased in all volunteers while the alcohol was infused, as compared to the pain threshold during an infusion with only saline solution.

The elevation in pain threshold occurred rapidly at first, and was followed by a slower increase. Some subjects experienced nausea, vomiting, and headaches toward the end of the experiment. In a subsequent study, the alcohol was infused at one-half the initial strength (0.75 ml/kg), which did not significantly alter the analgesic action of the alcohol infusion but minimized unpleasant side-effects. In comparing the analgesic effect of the lower-dose alcohol infusion with the analgesia produced by 0.2 mg/kg of morphine diluted in the same volume and infused over the same period of time, alcohol, on the average, produced a greater increase in the pain threshold than did the morphine. All subjects distinguished readily between alcohol and morphine and all expressed a strong preference for alcohol, both during the time of the experiment and during recovery.

The investigators remark that these results demonstrate the value of alcohol when applied for relief of somatic pain and caution against extrapolating the results to include pain of visceral origin, against which alcohol may be less effective. They suggest that the use of intravenous alcohol may decrease or even eliminate the need for opiates in certain circumstances (e.g., when maintenance of renal output and enhancement of peripheral perfusion may be of particular concern).

Intravenous Anesthesia

In the development of the method of intravenous alcohol anesthesia, various investigators who conducted trials in laboratory animals and in humans reported different doses of alcohol required to produce loss of consciousness and anesthesia.[15,32,33] Also, opinions differ regarding the optimal rate of alcohol infusion. The original method of intravenous alcohol anesthesia, as proposed by Marin, consisted of administering a 25% alcohol solution at a rate of 20 to 40 ml/minute to reach a total dose of 2 to 3 ml/kg within 20 to 25 minutes.[6] A similar technique was employed by another researcher who administered 10 to 15 mg of morphine sulfate approximately 1 hour before surgical intervention to reduce post-anesthetic excitement.[12,13] A total dose of 2.5 ml/kg of alcohol to induce "alcohol coma" has been suggested.[34] Also, infusion of approximately 300 ml of a 5% alcohol solution was recommended to produce a blood alcohol concentration of 2.5 to 3.0 ml/kg, after which thiopental (50 mg intravenously) was administered. Consciousness is then lost in approximately 75% of all groups of patients.[35]

Dundee found that this latter dosage, which is based on total blood volume and does not allow for the intracellular fluid volume, was insufficient to always produce sleep in normal subjects, even with the use of a more concentrated alcohol solution and heavier premedication.[17] This investigator arrived at an entirely new approach to the administration of appropriate intravenous doses of alcohol for the safe induction of sleep and anesthesia. An 8% w/v alcohol solution is prepared by diluting 55 ml of absolute alcohol (44 mg) in 400 ml of lactated Ringer's solution or isotonic saline solution. This solution is rapidly infused in 4 to 5 minutes, to a total administered dose of 550 ml, if required.

An average dose of 0.8 to 1.0 mg/kg of alcohol (approximately 1 ml/kg of absolute alcohol) is needed to render the patient unconscious. There is marked individual variation in response to alcohol; in this study, some patients remained wide awake at doses that induced sleep in other patients.

The significance of these findings is seen in the documentation that rapid infusion produces loss of consciousness at lower doses and lower blood alcohol concentration than was reported previously. The effectiveness of the lower dosage may be explained by the rapidity with which adequate cerebral alcohol concentrations are established before the drug reaches equilibrium with various body fluid compartments. The inducement of sleep with low blood alcohol levels may be the result of a possibly high blood-brain gradient that is not present, or is present to a lesser degree, with a prolonged infusion time.[18]

Achieving anesthetic effects with lower blood alcohol concentrations renders intravenous alcohol anesthesia a safe method. In the event of an inadvertent overdose, the alcohol diffuses rapidly from the brain, and vital functions recover quickly. In contrast, overdose that occurs with slower rates of alcohol infusion result in higher total amounts of alcohol, from which the patient may not recover as rapidly. One potential disadvantage of the lower-dose, fast-infusion technique is the frequent need for small doses of a barbiturate to maintain an adequate level of anesthesia.

Interaction with Sedatives

A synergism exists between alcohol and sedatives.[36,37] In one study, sleep occurred in subjects with a significantly lower blood alcohol content after premedication with pentobarbital (100 to 200 mg intramuscularly). In contrast, with chlordiazepoxide (100 to 140 mg intramuscularly) used as a premedicant, considerably higher blood alcohol concentrations were required to produce loss of consciousness. This finding was indicative of an antagonistic action of chlordiazepoxide on the cerebral effects of alcohol.

A synergism also exists between methohexital and alcohol, as evidenced by an increased incidence of emergence delerium reactions when methohexital is used during recovery from intravenous alcohol anesthesia.[38]

SIDE-EFFECTS AND COMPLICATIONS

Occasional failure to induce sleep with the rapid infusion of the "standard" 8% w/v alcohol solution may not be considered a serious complication, because small amounts of barbiturate given by rapid intravenous injection enhance the soporific action of the alcohol and induce sleep. Similarly, the occurrence of excitement and delirium immediately before the loss of consciousness can be promptly controlled with a small intravenous dose of a barbiturate.

A more serious problem is the relatively high incidence of emergence reactions, including "hangover," associated with headaches, nausea, vomiting, thirst, and dizziness. The administration of chlordiazepoxide may reduce the incidence and intensity of these reactions, but the drug, as previously mentioned, can adversely affect the anesthetic properties of the alcohol.

Pain may be severe during the rapid infusion of 8% w/v alcohol solution, but usually subsides within 1 minute of the start of the infusion. With regard to venous complications, phlebitis reportedly occurred in 18 patients, localized thrombosis occurred in 2 patients, and localized thrombophlebitis was noted in 3 of 233 patients. This rate of occurrence is somewhat higher than that encountered with clinical doses of thiopental or methohexital but is similar to that observed with the use of propanidid.[39]

Whether erythrocytic lysis may occur with the more concentrated alcohol solutions is doubtful. Findings of in vitro studies showed that the addition of 2 to 2.5 mg of alcohol in compound lactate sodium BP (Hartmann's solution) to the blood caused less lysis than did the solvent alone.[40]

Any value for the use of alcohol as a general anesthetic or anesthesia induction agent is difficult to establish. Even with adequate sedative or analgesic premedication, which reduces some of the undesirable effects of alcohol, the drug is not as reliable and predictable as the ultra-short-acting barbiturates or nonbarbiturate compounds, such as ketamine, propanidid, althesin, and etomidate. Because of its remarkable analgesic properties and cardiovascular stabilizing action, however, intravenously administered alcohol may find a useful place as a basal narcotic, as an adjunct to general anesthesia, and in postoperative pain control.[35]

In its ability to reduce intracranial pressure, alcohol may be an appropriate anesthetic in patients with elevated intracranial tension.[41] Because of its peripheral vasodilating action, intravenous alcohol may facilitate the induction of hypothermia.[42] Alcohol may protect against arrhythmias encountered at low body temperatures.[43] Intravenous alcohol can be most beneficial in the anesthetic management of the alcoholic patient in whom pre- or postoperative alcohol deprivation may precipitate acute withdrawal symptoms.[44] The successful use of intravenous alcohol in the treatment of barbiturate poisoning was also reported.[45] The authors of this study based their work on clinical and experimental evidence of an antagonistic action of alcohol on barbiturates.

Whether the calorific value of intravenous alcohol is of clinical significance is debatable. As mentioned previously, almost all alcohol that enters the body is oxidized, and approximately 6 cal/ml are liberated. The standard w/v alcohol solution provides 267 cal/500 ml.[46] The use of alcohol for its high calorific value carries the risk of potential toxic effects when administered in combination with fructose and the sugar alcohols, which may result in serious lactic acidosis.[47]

REFERENCES

1. Keys, T.E.: The History of Surgical Anesthesia. New York, Dover Publications, 1945.
2. Macht, D.E.: The history of intravenous and subcutaneous administration of drugs. JAMA, 66:856, 1916.
3. Nakagawa, K.: Experimentelle Studien ueber die intravenoese Infusionsnarkose mittels Alkohols. (Mitteilung der Ergebnisse der Tierversuche). Tohoku J. Exp. Med., 2:81, 1921.
4. Cardot, H., and Laugier, H.: Anesthesie par intraveineuse d'un melange alcool-chloroforme-solution physiologique chez le chien. C. R. Soc. Biol. (Paris), 87:889, 1922.
5. Behan, R.J.: Ethyl alcohol intravenously as postoperative sedative. Am. J. Surg., 69:227, 1920.
6. Marin, M.G.: Application des alkohol ethilico como anesthetico general por via endovenosa. Mexico City, F. Mesones, 1929.
7. Ocaranza, F., Ramirez, E., and Villagrana, J.C.: Dictamen de la consulta que formule la Universidad Nacional, para conocer el criterio de la Academia Nacional de Medicina, sobre la anesthesia general por el alcohol etilico inyectado pro via endevenosa. Gac. Med. Mex., 61:462, 1930.
8. Charpy, P.: L'anesthesie par l'alcool ethylique par voie endoveineuse. Paris, Clinique, 25:89, 1930.
9. Kuss, G.: L'anesthesie generale par injection intravenineuse d'alcool ethylique. Bull Mem. Soc. Nat. Chir., 56:587, 1930.
10. Gaudenz, I.: Kleine diagnostische und therapeutishce Mitteilungen. Totalanaesthesie durch Intravenoesinjektion von Aethylalkohol. Schweiz. Med. Wochenschr., 59:770, 1929.
11. Fohl, T.H.: Der Athylalkohol als Narkoticum und Therapeuticum bei intravenoeser Darreichung. Arch. Klin. Chir., 165:641, 1931.
12. Constantin, J.D.: General anaesthesia by the intravenous injection of ethyl alcohol. Lancet, 1:1247 1929.
13. Constantin, J.D.: General anaesthesia by the intravenous injection of ethyl alcohol. Lancet, 1:1393, 1930.
14. Adams, R.C.: Intravenous Anesthesia. 1st Ed., New York, Hoeber, 1944.
15. Dundee, J.W., Isaac, M., and Clarke, R.S.J.: Alcohol in anesthetic practice. Anesth. Analg., 48:665, 1969.
16. Dundee, J.W., and Wyant, G.M.: Alcohol. *In* Intravenous Anaesthesia. Edited by J.W. Dundee and G.M. Wyant. Edinburgh, Churchill Livingstone, 1974.
17. Dundee, J.W.: Intravenous ethanol anaesthesia: a study of dosage and blood levels. Anesth. Analg., 49:467, 1970.
18. Dundee, J.W., Isaac, M., and Taggart, J.: Blood ethanol levels following rapid intravenous infusion. Q. J. Stud. Alcohol, 32:741, 1971.
19. Gostomzyk, J.G., Dilger, B., and Dilger, K.: Untersuchungen ueber die Verteilung intravenoes applizierter Substanzen im Organismus am Beispiel des Aethylalkohols. Blutalkohol, 6:340, 1969.
20. Newman, H.W., Wilson, R.H.L., and Newman, E.J.: Direct determination of maximal daily metabolism of alcohol. Science, 116:328, 1952.
21. Dundee, J.W., Knox, J.W.D., and Isaac, M.: Blood urine and breath levels after rapid intravenous infusion of ethanol. Br. Med. J., 3:552, 1972.
22. Goodman, L.S., and Gilman, A.: The Aliphatic Alcohols. *In* The Pharmacological Basis of Therapeutics. Edited by L.S. Goodman and A. Gilman. New York, MacMillan, 1980.
23. Battey, L.I., Heyman, A., and Patterson, Jr., J.L.: Effects of alcohol on cerebral blood flow metabolism. JAMA, 152:6, 1953.
24. Haggard, H.W., Greenberg, L.A., and Lolli, G.: The absorption of alcohol with special reference to its influence on the concentration of alcohol appearing in the blood. Q. J. Stud. Alcohol, 1:684, 1941.
25. Hitchock, F.A.: Alteration in respiration caused by alcohol. Q. J. Stud. Alcohol, 2:641, 1942.

26. Dragstedt, C.A., Gray, J.S., Lawton, A.H., and deArellano, M.R.: Does alcohol stimulate gastric secretion by liberating histamine? Proc. Soc. Exp. Biol. Med., 43:26, 1940.
27. Beazell, J.M., Berman, A.L., Hough, V.H., and Ivy, A.C.: The effect of acute alcoholic intoxication on hepatic function. Dig. Dis. Sci., 9:82, 1942.
28. Isaac, M.: Hepatic function following intravenous ethanol anaesthesia. Anaesthesia, 25:198, 1970.
29. Van Dyke, H.B., and Ames, R.G.: Alcohol diuresis. Acta Endocrinol. (Copenh.), 7:110, 1951.
30. James, M.F.M., Duthrie, A.M., Duffy, B.L., Mckeag, A.M., and Rice, C.P.: Analgesia effect of ethyl alcohol. Br. J. Anaesth., 50:139, 1978.
31. Dundee, J.W., and Moore, J.: Alterations in response to somatic pain associated with anaesthesia. I. An evaluation of a method of analgesimetry. Br. J. Anaesth., 32:396, 1960.
32. Gostomzyk, J.G., Dilger, B., and Dilger, K.: Alkoholkonzentration im Blut und Alkoholgehalt des Gehirns. Z. Klin. Chem., 7:162, 1969.
33. Gostomzyk, J.G., and Streffer, C.: Tierexperimentelle Undersuchungen zur Verteilung von Aethylalkohol in verschiedenen Organen, insbesondere im Gehirn, waehrend der Resorption-spase. Blut, 6:211, 1969.
34. Koppanyi, T., Canary, J.J., and Maengwyn-Davies, G.D.: Problems in acute alcohol poisoning. Q. J. Stud. Alcohol, [Suppl.], 1:24, 1961.
35. Schnelle, N.: Alcohol given intravenously for general anaesthesia. Surg. Clin. North Am., 45:1041, 1965.
36. Dundee, J.W., and Isaac, M.: Interaction of alcohol with sedatives and tranquillisers (a study of blood levels at loss of consciousness following rapid infusion). Med. Sci. Law, 10:220, 1970.
37. Dundee, J.W., and Isaac, M.: Interaction between intravenous alcohol and some sedatives and tranquillisers. Br. J. Pharmacol., 39:199, 1970.
38. Dundee, J.W., and Isaac, M.: Clinical studies of induction agents. XXIX: Ethanol. Br. J. Anaesth., 41:1063, 1969.
39. Isaac, M., and Dundee, J.W.: Clinical studies of induction agents. XXX: Venous sequelae following ethanol anaesthesia. Br. J. Anaesth., 41:1070, 1969.
40. Sanderson, F.M., Lappin, T.R.J., Isaac, M., and Dundee, J.W.: In vitro erythrocyte stabilisation by ethanol. Br. J. Anaesth., 42:606, 1970.
41. Duthie, A.M., Adams, J.S., and White, J.F.: The influence of ethyl alcohol on cerebro-spinal fluid pressure. Anaesthesia, 31:893, 1976.
42. Hewer, A.J.M.: Hypothermia for neurosurgery. Int. Anaesthesiol. Clin., 2:919, 1964.
43. Duthie, A.M., and White, J.F.: Cardiac arrest temperature: the effect of ethyl alcohol and carbon dioxide on rats, guinea-pigs and isolated rat hearts. Clin. Exp. Pharmacol. Physiol., 4:311, 1977.
44. Keilty, S.R.: Anesthesia for the alcoholic patient. Anesth. Analg., 48:659, 1969.
45. Carrier, H., and Willoquiet, P.: Role des injections intraveineuses d'alcool a 30 p. 100 dans le traitement du barbiturisme aigu. Bull. Acad. Natl. Med. (Paris), 111:655, 1934.
46. Dundee, J.W., and Isaac, M.: Intravenous ethanol. *In* Newer Intravenous Anesthetics. Edited by R.S.J. Clarke. Int. Anaesthesiol. Clin., 7:67, 1969.
47. Woods, H.F., and Alberti, K.G.M.: The dangers of intravenous fructose. Lancet, 4:1354, 1972.

Chapter 15

PROCAINE

HISTORY

Soon after the introduction of the alkaloid, cocaine, as a local anesthetic by Koller in 1884, Einhorn began an intensive search for a synthetic substitute.[1,2] The result was the introduction of procaine (Novocaine) in 1905.[2] This drug has been employed intravenously for analgesic and anesthetic purposes for more than 75 years, starting with a description by Bier in 1908 of the method of intravenous regional analgesia of the extremities.[3] Goyanes later anesthetized limbs by a similar method of intra-arterial injection of procaine.[4]

Lundy first proposed the intravenous use of procaine for general anesthesia in 1942, noting also its antipruritic effect.[5] Other investigators soon confirmed the safety and effectiveness of procaine as a general anesthetic, emphasizing its analgesic, antihistaminic, ganglionic blocking, and cardiovascular stabilizing actions.[6–9] Burstein found the drug effective in treating the arrhythmias frequently encountered during anesthesia with cyclopropane, and Gordon reported the value of procaine analgesia in the surgical treatment of burn victims.[10,11] Subsequently, Graubard, et al., used procaine intravenously for general anesthesia in a large group of patients and proposed as the "procaine unit" a 4-mg/kg dose of procaine (1%) administered intravenously within 20 minutes.[12,13] More reports of the intravenous use of procaine, both as the sole anesthetic and as a supplement to general anesthesia, soon followed.[14–18] Nevertheless, in the United States, interest in the use of procaine as a general anesthetic subsequently declined. Its use in South America, however, particularly in Argentina, and in some European countries, e.g., Spain, gained momentum. For example, the Fourth Argentinian Congress of Anesthesiology in 1953 devoted most of its scientific program to procaine-induced general anesthesia. Anesthesiologists now agree that the use of procaine intravenously as the sole agent to produce general anesthesia should be discouraged because the risk of severe circulatory depression resulting from overdosage far outweighs the general benefits of analgesia, the antiarrhythmic effects, and the suppression of troublesome autonomic reflexes during surgical procedures. On the other hand, procaine continues to be an acceptable adjuvant for pain control in surgical patients under general anesthesia with other agents.

CHEMISTRY AND PHYSICAL PROPERTIES

Procaine is an ester of para-aminobenzoic acid (PABA) and diethylaminoethanol (DEAE) (Fig. 15–1). Procaine hydrochloride is soluble in water, stable in solution, and withstands boiling without deterioration, thus facilitating sterilization. A 1% procaine solution has a pH of approximately 4.

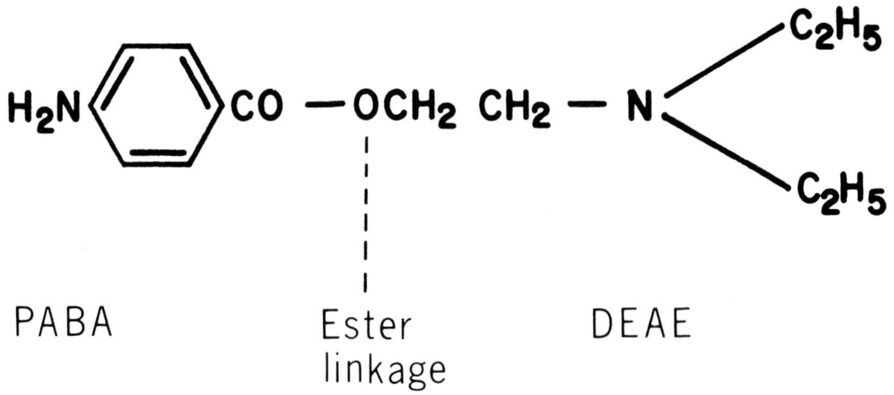

Fig. 15–1. Structural formula of procaine. PABA = para-aminobenzoic acid; DEAE = diethylaminoethanol.

Anesthetic Potency

Because only the non-ionized, unbound moiety of procaine can cross biologic membranes, such as the blood-brain barrier, the anesthetic potency of this drug depends on this fraction in the circulating blood. Peak plasma concentrations required for general anesthesia range from 6 to 20 µg/ml, and can be established by intravenous administration at a rate of 1.5 mg/kg/minute for 5 minutes. To maintain anesthesia, the average concentration of procaine in plasma is kept at 15 µg/ml.[19]

Metabolism and Excretion

Procaine, with a pK_a of 8.9, is 97% ionized at the pH of the blood. The degree of dissociation changes in tissues or other body fluids depends on the local pH encountered. Plasma protein binding accounts for only 5% of the total concentration; hence, pharmacologic activity is negligibly altered by hypoproteinemia. Similarly, although the binding does decrease with a decrease in pH, thereby theoretically increasing the amount of free drug available to reach sites of action in the CNS and the heart, this benefit too is negligible, because the initial amount bound (5%) is scant.[20]

Plasma concentrations of procaine depend on the physical state of the patient, the rate and amount of administration of the drug, and, most importantly, the speedy hydrolysis of procaine by plasma cholinesterase, first demonstrated by Brodie, et al.[21] This enzyme, also known as butyrylcholinesterase, nonspecific cholinesterase, or pseudocholinesterase, is a nonspecific drug-metabolizing enzyme synthesized in the liver and circulated in the plasma. It can attack and hydrolyze an ester linkage in any invading foreign substance, e.g., procaine or succinylcholine, at a rate of 1.2 mol/ml/hour or 1 mg/kg/minute.[21] This rapid reaction accounts for the normally short duration of action of succinylcholine and of intravenously administered procaine. Conversely, should the plasma cholinesterase inhibitor, hexafluorenium (Mylaxen), be administered, as advocated by Foldes and colleagues, to prolong the action of succinylcholine by retarding its hydrolysis, the same effect is applied to concurrently administered procaine.[19,22] Such anticholinesterase drugs as neostigmine, when used to antagonize the action of muscle relaxant drugs, also prolong the action of procaine.

The speedy hydrolysis of procaine by plasma cholinesterase limits the duration of its antiarrhythmic effect. This shortcoming was remedied by replacing the ester linkage of procaine by an amide group not susceptible to hydrolysis. The result was procaine amide (Pronestyl), the stable antiarrhythmic drug co-discovered by Mark and Brodie.[23]

If hepatic enzyme synthesis is impaired, as in chronic malnutrition, poisoning with organophosphates, cancer of the gastrointestinal tract, or advanced pregnancy, the hydrolysis of procaine and succinylcholine is hampered, with a resultant increase in their pharmacologic activity.[24] With procaine use, toxic levels may easily result. Despite this fact, if acceptable clinical doses are not exceeded, procaine can be safely administered intravenously for obstetric anesthesia.[25,26] Similarly, genetically determined variants, e.g., inherited abnormalities of the enzyme encountered in 1 of 2500 patients in a normal population, also prolong the effects of the drug.[27] A simple test to predict the rate of hydrolysis of procaine given intravenously in any patient involves the consideration of the duration of muscular paralysis induced by succinylcholine when given prior to endotracheal intubation.[19] Prompt recovery of muscular tone, indicating normal enzyme activity, verifies the adequacy of procaine hydrolysis in the bloodstream.

The passage of procaine across biologic membranes, such as the blood-brain barrier, is fairly prompt; peak CNS effects appear within 2 minutes of intravenous injection.[28] Similarly, procaine readily crosses the placenta, achieving plasma levels in the fetus that are 40 to 60% lower than in the mother, regardless of the sampling time; however, unless the maternal dose of procaine exceeds 4 mg/kg, the drug is difficult to detect in the fetal circulation.[29] Of the metabolic breakdown products of procaine, PABA is mainly (80%) excreted through the kidneys; DEAE is further metabolized, with only 25 to 30% appearing in the urine.[21] Rarely is more than 10% of the procaine administered excreted unchanged in the urine. Although PABA is pharmacologically inert, the DEAE moiety is weakly active as an antiarrhythmic agent (equipotent intravenous doses are 100 mg procaine versus 2.5 g DEAE).[30] PABA also inhibits the action of sulfonamides, which may affect patient care.[31]

PHARMACODYNAMICS

Central Nervous System (CNS)

Although procaine is a well-known convulsant agent, lower doses exert centrally mediated analgesic and depressant actions, providing the basis for its use as a general anesthetic or supplement. In unpremedicated subjects, mental confusion appears initially, followed by hallucinations and delirium before sedation and sleep occur.[19] If the undesirable subjective effects are suppressed by prior administration of thiopental, more appropriate anesthetic effects ensue in sequence (Table 15–1).[19] The eyeballs deviate and then become centered and fixed; lacrimation diminishes and then ceases; the pupils constrict and then dilate; and the pupillary and corneal reflexes, initially brisk, become sluggish or cease, as does the response to surgical stimulation, indicative of analgesia.

Cardiovascular System

Procaine exerts a quinidine-like action on the heart, with prolongation of conduction time, widening of QRS complexes, and deepening of the S waves.[9,19,32] Large doses can cause myocardial depression and hypotension, although hypertension may occur.[31,33,34] A vasoconstrictor effect of procaine was described in one

Table 15–1. Depth of Anesthesia with Intravenously Administered Local Anesthetic Agents

	Light	*Medium*	*Deep*
Eyeballs	Deviated	Centered, immobile	Centered, immobile
Lacrimation	Present	Diminished	Absent
Pupils	Medium size	Miotic	Mydriatic
Pupillary reflex to light	Very active	Sluggish	Absent
Corneal reflex	Present	Sluggish or absent	Absent
Response to surgical stimulation	Yes	No	No
Arterial blood pressure	Normal	Normal to moderate hypotension	Moderate to severe hypotension
Spontaneous respiration	Tachypnea	Tachypnea	Hypoventilation, apnea

report, but this action seems unlikely because procaine is an excellent vasodilator.[35,36] Indeed, the widespread vasodilation produced by the intravenous use of procaine is beneficial to patients suffering from a variety of vasomotor disturbances, including acrocyanosis and Raynaud's disease.[37]

Respiratory System

Procaine initially causes tachypnea, which progresses with excessive dosage to hypoventilation and apnea (Table 15–1).

Musculoskeletal System

Skeletal muscle tone is somewhat decreased by procaine, with slight enhancement of the action of nondepolarizing muscle relaxant drugs.[32] Fasciculations produced by succinylcholine are prevented by the intravenous administration of procaine.[38] Smooth muscle activity is suppressed and antispasmodic activity is pronounced as the result of an atropine-like action.[32]

Antiallergic Activity

The trivalent nitrogen configuration in the DEAE portion of the procaine molecule (Fig. 15–1) imparts an antihistaminic property to the drug, which relieved the pruritus of jaundice and the urticaria of serum sickness.[5,39]

TOXICITY AND SIDE-EFFECTS

Unpremedicated subjects may exhibit mental confusion, hallucinations, and delirium before sedation and sleep ensue. Apart from tachycardia and tachypnea (Table 15–1), mydriasis, muscular hypertonia, and myoclonia then appear in rapid succession, followed by generalized convulsion.[40] These effects occurred in patients in an experimental study series at intravenous procaine dose levels of 23 to 29 mg/kg; much higher doses of procaine (36 to 55 mg/kg intravenously) are required for toxicity after induction of anesthesia with thiopental.[40] Note that the rates of procaine administration to produce convulsions (3 to 5 mg/kg/minute intravenously without premedication, but as much as 14 mg/kg/minute after thiopental) are much higher than the 1 to 1.5 mg/kg/minute rate suggested for clinical intravenous use of procaine.[19,40]

How do convulsions harm patients? If sustained, they may result in severe hypoxia, due to prolonged incoordinate contraction of the muscles of respiration. Adequate artificial respiration cannot be accomplished until the uncontrolled activity of the respiratory muscles subsides. Thiopental or benzodiazepines, such as diazepam and succinylcholine, terminate the convulsive movements, but by different mechanisms. Thiopental and diazepam suppress the underlying electric seizure activity seen in the EEG; succinylcholine blocks the hyperactive muscles, but convulsive discharges continue in the EEG. Studies in dogs have shown that, provided hypoxia is promptly interrupted, continued electric seizure activity of the brain is not detectably harmful.[28]

CLINICAL APPLICATIONS

Administration of Anesthesia

Usual preanesthetic medication with an opiate and a belladonna agent may be usefully augmented by the administration of a benzodiazepine drug (diazepam, lorazepam, or flunitrazepam). Anesthesia is induced with thiopental (propanidid may be substituted), succinylcholine is given intravenously to facilitate endotracheal intubation and administration of a 50:50 mixture of nitrous oxide and oxygen is instituted.[41] Procaine (1%) is then administered in a "priming" dose of 60 to 80 mg/minute (1 to 1.5 mg/kg/minute) over a 5-minute period. By this time, a stable level of anesthesia is usually reached. The rate of procaine infusion is then decreased to 20 to 40 mg/minute to maintain plasma concentrations below 30 mg/L (note that the convulsant threshold is 60 mg/L).[19]

Because only a light to moderate depth of anesthesia is intended, close monitoring of clinical signs is essential (Table 15–1). Light anesthesia is indicated by lacrimation, active pupillary and corneal reflexes, sinus tachycardia, and occasional slight muscle movements in response to surgical stimulation. In the nonparalyzed patient, tachypnea may be present. Increased bleeding in the surgical field is common. Deep planes of anesthesia are characterized by mydriatic pupils unresponsive to light, the absence of the corneal reflex, and moderate to severe hypotension, with the possibility of an irregular heart rate and apnea in the nonparalyzed patient.

The total consumption of procaine varies from 0.2 to 1.7 mg/kg/minute, with an average total dose of 0.5 mg/kg/minute. Muscle relaxant drugs are used as needed, although perhaps in somewhat reduced dosage. When propanidid instead of thiopental is used for speedy induction of procaine anesthesia, the action of succinylcholine on the myoneural junction may be further enhanced.[42] If procaine administration precedes tracheal intubation, prophylactic use of a curare drug to reduce or eliminate the muscular fasciculations produced by succinylcholine is not needed because procaine fulfills this function.[38] Finally, because the analgesic action of procaine is only moderate, concomitant administration of nitrous oxide and other analgesics is essential to ensure adequate pain control during surgical procedures.[43]

Obstetrics

Procaine administered intravenously can provide satisfactory obstetric analgesia and anesthesia.[25,26] At a rate of infusion sufficiently slow to avoid dizziness or other subjective symptoms, the second stage of labor can be made more endurable for the mother. For delivery, the rate is increased to maintain a state of dim consciousness in which the patient is more or less unresponsive and painfree but retains some memory of the events. Anesthesia is flexible and can be rapidly controlled; uterine contractions are not impaired. Awakening is quick, with no headache, nausea, or disorientation. Prior administration of barbiturates reduces the incidence of side-effects.

Surgical Treatment of Pheochromocytoma

The intravenous use of procaine is a valuable component of anesthesia in the surgical treatment of pheochromocytoma.[44] Its antiarrhythmic properties, together with its suppressant action on the autonomic responses periodically activated by the manipulation of the tumor, are important contributions to a relatively smooth and uneventful course of anesthesia. Additional advantages are a reasonable margin of safety and minute-to-minute control of the circulation.

Chronic Pain

Procaine delivered intravenously can benefit patients suffering from painful disorders, such as thrombophlebitis, arthritis, and neuralgia of varied causes.[45,46] Because of the combined centrally mediated analgesia and vasodilating properties of procaine, the drug may offer advantages over non-narcotic and narcotic analgesics in the treatment of patients in whom the painful condition is caused by or is associated with peripheral vascular insufficiency.

Debilitating Conditions

A review of many enthusiastic reports, including those of Aslan, concerning procaine use in the treatment of debilitating conditions associated with aging revealed that relief of pain was the only relevant factor. Procaine does not produce curative or "rejuvenating" effects on the aging process.[47,48]

REFERENCES

1. Koller, K.: Ueber die Verwendung des Cocain zur Anaesthesierung am Auge. Wien. Med. Wochenschr., 7:1352, 1884.
2. Einhorn, A.: Ueber einige neue oertliche Anaesthetika (Stovain, Alypin, Novocain). Dtsch. Med. Wochenschr., 31:1667, 1905.
3. Bier, A.: Ueber einen neuen Weg Lokalanesthesie an den Gliedmassen zu erzeugen. Verh. Dtsch. Ges. Chir., 37:204, 1908.
4. Goyanes, J.: El metodo ideal o conservador aplicado al tratamiento de los aneurismos de la arteria subclavia. Rev. Clin. Esp., 9:287, 1913.
5. Lundy, J.S.: Clinical Anesthesia. Philadelphia, W.B. Saunders, 1942.
6. Barbour, C.M., and Tovell, R.M.: Experiences with procaine administered intravenously. Anesthesiology, 9:514, 1948.
7. Fraser, R.J., and Kraft, K.: Pentothal-procaine analgesia. Anesth. Analg., 27:282, 1948.
8. Bittrich, N.M., and Powers, W.F.: Intravenous procaine in thoracic surgery. Anesth. Analg., 27:181, 1948.
9. Allen, F.M., Crossman, L.W., and Lyons, L.: Intravenous procaine analgesia. Anesth. Analg., 25:1, 1946.
10. Burstein, C.L.: Treatment of acute arrhythmias by intravenous procaine. Anesthesiology, 7:113, 1946.
11. Gordon, R.A.: Intravenous Novocaine (procaine hydrochloride) for analgesia in burns. Preliminary report. Can. Med. Assoc. J., 49:478, 1943.
12. Graubard, D.J., Robertazzi, R.N., and Peterson, M.C.: Microdetermination of blood levels of procaine hydrochloride after intravenous injection. Anesthesiology, 8:236, 1947.
13. Graubard, D.J., and Peterson, M.C.: Clinical uses of Intravenous Procaine. Springfield, IL, Charles C Thomas; Oxford, Blackwell, 1950.
14. Doud, E.A.: Intravenous procaine anesthesia. Anesth. Analg., 30:147, 1951.
15. Frazer, R.J.: Intravenous pentothal procaine analgesia. Anesth. Analg., 27:159, 1948.
16. Frazer, R.J., and Kraft, K.: Pentothal procaine analgesia. Anesth. Analg., 27:282, 1948.
17. Taylor, I.B., Stearne, A.B., Kurtz, H.C., Henderson, J.C., Sigler, L.E., and Nolte, E.C.: Intravenous procaine—an adjuvant to general anesthesia: a preliminary report. Anesthesiology, 11:185, 1950.
18. Turner, F.L., and Leaming, H.L.: Intravenous procaine hydrochloride in anesthesia for thoracic surgery. A preliminary report on 50 cases. Anaesthesia, 6:8, 1951.

19. Wikinski, J.A., Wikinski, R.L.W., Ceraso, O., Areia, R., and Torrieri, A.: General anesthesia with intravenous procaine. *In* Trends in Intravenous Anesthesia. Edited by J.A. Aldrete and T.H. Stanley. Miami, Symposia Specialists, 1980.
20. Burney, R.G., DiFazio, C.A., and Forster, J.A.: Effect of pH on protein binding of lidocaine. Anesth. Analg., 57:478, 1978.
21. Brodie, B.B., Lief, P.A., and Poet, R.: The fate of procaine in man following its intravenous administration and method for the estimation of procaine and diethylaminoethanol. J. Pharmacol. Exp. Ther., 94:359, 1948.
22. Foldes, F.F., Hillmer, N.R., Molloy, R.E., and Monte, A.P.: Potentiation of the neuromuscular effect of succinylcholine by hexafluorenium. Anesthesiology, 21:50, 1960.
23. Mark, L.C., Kayden, H.J., Steele, J.M., Cooper, J.R., Berlin, J., Rovenstine, E.A., and Brodie, B.B.: The physiological disposition and cardiac effects of procaine amide. J. Pharmacol. Exp. Ther., 102:5, 1951.
24. Shnider, S.M.: Serum cholinesterase activity during pregnancy, labor and the puerperium. Anesthesiology, 26:335, 1965.
25. Allen, F.M.: Intravenous obstetric anesthesia. Am. J. Surg., 70:283, 1945.
26. Johnson, K., and Gilbert, C.R.: Intravenous procaine for obstetrical anesthesia. Anesth. Analg., 25:133, 1946.
27. Kalow, W., and Gunn, D.R.: Some statistical data on atypical cholinesterase of human serum. Ann. Hum. Genet., 23:239, 1959.
28. Mark, L.C., Brand, L., and Goldensohn, E.S.: Recovery after procaine-induced seizures in dogs. Electroencephalogr. Clin. Neurophysiol., 16:280, 1964.
29. Usubiaga, J.E., LaTuppa, M., Moya, F., Wikinski, J.A., and Velazco, R.: Passage of procaine hydrochloride and paraaminobenzoic acid across the human placenta. Am. J. Obstet. Gynecol., 100:918, 1968.
30. Rosenberg, B., Kayden, H.J., Lief, P.A., Mark, L.C., Steel, J.M., and Brodie, B.B.: Studies on diethylaminoethanol. 1. Physiological disposition and action on cardiac arrhythmia. J. Pharmacol. Exp. Ther., 95:18, 1949.
31. Ritchie, J.M., and Greene, N.M.: Local anesthetics. *In* The Pharmacologic Basis of Therapeutics. Edited by A.G. Gilman, L.S. Goodman, and A. Gilman. New York, Macmillan, 1980.
32. Doenicke, A.: Klinische Pharmakologie, Lokalanaesthetika. *In* Lehrbuch der Anaesthesiologie, Reanimation und Intensivtherapie. Edited by H. Benzer, R. Frey, W. Huegin, and O. Mayrhofer. Berlin, Springer 1977.
33. Wikinski, J.A., Docovsky, C., Torrieri, A., and Usubiaga, J.E.: Modificaciones electrocardiograficas de la presion arterial y la frecuencia cardiaca producidas por altas dosis de procaina y lidoccaina administradas por via intravenous en el hombre. XIII Congresso Argentino de Anesthesiologia, Tomo, 1, 1971,
34. Foldes, F.F., Davidson, G.M., Deryck, D., and Kuwabara, S.: The intravenous toxicity of local anesthetic agents in man. Clin. Pharmacol. Ther., 6:328, 1965.
35. Sanders, H.D.: The vasoconstrictor and vasodilator effects of procaine. Can. J. Physiol. Pharmacol., 43:31, 1965.
36. Beutner, R.: Vasodilating action of some local anesthetics. Anesth. Analg., 27:192, 1948.
37. Leriche, R.: Petits moyens pour sottlager facilement les douleurs des extremities chez les arteritiques et dans certains trouble vaso-moteurs. Presse Med., 49:641, 1941.
38. Usubiaga, J.E., Wikinski, J.A., Wikinski, R.L.W., and Usubiaga, L.E.: Prevention of succinylcholine fasciculation by local anesthetic agents. Anesthesiology, 26:3, 1965.
39. State, D., and Wangensteen, O.H.: Procaine intravenously in treatment of delayed serum sickness. JAMA, 147:1761, 1951.
40. Usubiaga, J.E., Wikinski, J.A., Ferrero, R., Usubiaga, L.E., and Wikinski, R.: Local anestheticinduced convulsions in man. An electroencephalographic study. Anesth. Analg., 45:611, 1968.
41. Parada, J.F.: Propanidid mit Diazepam zur Einleitung der Procaine bzw. Lachgasnarkose. Anaesthesist, 8:267, 1968.
42. Clarke, R.S.J., Dundee, J.W., and Hamilton, R.C.: Interactions between induction agents and muscle relaxants. Anaesthesia, 22:235, 1967.
43. Keats, A.S., D'Alessandro, G.L., and Beecher, H.K.: A controlled study of pain relief by intravenous procaine. JAMA, 147:1761, 1951.
44. Usubiaga, J.E., Wikinski, J.A., and Usubiaga, L.E.: Use of lidocaine and procaine in patients with pheochromocytoma. Anesth. Analg., 48:443, 1969.
45. Corssen, G., and Rausch, F.: Intravenoese Novocaintherapie bei inneren Krakheiten. Ther. Gegenw., 10:368, 1951.
46. Edmonds, G.W., Corner, W.H., Kennedy, J.D., and Taylor, I.B.: Intravenous use of procaine in the management of arthritis. JAMA, 141:761, 1949.
47. Chiu, G.C.: "Rejuvenating" effect of procaine. A clinical review of reports. JAMA, 175:502, 1961.
48. Aslan, A.: Eine neue Methode zur Prophylaxe und Behandlung des Alters mit Novocain-Stoff H-3—entrophische und verjuengende Wirkung. Ther. Woche, 7:14, 1956.

Chapter 16

GAMMA-HYDROXYBUTYRIC ACID

HISTORY

In the search for a naturally occurring neuroinhibitor with anesthetic properties Appleton and colleagues explored the suitability of γ-aminobutyric acid, also called GABA (Fig. 16–1), as an anesthetic.[1] Subsequently, Laborit and colleagues searched for substances that could bring about "biochemical rest" and a diminution of cellular response to stress; they reported the usefulness of butyric acid.[2] This agent was studied previously by Jovany and colleagues with regard to its sleep-producing properties.[3] Butyric acid was presumed to be a central inhibitory substance with an action similar to that of GABA. Butyric acid was found to traverse the blood-brain barrier freely. Although butyric acid, a natural product of lipid metabolism, induced "natural" sleep and anesthesia with some degree of muscular relaxation, its administration in sufficient quantity to produce anesthesia caused the formation of ketone bodies.

The continuing search for an appropriate anesthetic neuroinhibitor resulted in the synthesis of γ-hydroxybutyric acid (gamma-OH, gamma-hydroxybutyrate) (Fig. 16–2) from γ-butyrolactone (Fig. 16–3). Gamma-OH also crosses the blood-brain barrier and has general central nervous system (CNS) depressant effects, but it does not cause the formation of ketone bodies. The apparent ability of the drug to act as an energy-producing substrate was particularly interesting to researchers. Although evidently affecting intracellular metabolism, gamma-OH proved to be truly nontoxic. When employed clinically, however, gamma-OH had significant drawbacks, including lack of analgesia, prolonged recovery often associated with emergence delerium reactions, frequent occurrence of extrapyramidal-type muscle movements, and venous irritant properties. As a result, the United States Food and Drug Administration refused to release the drug for general use. It is unlikely that gamma-OH will ever be marketed in the United States.

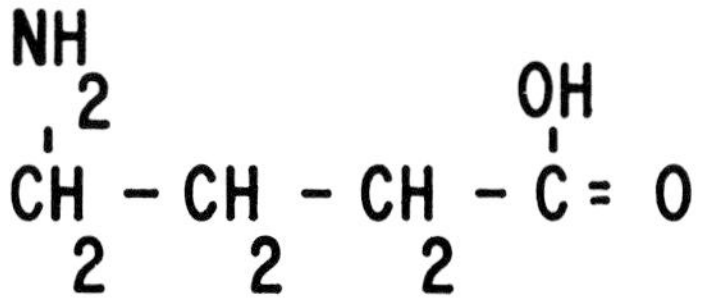

$$CH_2 - CH_2 - CH_2 - C = O$$

with NH_2 on the first carbon and OH on the final carbon

Fig. 16–1. Structural formula of γ-aminobutyric acid (GABA).

313

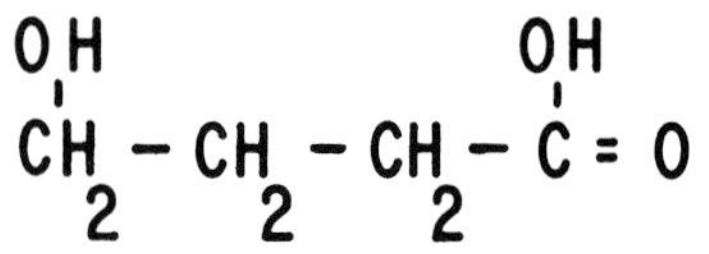

$$CH_2 - CH_2 - CH_2 - \overset{OH}{\underset{}{C}} = O$$

Fig. 16–2. Structural formula of γ-hydroxybutyric acid (gamma-OH).

CHEMISTRY AND PHYSICAL PROPERTIES

The chemical structure of gamma-OH is shown in Figure 16–2. Gamma-OH is a white to off-white, crystalline, hygroscopic solid, which is freely soluble in water. The molecular weight of gamma-OH is 126.1. Gamma-OH has the alkalizing properties of sodium lactate; however, sodium lactate does not possess the anesthetizing properties of gamma-OH. Gamma-OH is a normal constituent of the human body. When acidified, gamma-OH is recycled into gamma-lactone; this is a common property of gamma-hydroxy fatty acids. The pH of gamma-OH ranges from 8.2 to 8.9. Gamma-OH is also active orally and is available as a syrup (15 g of gamma-OH in 100 ml of water).[4]

Metabolism

The sites of metabolic breakdown of gamma-OH are the liver, kidney, and brain. The process of metabolic degradation is caused primarily by β-oxidation and also possibly by reduction in lactic dehydrogenase, which involves the tricarboxylic cycle without forming lactic acidosis. Ultimately, gamma-OH is metabolized to carbon dioxide and water, with 80 to 90% of the drug being eliminated through the lungs; most of the remaining 10 to 20% is excreted in urine.

The initial enthusiasm generated for the use of gamma-OH and, in fact, the rationale for its introduction into clinical anesthesia by Laborit were based on the assumption that gamma-OH would modify the catabolic responses to surgical intervention. Laborit postulated that an intracellular shift of potassium would initiate a shift to anabolic metabolic activity.[5] At clinically useful dosages, however, gamma-OH does not seem to modify such responses.[6] A positive nitrogen balance may be achieved with larger doses of gamma-OH administered along with intravenous amino acids and other nutritional substances that provide caloric input.

Whether there is an adequate indication for the use of gamma-OH on metabolic grounds may, therefore, be debatable, particularly because the drug causes a rise in serum cortisol levels during surgical procedures. This increase may be associated with other metabolic effects, including moderate metabolic alkalosis, a slight rise in the level of blood glucose, and a marked increase in the level of serum sodium as a result of the sodium content of gamma-OH.

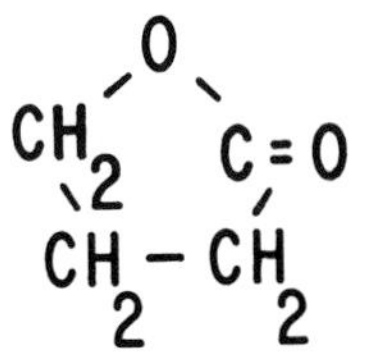

$$\begin{array}{c} \overset{O}{\diagup\diagdown} \\ CH_2 \quad C = O \\ \diagdown \quad \diagup \\ CH_2 - CH_2 \end{array}$$

Fig. 16–3. Structural formula of γ-butyrolactone.

Mode of Action

Findings of initial laboratory studies suggested that γ-butyrolactone, which is readily formed from gamma-OH, was the active substance that produced general anesthesia.[7] The slow onset of action of gamma-OH and the documentation that maximal blood levels of the drug precede peak CNS depressant effects indicate that biotransformation occurs, which favors the aforementioned assumption.[8] Because gamma-OH-induced coma is not associated with a higher level of GAMA in the brain, researchers now assume that gamma-OH is the active substance that produces general anesthesia. Whether the anesthetic effects of gamma-OH are the result of intracellular penetration rather than the result of cell membrane interaction remains unclear. Laborit proposed a biochemical, intracellular mode of acion, postulating that the CNS effects of gamma-OH are caused by neuronal hyperpolarization rather than by synaptic block.[5] This researcher traced the cellular effects of gamma-OH to interferences with the two metabolic pathways for energy, and hypothesized that changes in the cellular mode of activity are dependent on the relative quantities of reduced and nonreduced triphosphonucleotides.

Onset and Duration of Action

Gamma-OH, intravenously administered as a sodium salt in a 20% solution in doses of 40 to 50 mg/kg, produces a somnolent state within 5 to 15 minutes. If left undisturbed, the patient will subsequently lapse into sleep, from which arousal is possible. Larger doses of gamma-OH (60 to 70 mg/kg) deepen the sleep state, and the patient progresses into an unarousable coma that lasts from 1 to 2 hours. When administered orally, similar doses of gamma-OH result in essentially the same depth and duration of sleep and coma.[4] The drug produces no analgesia. Extrapyramidal muscle activity, including clonic movements of the extremities, are common, particularly during the induction of anesthesia. Emergence from a coma may be associated with psychic disturbances and agitation.[9]

PHARMACODYNAMICS

Electroencephalographic (EEG) Changes

The EEG activity associated with the use of gamma-OH is characterized by slow, high-voltage waves during the induction of anesthesia, which are followed by "burst suppression" activity similar to the EEG activity seen in barbiturate-induced coma (i.e., electric silence interspersed with bursts of activity). The drug-induced EEG changes clearly indicate that the principal sites of the depressant action of gamma-OH are the cerebral cortex and subcortical areas, including the limbic-hippocampal system. Evidence to suggest a depressant action on the reticular activating system is scant.

Excitatory Effects

During the induction of anesthesia, and particularly during emergence from gamma-OH-induced coma, periods of rapid eye movement (REM) sleep can be detected. Random clonic movements of the extremities and of the facial muscles are also frequently encountered during induction. Such muscle activities are not reflected as seizure discharges in the EEG. According to the hypothesis of Laborit, however, that gamma-OH tends to hasten neuronal repolarization, gamma-OH may facilitate an epileptic discharge. Gamma-OH does not sufficiently suppress brain stem centers and autonomic activity, which is often manifested by a vigorous and precipitous response to noxious surgical stimuli. Apparently as a result of the release of inhibition from the cerebral cortex, uterine activity during labor is enhanced; the frequency and intensity of uterine contractions are increased.

Cardiovascular System

Gamma-OH induces bradycardia, which may result in a moderate decrease in cardiac output and a slight, clinically insignificant fall in blood pressure level.[10] The administration of atropine sulfate reverses this phenomenon, which indicates that it may be vagal in origin.

Gamma-OH does not significantly depress autonomic nervous system activity. Therefore, surgical stimuli may result in marked cardiovascular responses, such as tachycardia, hypertension, and peripheral vasoconstriction associated with sweating. In laboratory animals, gamma-OH has shown some protective effects against various types of arrhythmias, but the antiarrhythmic properties of gamma-OH have not been confirmed in human subjects.

Respiratory System

Deepening of the comatose state is accompanied by slowing and deepening of respiration, which occasionally shows a Cheyne-Stokes pattern. Blood gas determinations are essentially unchanged or may show an insignificant rise in $PaCO_2$ similar to the rise that occurs during natural sleep.[4]

Miscellaneous Effects

Gamma-OH does not completely abolish pharyngeal and laryngeal reflexes, even in a state of deep coma. This sparing effect on reflex activity, however, should not lead to the assumption that a patent airway can always be secured during gamma-OH anesthesia and that aspiration of foreign material cannot occur. Liver and kidney function is not adversely affected by gamma-OH, nor have teratogenic effects been observed with the use of this drug.[4]

TOXICITY AND SIDE-EFFECTS

Acute toxicologic studies in animals yielded results that emphasized the low toxicity of gamma-OH, regardless of the route of administration. In laboratory animals, the LD_{50} is 5 to 15 times the dose that is necessary to produce coma. Chronic administration of gamma-OH does not lead to tolerance. No deaths in humans have been reported that can be attributed to acute drug toxicity. No ill effects were observed when the drug was administered at doses of 20 to 30 mg/kg within 24 hours for several days.[4] It should be recognized, however, that the injection of large doses of the sodium salt of gamma-OH may impose a significant sodium load.

Vomiting is common after oral administration of gamma-OH and is also occasionally observed during the awakening phase after intravenous use of the drug. Venous irritation, thrombophlebitis, and phlebothrombosis occur at essentially the same rate as that observed with most other intravenously administered anesthetic agents.

Because gamma-OH does not sufficiently suppress autonomic reflexes, the drug should not be used in patients with uncontrolled hypertension or those with toxemia associated with pregnancy. The use of gamma-OH in epileptic patients is discouraged.

CLINICAL APPLICATIONS

General Sedative

Gamma-OH may offer advantages over barbiturates for use in providing night sedation because the drug may interfere less with sleep patterns and, probably more importantly, is unlikely to cause habituation or emotional or physical dependence. Because of its low toxicity, gamma-OH may be particularly suitable when a drug is to be administered over a prolonged period, such as is required in the treatment of tetanus; when extended use of mechanical respiratory assistance is required; and when continuous synchronization of the patient with the automated ventilator is essential.[11,12]

When gamma-OH is employed as an oral premedicant in children, an unacceptably high incidence of vomiting has been observed during the first hour after the drug is administered. Reaction of such frequency may limit the usefulness of the drug as a preanesthetic medication.[13]

General Anesthetic

Gamma-OH does not block surgical stimuli and, therefore, has little to offer when employed alone as an anesthetic. To diminish undesirable brain stem responsiveness, which is predominantly revealed by brisk cardiovascular reactions, phenothiazines, such as promethazine, can be administered prior to the induction of anesthesia. Supplementary analgesia provided by narcotic analgesics or nitrous oxide-oxygen mixtures is also recommended.

Atropine sulfate premedication reduces the tendency for the recipient to develop bradycardia and salivation. Also, small intravenous doses of an ultra-short-acting barbiturate are effective in abolishing clonic muscle movements during the induction of anesthesia.

Anesthesia of acceptable quality can be obtained by using gamma-OH in combination with a variety of supplemental agents; the quantity of depressant drugs that is required is then significantly diminished, in turn reducing the potential for toxic side-effects to occur.[4] When properly supplemented, gamma-OH can be used satisfactorily in providing anesthesia for general and orthopedic surgical procedures, primarily when long operations are involved.

In Combination with Local and Regional Analgesics

Gamma-OH may be a satisfactory substitute for nitrous oxide in countries where either the nitrous oxide or well-trained personnel to administer the gas properly are not available. At an intravenous dose of approximately 50 mg/kg, basal sedation and sleep can be provided to supplement local or regional analgesia for abdominal and perineal surgery.[9] Gamma-OH anesthesia will not compensate, however, for an inadequate local or regional block.

Obstetrics

When gamma-OH was employed as a supplement to epidural anesthesia for cesarean section, it was inferior to other standard anesthetic methods.[14] In contrast, good results have been reported with gamma-OH in cesarean section when the drug is combined with a sleeping dose of an ultra-short-acting barbiturate that is given before the administration of the initial dose of gamma-OH. Positive results have also been recorded when the gamma-OH is supplemented by nitrous oxide-oxygen mixtures that are subsequently administered to maintain anesthesia.[15] Gamma-OH is advantageous in anesthesia for cesarean section because the drug has no respiratory depressant effects, does not interfere with cardiovascular homeostasis, and preserves the protective laryngeal and pharyngeal reflexes. Restlessness during the induction of anesthesia is a disadvantage, although this complication can be controlled by administering small incremental doses of a barbiturate. Other investigators reported equally satisfactory results with the use of gamma-OH in anesthesia for cesarean section.[16,17]

Trauma

The use of gamma-OH and ketamine in trauma patients has yielded satisfactory results.[18] An initial dose of gamma-OH (1 to 4 g intravenously) renders the patient unconscious and preoperative preparations can proceed. Ketamine (2 mg/kg intravenously) is delivered when the operation begins. If the surgical procedure can be completed within 10 to 20 minutes, no further drug administration is necessary. To provide anesthesia for procedures of longer duration, ketamine is administered by the fractional method or by the continuous drip method. Emergence delerium reactions, which may be encountered in adult patients receiving ketamine as a single anesthetic agent, are rarely observed when gamma-OH and ketamine are used together.

Cardiac Catheterization and Angiography

Because gamma-OH interferes minimally with cardiovascular homeostasis, the drug can be successfully administered to patients, predominantly children, in whom cardiac catheterization and angiographic evaluation are to be performed. It may be advisable to administer small doses of phenothiazines and narcotic analgesics to the patient in gamma-OH sleep to minimize undesirable autonomic responses to surgical stimuli. Also, slightly higher intravenous doses (80 to 100 mg/kg) are needed to achieve satisfactory anesthesia in children.

Cardiac Surgery

Aldrete and Barnes compared the effectiveness and safety of gamma-OH with those of halothane in the anesthetic management of patients undergoing cardiac and major vascular surgical procedures.[19] With gamma-OH and gallamine used as a muscle relaxant, the arterial blood pressure of the patient remained within 10 to 40% of preanesthetic values, as opposed to a relatively high incidence of hypotension observed in patients who were anesthetized with halothane. These favorable results with use of gamma-OH in surgical patients, the majority of whom were high-risk patients, confirmed findings from previous studies concerning the effects of gamma-OH on various cardiovascular conditions; also mentioned was the remarkable degree of cardiovascular stability provided by gamma-OH.[20,21]

Neurosurgery

Satisfactory results were reported with gamma-OH-induced anesthesia in patients undergoing various minor and major neurosurgical procedures.[22]

Gamma-OH occupies a unique position among the intravenously employed anesthetics. The drug has potent hypnotic properties, and at the same time is fully metabolized as an energy-producing substrate. Gamma-OH is a basal hypnotic. The drug produces a nontoxic coma and markedly reduces the quantity of supplemental agents required to achieve a satisfactory surgical anesthetic state. The disadvantages of gamma-OH are that its onset of hypnotic action is slow, its recovery period is long, and it lacks analgesic properties.

REFERENCES

1. Appleton, P.J., and Burns, J.M.B.: A neuroinhibitory substance: gamma-hydroxybutyric acid. Anesth. Analg., *97*:164, 1968.
2. Laborit, H., Savany, J.M., Gerard, J., and Fabiani, F.: Generalites concernant l'etude experimentale de l' emploi clinique du gamma-hydroxybutyrate de Na. Agressologie, *1*:407, 1960.
3. Jovany, J.M.: Pharmacologic comparee des sals de l'acide butyrique et l'acide 4-hydroxybutyrique. Agressologie, *1*:417, 1960.
4. Vickers, M.D.: Gamma-hydroxybutyric acid: clinical pharmacology and current status. Proc. R. Soc. Lond. [Biol.], *61*:821, 1968.
5. Laborit, H.: Equilibre hydro-electrolytique et metabolisme cellulaire. Agressologie, 2:439, 1961.
6. Robinson, J.S., Tomlin, P.J., and Morris, L.: The metabolic responses following gammahydroxybutyric acid. Proc. R. Soc. Lond. [Biol.], *61*:824, 1968.
7. Bessman, S.P., and Skolnik, S.: Gamma-hydroxybutyrate and gamma-butyrolactone: concentrations in rat tissue during anesthesia. Science, *143*:1045, 1965.
8. Helrich, M., McAslan, T.C., Skolnik, S., and Bessman, S.P.: Correlation of blood levels of 4-hydroxybutyrate with state of consciousness. Anesthesiology, *25*:771, 1964.
9. Steel, G.C.: Clinical application of gammahydroxybutric acid as a sleep cover in lumbar epidural block. Proc. R. Soc. Lond. [Biol,], *61*:825, 1968.
10. Virtue, R.W., Lund, L.O., Beckwitt, H.J., and Vogel, J.H.K.: Cardiovascular reactions to gamma-hydroxybutyrate in man. Can. Anaesth. Soc. J., *13*:119, 1966.
11. Dundee, J.W.: Discussion. Proc. R. Soc. Lond. [Biol.], *61*:830, 1968.
12. Hassenstein, J.: Discussionsbeitrag. *In* Anaesthesie mit Gamma-Hydroxibuttersaeure. Edited by W. Bushart and P. Rittmeyer. Berlin, Springer, 1973.
13. Root, B.: Oral premedication of children with 4-hydroxybutyrate. Anesthesiology, *26*:259, 1965.
14. Tunstall, M.E.: Useful narcotic agent. Br. Med. J., *1*:315, 1968.
15. Janecek, P.: Klinische Erfahrungen mit Gamma-Hydroxibuttersaeure bei Sectio Caesarea. *In* Anaesthesie mit Gamma-Hydroxibuttersaeure. Edited by W. Bushart and P. Rittmeyer. Berlin, Springer, 1973.
16. Laget-Corsin, L., and Baroche, J.: L'Anesthesie au Gamma-hydroxybutyrate de Sodium Dans L'Operation Cesarienne. Anaesth. Anal., *20*:43, 1972.
17. Youssef, A.R.M.: Gamma-hydroxybutyrate anaesthesia in caesarean section. Middle East J. Anaesthesiol., *3*:691, 1973.
18. Guertner, T.: Praktische Erfahrungen mit Gamma-Hydroxibuttersaeure in Kombination mit Ketamine in der Unfallchirurgie (205 Faelle). *In* Anaesthesie mit Gamma-Hydroxibuttersaeure. Edited by W. Bushart and P. Rittmeyer. Berlin, Springer, 1973.
19. Aldrete, J.A., and Barnes, D.P.: 4-Hydroxybutyrate anaesthesia for cardiovascular surgery. Anaesthesia, *23*:558, 1968.
20. Solway, J., and Sadove, M.S.: 4-Hydroxybutyrate: a clinical study. Anesth. Analg., *44*:532, 1965.
21. Blumenfeld, M., Suntay, R.G., and Harmel, M.H.: Sodium gamma-hydroxybutyric acid: a new anesthetic adjuvant. Anesth. Analg., *41*:721, 1962.
22. Laborit, H., Kind, A., and Regil, E.L.: 220 Cas d'anesthesie en neurochirurgie avec le 2-hydroxybutyrate de sodium. Presse Med., *69*:1216, 1961.

INDEX

Page numbers in *italics* indicate figures; page numbers followed by "t" indicate tables.